Oncogenes and Growth Factors

Edited by

Ralph A. Bradshaw and Steve Prentis

1987
ELSEVIER SCIENCE PUBLISHERS
Amsterdam—New York—Oxford

© 1987 Elsevier Science Publishers

ISBN: 0 444 80827 2

Published by
Elsevier Science Publishers
PO Box 1527
1000 BM Amsterdam
The Netherlands

Sole distributors worldwide except for the USA and Canada
Elsevier Science Publishers Cambridge
68 Hills Road
Cambridge CB2 1LA
UK

Sole distributors for the USA and Canada
Elsevier Science Publishing Company Inc.
52 Vanderbilt Avenue
New York, NY 10017
USA

Printed in England by
The Burlington Press (Cambridge) Ltd.
Station Road, Foxton, Cambridge. Tel: (0223) 870266

This book is dedicated to

Steve Prentis

who was tragically killed in a road accident just
before this book was printed.

Contents

Receptors and second messengers

Preface

It has been clear for many decades that the phenomenon called 'cancer' is in some way related to defects in the normal mechanisms that control cell growth. It is only in the last few years, however, that the precise molecular mechanisms involved in some forms of uncontrolled cell proliferation have begun to be elucidated. The discovery of a link between many known oncogenes and growth factors, their receptors and their signalling mechanisms has renewed hopes that the underlying features of the cancerous process can be understood. Such an understanding seems likely to lead eventually to novel means of treating and diagnosing cancer. The articles in this book illustrate just how rapidly knowledge of these aspects of cancer has grown and how this knowledge may come to be applied. The variety of scientific disciplines that are now contributing fundamental information about cancer is demonstrated by the fact that the articles in this book were first published in three of Elsevier's monthly review publications: *Trends in Biochemical Sciences, Trends in Genetics* and *Immunology Today.*

We should like to thank the authors of these articles for granting permission to have their work reproduced in this collection. We hope that the juxtaposition of these articles will help stimulate new and even more productive research into the mystery of cancer.

STEVE PRENTIS

Introduction

The control of cell growth: The role of polypeptide growth factors and oncogene products

Ralph A. Bradshaw

Polypeptide growth factors (PGF) are a diverse group of regulatory agents that act to control cell viability and proliferation in a hormone-like receptor-dependent fashion[1]. Although the mechanism of action is not well understood for any of them, there is an emerging view that they initiate a cascade of responses involving a variety of key proteins, in addition to the PGFs and their receptors, and that the alteration and/or amplification of one or more of these proteins leads to transformation and the accompanying loss in growth control[2]. At least some of these proteins are now recognized to be the products of oncogenes; their structure, function and relationship to PGFs as well as the PGFs themselves is the subject of this book.

Identification and cataloging

As with many natural processes, the origins of the discovery of cellular growth control are diffuse and diverse. Certainly it has been appreciated for a long time that extracts and homogenates of various tissues could cause cell division in culture. However, the causative mitogenic substances remained poorly defined even into the last decade. Curiously, the first protein for which the designation *growth factor* became a permanent part of biological nomenclature was nerve growth factor (NGF; and even this started as nerve growth-stimulating factor[3]), which is widely held to be non-mitogenic, although it may have such an activity on certain established cells or during short periods of development[4,5]. Studies on NGF in turn led to the discovery of epidermal growth factor (EGF), also present in the adult male mouse submandibular gland[6], which proved to be a potent mitogen and ultimately the source of a number important observations regarding PGFs, with a goodly number emanating from Stanley Cohen's laboratory at Vandebilt University.

Since the early 1970s, the identification and characterization of PGFs has accelerated[1,7]. Platelet-derived growth factor (PDGF), the insulin-like growth factors [IGFs; which were initially identified by the less elegant but certainly highly descriptive non-suppressible insulin-like activity (NSILA)[8] and the perhaps biologically more relevant somatomedin[9]] and the fibroblast growth factors (FGFs) were and are among the more popular, and all have been defined in some detail. The identification of the transforming growth factors (TGFs) led to the development of the autocrine hypothesis which expanded the already growing realization that many PGFs did not depend on systemic transport alone[10,11]. At the same time, research in hemopoietic development and immunology were revealing rich sources of PGFs and many colony stimulating factors (CSFs) (including erythropoietin) and interleukins (ILs) have now been well defined. A representative listing of PGFs can be found in Ref. 1. Many of these are also discussed in this volume.

It is also clear that there are many more PGFs awaiting identification and detailed characterization. In the area of neurotrophic substances alone (which clearly should be considered as growth factors), there have been many reports[12] and further definitions are expected soon. The same can be said for many other activities. However, it is also true that some substances have been independently discovered (using different species or assays) that apparently will turn out to be the same. The aforementioned case of IGF I and II, where the human and rat proteins were also called somatomedins and/or multiplication stimulating activity[13,14], and the identification of human EGF as urogastrone[15] illustrate the species problem. The occurrence of the same protein with different names (usually reflecting different assays) is well illustrated by the various substances (listed in Table 1, p. 150) that are apparently identical with the acidic and basic FGFs. Conversely, further characterization may yield examples of closely related but genetically or structurally distinct PGFs that will require separate consideration (and independent listings).

A final problem confronting cataloging efforts is the matter of definition. It is quite clear that a number of 'classical' hormones are involved in growth regulation, as well as other substances that are clearly not even endocrine in nature[1]. Thus, it is difficult to exclude insulin, growth hormone and prolactin from any list of growth factors (for a variety of compelling reasons, some of which are discussed below) and thrombin almost certainly is a physiologically important mitogen under appropriate conditions[16]. Probably the best approach to this problem is to resist the urge to have all things properly tagged, identified and archived and to continuously compare all findings with these molecules for their relevance to PGFs; they will likely be germane.

The endocrine connection

It is now doubtful whether anyone would seriously put forward a functional definition of PGFs that did not include receptor interaction as the initiating event. However, growth factors were not always viewed as hormone-like and one need only scan early discussions* regarding NGF and EGF to grasp the initial, rather pronounced resistance to this concept. (It might be fairly pointed out that some of these skeptics viewed the whole relevance of these newly discovered factors with considerable askance thus leaving little room for them to even contemplate let alone accept them as a new endocrine subgroup. The comments of Stanley Cohen to the press when he was jointly awarded the 1986 Nobel prize in Physiology and Medicine are illustrative). Clues regarding the similarity of PGFs and polypeptide hormones probably abound in the early literature; many are now more visible with the advantage of hindsight. However, one that was unmistakable was the discovery of the structural, and therefore apparently evolutionary, relationship of NGF and insulin[17]. By 1972, it had become a well-established principle that proteins with related function often showed such homology and, conversely, structural relatedness strongly implied some similarity in function. Although there are a few exceptions, or at least examples for which there are not as yet explanations e.g. α-lactalbumin and lysozyme[18], this has proven to be, and still is[19] a useful concept.

A more convincing connection between PGFs and hormones was revealed by their common dependency on surface membrane receptors located on responsive cells. Initially, receptors for NGF and EGF were identified by equilibrium and kinetic binding studies using suitably labeled ligands as had been done for several

---

*Fortunately or not, depending on your viewpoint, much of this criticism was verbal making it difficult to trace the history of this part of PGF research. Many of us, however, remember it well.

polypeptide hormones. The characteristic parameters deduced for these and other PGFs were entirely similar to the hormones. Indeed, unusual binding phenomena, such as apparent occupancy-dependent negative cooperativity found with some hormones (most notably insulin[20]), were also observed with some PGF receptors, further emphasizing the relationship of these two groups of extracellular regulators.

In due course, molecular characterization of receptors for both hormones and PGFs revealed substantial similarities in structural organization and functional properties. Covalent cross-linking (of labeled ligand and receptors), monoclonal antibodies and finally, and most definitively, cloning and sequencing of corresponding cDNAs established similarities in size, subunit structure, domain architecture and sequence homology. These data indicate both similarities and distinctive features. These may be briefly summarized as follows.

(1) There are two broad classes of PGF receptors, distinguished by the presence or absence of an intracellular tyrosine kinase domain; polypeptide hormone receptors also exist with and without this activity.

(2) Most receptors are composed of a single polypeptide, divided into three domains: extracellular, transmembrane and intracellular. (The receptor for insulin and IGF I have four polypeptides; however, they are symmetrical dimers of two α- and two β-chains with each type derived from a single chain precursor. This precursor has the same three-domain organization found in other PGF receptors[21,22]).

(3) The extracellular domain is glycosylated (both N- and O-linked have been observed), is generally rich in disulfide bonds (often clustered in subdomains) and contains the ligand binding site.

(4) The transmembrane segment is composed of a simple polypeptide segment, followed by a polar, basic sequence which presumably blocks further extrusion through the membrane.

The presence of tyrosine kinase in receptor structures was first observed with the EGF receptor by Ushiro and Cohen[23]. This observation provided an important insight into the mechanistic properties of some PGFs, provided a major link to oncogenes and their products and solidified the relationship of PGFs and hormones (with the subsequent finding that the insulin receptor contained a similar function[24]). Although the relationship of this activity to PGF mechanism and to transforming potential remains to be elucidated definitively, it is of unquestionable importance. Several of the articles in this volume deal extensively with this aspect of the PGF/oncogene relationship.

Mechanistic considerations

Although the functional responses of PGFs with respect to their individual target cells are generally appreciated in some detail, the molecular mechanisms that produce these responses are more poorly understood. It is clear that PGF/receptor complexes are capable of inducing a transmembrane signal(s) which is undoubtedly amplified as it is processed intracellularly. Eventually this results in a clear effect on gene expression at either a transcriptional or translational level[1]. However, a number of other metabolic processes are also affected, usually on a more rapid time scale, implying the existence of a second messenger system, similar to the adenyl cyclase cascade that characterizes certain rapidly acting hormones. The adenyl cyclase system uses a complex family of G (GTP binding) proteins which connect the occupied receptor to the effector enzyme (adenyl cyclase)[1,11]. Among the more popular candidates for second messengers of polypeptide growth factors are the products of the cleavage of phosphoinositides by a phospholipase C[25]. In this pathway, diacylglycerol (DAG) is generated, which is thought to act primarily on protein kinase C, along with phosphorylated inositols, which act to release calcium from the endoplasmic reticulum. The combination of these two stimuli may account for a significant portion of the PGF mechanism. The protein kinase C molecule, in turn, phosphorylates a number of other substrates although as yet none have been identified as being crucial for the growth response in any system[26]. The same enzyme also acts as the receptor for phorbol esters, well characterized tumor promoters, that enhance but do not initiate tumor formation.

In analogy to the G proteins that characterize adenyl cyclase systems, it has been suggested that the *ras* oncogene products may serve in this capacity connecting growth factor receptors with phospholipase C. The best evidence for such an involvement has arisen from studies with NGF and PC12 cells[27,28]. Whether or not *ras* acts to stimulate phospholipase C, it almost certainly connects at least some polypeptide growth factor receptors to appropriate effector molecules. As such, the viral forms of *ras* would act to interrupt the normal flow of information transfer from the exterior to the interior of the cell resulting in the transformed phenotype.

A second major consequence of the interaction of PGFs with their receptors is to induce the endocytic uptake of both receptors and their ligands, which ultimately leads to the destruction of both. It remains a strong possibility that either one or both (directly, or in some altered form) also plays a role in the signal transmission. The most likely target is the nucleus with resultant effects on the transcriptional processes that are characteristic of each PGF response. In this regard, several PGF receptors have been identified as components of the nuclear matrix/envelope of responsive cells[29]. For the most part, these identifications have been primarily based on ligand recognition assays and in no case has a genuine receptor function been attributed to any. It is also important to note that the origin of these molecules is uncertain. They may arise at the nucleus as a result of translocation from the plasma membrane or they may be directly inserted into the matrix structure as part of the biosynthetic process and avoid the plasma membrane entirely. The role of receptor-mediated endocytosis or of internal receptors (or ligands), regardless of their origin, in the mechanism of PGFs remains one of the intriguing aspects of PGF function.

Oncogene involvement

Although a few of the oncogene products have been clearly associated with polypeptide growth factors or their receptors, the majority appear to be related to proteins involved in the transfer of the stimulus from the cell surface to the intracellular machinery[30]. As noted above, *ras* almost certainly plays some role in connecting occupied receptors with appropriate effector molecules. By the same token, those oncogenes which possess tyrosine kinase activities may well act to mimic the tyrosine kinase functions associated with growth factor receptors[31]. Alternatively, they may deregulate other tyrosine kinase-dependent processes that can also lead to the transformed state. A particularly interesting set of oncogenes that have not yet been directly related to growth factor mechanisms are those that are associated with the nucleus. The products of *myc, myb* and *fos* have all proven to be effective markers in following growth factor stimulation, but their role in the nucleus is still enigmatic. The elucidation of their function is certain to be of great significance in understanding the mechanism of action of PGFs. A major portion of this book deals with oncogenes and their products and their role in both cancer and normal cellular growth. Although much remains to be determined, the importance of the interralationships of PGFs on the one hand and oncogene products on the other can already be inferred.

Concluding remarks

Before leaving the reader with many interesting and stimulating chapters to read and contemplate, it is appropriate to issue a few caveats. First, and certainly most importantly, all of the material related to this topic cannot possibly be contained in one volume. Restrictions imposed by the sources of these materials has contributed to some of the more obvious deficits, but even if the contents could have been more broadly orchestrated, it still would not have been possible to cover all germane material completely. This situation is, of course, exacerbated by the rapid developments of the field and the changes that occur in our knowledge in this area almost daily. Thus there are shortfalls and inadequacies in this collection that are clearly recognizable even to the unitiated. Nonetheless this group of articles has surprising breadth and emphasizes, to a very real degree, the important thoughts and concepts that are presently held. Hopefully it will have the desired effect of leading the interested reader back to the primary literature including articles that will have appeared since this collection was assembled. At the least, this volume should provide its readers with some new insight and feeling for the molecular basis of cancer and the underlying principles that regulate the growth, development and differentiation of eukaryotic organisms.

References

1 James, R. and Bradshaw, R. A. (1984) *Annu. Rev. Biochem.* 53, 259–292
2 Land, H., Parada, L. F. and Weinberg, R. A. (1983) *Nature* 304, 596–602
3 Cohen, S., Levi-Montalcini, R. and Hamburger, V. (1954) *Proc. Natl Acad. Sci. USA* 40, 1014–1018
4 Lillien, L. E. and Claude, P. (1985) *Nature* 317, 632–634
5 Burstein, D. E. and Greene, L. A. (1982) *Dev. Biol.* 94, 477–482
6 Cohen, S. (1962) *J. Biol. Chem.* 237, 1555–1562
7 Heldin, C-H. and Westermark, B. (1984) *Cell* 37, 9–20
8 Rinderknecht, E. and Humbel, R. E. (1976) *Proc. Natl Acad. Sci. USA* 73, 2365–2369
9 Daughaday, W. H., Hall, K., Raben, M. S., Salmon, W. D. Jr, Van den Brande, J. C. and Van Wyk, J. J. (1972) *Nature* 235, 107–109
10 Sporn, M. B. and Todaro, G. J. (1980) *N. Engl. J. Med.* 303, 878–880
11 Bradshaw, R. A. and Niall, H. D. (1978) *Trends Biochem. Sci.* 3, 274–278
12 Perez-Polo, J. R. and de Vellis, J., eds (1982) *J. Neurosci. Res.* 8, 127–567
13 Rubin, J. S., Mariz, I., Jacobs, J. W., Daughaday, W. H. and Bradshaw, R. A. (1982) *Endocrinology* 110, 734–740
14 Marquardt, H., Todaro, G. J., Henderson, L. E. and Oroszlan, S. (1981) *J. Biol. Chem.* 256, 6859–6865
15 Gregory, H. (1975) *Nature* 257, 325–327
16 Cunningham, D. D., Carney, D. H., Baker, J. B., Low, D. A. and Glenn, K. C. (1982) in *Proteins in Biology and Medicine* (Bradshaw, R. A., Hill, R. L., Tang, J., Liang, C-C. and Tsou, C.I., eds), pp. 43–59, Academic Press
17 Frazier, W. A., Angeletti, R. H. and Bradshaw, R. A. (1972) *Science* 176, 482–488
18 Hill, R. L., Brew, K., Vanaman, T. C., Trayer, I. P. and Matlock, P. (1969) *Brookhaven Symp.* 21, 139–152
19 Doolittle, R. F. (1981) *Science* 214, 149–159
20 De Meyts, P. (1980) *Hormone Cell Regul.* 4, 107–121
21 Ullrich, A., Bell, J. R., Chen, E. Y., Herrera, R., Petruzzelli, I. M., Dull, T. J., Gray, A., Coussens, L., Liao, Y-C., Tsubokawa, M., Mason, A., Seeburg, P. H., Grunfeld, C., Rosen, O. M. and Ramachandran, J. (1985) *Nature* 313, 756–761

R. A. Bradshaw is at the Department of Biological Chemistry California College of Medicine, University of California Irvine, CA 92717, USA.

22   Ebena, Y., Ellis, L., Jarnagin, K., Edery, M., Graf, L., Clauser, E., On, J., Masiarz, F., Kan, Y. W., Goldfine, I. D., Roth, R. A. and Rutter, W. J. (1985) *Cell* 40, 747–758
23   Ushiro, H. and Cohen, S. (1980) *J. Biol. Chem.* 255, 8363–8365
24   Kasuga, M., Zick, Y., Blithe, D. C., Crettaz, M. and Kahn, C. R. (1982) *Nature* 298, 667–669
25   Nishizuka, Y. (1984) *Nature* 308, 693–698
26   Woodgett, J. R., Hunter, T. and Gould, K. L. in *Cell Membranes: Methods and Reviews* (Elson, E., Frazier, W. A. and Glaser, L., eds) Plenum Press (in press)
27   Hagag, N., Halegoua, S. and Viola, M. (1986) *Nature* 319, 680–682
28   Bar-Sagi, D. and Feramisco, J. R. (1985) *Cell* 42, 841–848
29   Goldfine, I, (1981) *Biochim. Biophys. Acta* 650, 53–67
30   Bishop, J. M. (1983) *Annu. Rev. Biochem.* 52, 301–354
31   Hunter, T. and Cooper, J. A. (1985) *Annu. Rev. Biochem.* 54, 897–930

Oncogenes

Trends in oncogenes

J. Michael Bishop

The search for genetic damage in neoplastic cells has become a central theme of contemporary cancer research. Diverse examples of such damage are now in hand, and they in turn hint at biochemical explanations of why cancer cells run amok.

In 1820, Sir William Norris used the *Edinburgh Medical and Surgical Journal* to report the occurrence of malignant melanomas in a family[1]. 'The facts', he said, 'incline me to believe that this disease is hereditary'. To this day, we cannot explain familial tendency to cancer of the sort that Sir William observed, but the belief that cancer is, at its heart, a genetic disease is now stronger than ever. The belief arose from at least three sources: the perception of hereditary diatheses to cancer – Sir William was only one of many to sound this theme; the presence of damaged chromosomes in at least some cancer cells; and the emerging evidence that relates mutagenic potential to carcinogenicity. Now the belief has acquired the substance of experiment. A growing number of vertebrate genes have been implicated in tumorigenesis. In their normal guise, we call these genes 'proto-oncogenes'. They are thought to be substrates for carcinogenic influences of various sorts, a keyboard on which various carcinogens can play. Abnormal alleles of these genes can be found in retroviruses, where they first came to our attention[2]; or in tumors, where they often arise without the intervention of viruses, and where they include genes not represented in retroviruses[3]. In either setting, we know the malefactors as 'oncogenes'.

How have proto-oncogenes and oncogenes been found? How large is their roster at present? How do they work? What are the purposes of proto-oncogenes in normal cells and organisms? And how certain are we now that oncogenes have a role in carcinogenesis?

Lessons from viruses

We first learned of oncogenes from the study of tumor viruses. Diverse sorts of viruses can cause cancer, in either their natural hosts or experimental animals. In many instances, tumorigenesis can be attributed to one or more genes within the DNA or RNA of the viral genome[4]. Every viral oncogene promises valuable lessons in the molecular mechanisms of carcinogenesis, but the most decisive explication of oncogenes to date has come from the study of retroviruses.

Retroviruses are remarkably versatile carcinogens: in the aggregate, they cause virtually every major form of neoplasia known to plague humankind. They can do so in at least two ways:

(1) Some retroviruses carry oncogenes whose protein products can convert cells to cancerous growth by attacking crucial cellular machinery. The diversity of retroviral oncogenes is remarkable (Table 1). We know of nearly 20 oncogenes that are carried by retroviruses, isolated from numerous species. Each oncogene induces specific forms of neoplasia; each encodes a protein whose action wreaks the mischief. Every retroviral oncogene represents a cellular proto-oncogene as well, since it is by transduction from the genome of the host cell that retroviruses

Table 1. Proto-oncogenes that have appeared in retroviruses[a]

Proto-oncogene/oncogene[b]	Possible subcellular location(s) of gene product	Possible function of gene product
abl	Plasma and cytoplasmic membranes[c]	Protein-tyrosine kinase
erb-A	Cytoplasm	?
erb-B	Plasma and cytoplasmic membranes[c]	Protein-tyrosine kinase
ets	Nucleus (fused with product of v-*myb*)	?
fes/fps	Plasma and cytoplasmic membranes[c]	Protein-tyrosine kinase
fgr	Plasma and cytoplasmic membranes[c]	Protein-tyrosine kinase
fms	Plasma and cytoplasmic membranes[c]	Protein-tyrosine kinase
fos	Nucleus	?
kit	?	?
mil/raf	Cytoplasm	Protein-serine/threonine kinase
mos	Cytoplasm	Protein-serine/threonine kinase
myb	Nucleus	?
myc	Nucleus	?
ras	Plasma membrane	Regulator of adenylate cyclase
rel	Cytoplasm	?
ros	Plasma and cytoplasmic membranes[c]	Protein-tyrosine kinase
sis	Cytoplasm/secreted	Analogue of PDGF-B/2
ski	Nucleus	?
src	Plasma and cytoplasmic membranes[c]	Protein-tyrosine kinase
yes	Plasma and cytoplasmic membranes[c]	Protein-tyrosine kinase

[a] For details, see Refs 2 and 3.
[b] Normal and pathogenic alleles of each gene have been identified, the former (proto-oncogene) in metazoan genomes, the latter (onco-genes) in retroviruses.
[c] The products of v-*fms* and v-*src* reside on both the plasma membrane and juxta-nuclear cytoplasmic membranes (summarized in Ref. 4). Other proteins of the same family (products of v-*abl*, v-*fes/fps*, v-*fgr*, v-*ros* and v-*yes*) have not been localized so explicitly but are presumed to occupy analogous sites.

acquire their oncogenes – an accident of nature that brings to view potential seeds of cancer within our DNA[2].

(2) Retroviruses that do not carry oncogenes may nevertheless finger cancer genes for us. When retroviruses infect cells, the RNA of their genome is copied into DNA by reverse transcriptase. The viral DNA is then ensconced in the cell by integration into the chromosomal DNA of the host. Integration is potentially mutagenic and thus potentially carcinogenic: it might disrupt vital cellular genes, or bring them under the sway of powerful viral regulatory signals[3]. The cellular genes so affected are potential proto-oncogenes; the integration of viral DNA may convert them to oncogenes. The insertion of retroviral DNA in the vicinity of a proto-oncogene is apparently accidental, arising from the promiscuity with which integration occurs at different positions in host DNA. The insertions come to our attention because they are found in tumor cells, and because they violate expectation by being clustered in a limited domain of cellular DNA. Since viral DNA can be tracked to its residence in the genome of tumor cells, the harried proto-oncogene can be uncovered. Once incriminated, the cellular gene sometimes proves to be an old acquaintance – a proto-oncogene already known to us from the study of retroviral oncogenes; in other instances, new suspects are brought to light (see Table 2 for examples).

Oncogenes detected by gene-transfer

DNA taken from a variety of tumor cells can transform select cells in culture, as if it contained an active oncogene of the sort we were once accustomed to finding only in viruses[5]. The procedure has detected active transforming genes in perhaps 20% of all specimens tested, irrespective of their histiotype. It seemed at first as if this experimental strategy was destined to uncover only genes of the *ras* family, but now almost a dozen candidates not found previously in retroviruses have been uncovered (Table 2).

Oncogenes identified by gene-transfer are typically mutated in ways that alter the functions of the proteins they encode[5]. The mutations account for the ability of the genes to transform cells in culture; they have so far proved to be somatic lesions, restricted to tumor tissue; they presumably arise from either the original onslaught of a carcinogen or a misstep by cellular machinery during the evolution of the cancer cell; and they seem likely to be fuel for the engine that propels neoplastic growth. The occurrence of mutant genes in human cancer has so far been sporadic, but there are now diverse examples in which experimental carcinogenesis has reproducibly evoked the same neoplasm, carrying the same mutant gene (see Table 3). These findings have greatly enhanced the credibility of two themes in contemporary cancer research: first, that at least some of the proto-oncogenes discovered originally by the study of retroviruses may play a role in the genesis of human cancer; and second, that mutations may brook large in the pathogenesis of malignancy.

The use of gene-transfer (or 'transfection') to identify oncogenes has been criticized because the mouse 3T3 cell commonly used in the assays is itself abnormal. But the 3T3 cell should be viewed in this setting as nothing more than a sensitive indicator that can be used to ferret out genetic lesions. The mounting abundance of these lesions, their restriction to neoplastic cells, their reproducible occurrence in diverse experimental tumors, their phenotypic effects on both established and primary cultures of cells, and the evidence of biological selection for specific mutations all conjoin to make a powerful argument: it seems likely that mutant oncogenes are more than innocent by-standers or mere pawns in the tumors where they are found.

Table 2. *Proto-oncogenes that have not appeared in retroviruses*[a]

Proto-oncogene	Method of identification	Original source
bcl-1	Translocation	B-cell leukemia
bcl-2	Translocation	B-cell lymphoma
bcr	Translocation	Chronic myelogenous leukemia
B*lym*	Transfection	B-cell lymphoma
dil	Transfection	B-cell lymphoma
int-1	Insertional mutagenesis	Mammary carcinoma
int-2	Insertional mutagenesis	Mammary carcinoma
L-*myc*	Amplification	Lung carcinoma
*mcf*2	Transfection	Mammary carcinoma
*mcf*3	Transfection	Mammary carcinoma
met	Transfection	Chemically transformed osteosarcoma cells
Mlvi-1	Insertional mutagenesis	T-cell lymphoma
Mlvi-2	Insertional mutagenesis	T-cell lymphoma
Mlvi-3	Insertional mutagenesis	T-cell lymphoma
neu	Transfection	Neuroblastoma
N-*myc*	Amplification	Neuroblastoma
N-*ras*	Transfection	Neuroblastoma
onc-D	Transfection	Colon carcinoma
pim-1	Insertional mutagenesis	T-cell lymphoma
pvt-1	Translocation/insertional mutagenesis	Plasmacytoma
RMO-*int*-1	Insertional mutagenesis	T-cell lymphoma
tcl-1	Translocation	T-cell leukemia
T*lym*-1	Transfection	T-cell lymphoma
T*lym*-2	Transfection	T-cell lymphoma
T_KNS-1	Translocation	Plasmacytoma
tx-1	Transfection	Mammary carcinoma
tx-2	Transfection	PreB-cell leukemia
tx-3	Transfection	Myeloma/plasmacytoma
tx-4	Transfection	T-cell lymphoma
Uncharacterized relative of *ras*	Transfection	Melanoma

[a] There is presently no generally accepted taxonomic convention by which proto-onco-genes and oncogenes are recognized. I have chosen to list genetic loci that have been found as abnormal alleles in one or more tumors or tumor-cell lines, irrespective of how the damage might have arisen, and without regard for whether or not the loci encode proteins – some clearly do, others have yet to be sufficiently characterized. Literature citations and further information for most of the loci can be found elsewhere[3].

Chromosomal translocations and oncogenes

Many cancer cells contain chromosomal translocations[6]. These were once viewed with disdain, as mere amusements for the myopic microscopist. Now they have come to center stage, because they too bedevil proto-oncogenes[7]. The breakpoints that join portions of two chromosomes together in translocations tell the molecular biologist where to look for trouble: dissection of DNA in the vicinity of breakpoints can uncover proto-oncogenes, both old and new. The proto-oncogene may be moved to another chromosome, or it may remain in place, but be in the vicinity of the breakpoint[8]. In the first examples studied – the translocations that typify Burkitt's lymphoma (8;14) and chronic myelogenous leukemia (9;22) – the translocations affect a known proto-oncogene. In other instances, previously unknown genetic loci have been found at or near the breakpoints (see Table 2).

Translocations might affect either the expression or the protein products of proto-oncogenes. In Burkitt's lymphoma, translocation juxtaposes c-*myc* to one or another immunoglobulin gene[8]. In some cases, c-*myc* suffers mutations; in others, it does not. But inevitably, c-*myc* is unleashed: it cannot be silenced when it ought to be[9]. By contrast, the translocation in chronic myelogenous leukemia creates a chimeric coding domain that replaces the aminoterminal portion of the c-*abl* protein with a portion of another protein (encoded by a domain presently known as the 'breakpoint cluster region')[10]. The chimeric protein apparently has protein-tyrosine kinase activity that is more robust than normal[11].

At present, there is no decisive evidence to implicate chromosomal translocations in turmorigenesis. But their role in pathogenesis is strongly hinted by the consistency with which specific translocations occur in particular tumors, the abnormalities of gene structure and function the translocations impose, and the fact that at least two of the previously known proto-oncogenes are affected by translocations.

Amplification of proto-oncogenes

It now appears that amplification of proto-oncogenes can figure in the pathogenesis of human tumors. Amplification of proto-oncogenes has been observed in two patterns[12]: as a sporadic feature of diverse tumors; and as a common feature of particular tumors. In either instance, we suspect but cannot yet prove that gene amplification has contributed to tumorigenesis because the amplified DNA has survived countless generations of tumor cell growth, as if a selective advantage were in force. We presume that trouble arises because amplification enforces inordinate expression of the overgrown gene, and this imposes a pathogenic burden on the cell. Some of the amplified genes had been known to us before as proto-oncogenes for retroviral oncogenes; others are new to us – singled out merely because they are part of the amplified DNA in tumor cells (see Table 2). A cardinal example of the latter case is the gene presently dubbed N-*myc* because of its kinship with c-*myc*[13,14]. Amplification and the consequent increased expression of N-*myc* may be one of the factors that can evoke progression of both human neuroblastomas and small cell carcinoma of the lung to advanced malignancy[15,16]. N-*myc* can also be amplified and abnormally expressed in retinoblastomas[17]. The amplification of N-*myc* may have practical implications, since it apparently marks those neuroblastomas whose course will be rapid and refractory to therapy (Ref. 15; and R. Seeger). Here is a cameo example of how our burgeoning knowledge of oncogenes might be brought to bear on the care of the cancer patient.

Table 3. Reproducible oncogenes

Source of oncogene	Carcinogen(s)	Oncogene	Reference
Mouse papilloma/carcinoma	Dimethylbenzanthracene	c-Ha-*ras*	Balmain, A. *et al.* (1984) *Nature* 307, 658–660
Mouse breast carcinoma	Nitrosomethylurea	c-Ha-*ras*	Sukumar, S. *et al.* (1983) *Nature* 306, 658–661
Rat neuro/glioblastomas	Ethylnitrosourea	c-*neu*	Schechter, A. L. *et al.* (1984) *Nature* 312, 513–517
Mouse thymic lymphoma	Nitrosomethylurea	N-*ras*	Guerrero, I. *et al.* (1984) *Science* 225, 1041–1043
Mouse thymic lymphoma	γ-radiation	c-Ki-*ras*	Guerrero, I. *et al.* (1984) *Science* 225, 1159–1162
Chemically transformed fetal guinea pig cells	S-methylcholanthrene Benzo (a) pyrene N-methyl-N-nitrosoguanidine Diethylnitrosamine	c-*ras* (same unidentified allele in every instance)	Sukumar, S. *et al.* (1984) *Science* 223, 1197–1199

The biochemical functions encoded by proto-oncogenes and oncogenes

By the various devices outlined above, more than 40 possible proto-oncogenes/ oncogenes have been uncovered (see Tables 1 and 2). How do the proteins encoded by these genes act? We can answer this question in some detail for only a few of the genes, and in far more numerous instances, we can provide no answer whatsoever. Other chapters in this volume carry detailed accounts of where we stand with several prominent proto-oncogenes/oncogenes. As introduction, I point out that the products of these genes are characterized by a provocative diversity. Some attack in the nucleus of the cell, some in the cytoplasm, some at the plasma membrane. For the moment, we can perceive three biochemical strategies by which these proteins might act:

(1) Phosphorylation of proteins and polyphosphoinositides[18]: the oncogene product may itself be the enzymatic agent of phosphorylation, or it may be a factor that elicits phosphorylation – such as the subunit of platelet-derived growth factor encoded by the *sis* gene[19].

(2) Regulation of adenylate cyclase (in reality, regulation of protein phosphorylation at a distance): the products of RAS1 and RAS2 in yeast stimulate adenylate cyclase[20], but it appears unlikely that the products of metazoan *ras* genes do the same.

(3) Regulation of transcription: provisional evidence suggests that the product of *myc* may augment transcription from other genes[21], and there are reasons to suspect that other oncogenes/proto-oncogenes may act in the same manner[4,21]; but there is no direct evidence that this is the means by which these genes function in normal cells or induce neoplastic growth.

(4) Regulation of DNA replication: no product of a normal proto-oncogene or its pathogenic allele has yet been implicated in this function, but the possibility bears watching because of the precedent set by oncogenes of DNA tumor viruses[4].

The simplicity of the preceding summary is more likely a reflection of our ignorance than of cellular design. It derives in part from the fact that a substantial number of the proteins encoded by proto-oncogenes can be arranged in three families: the protein-tyrosine kinases[18], exemplified by *src* (which encodes a peripheral membrane protein) and by *erb*-B (encoding the transmembrane receptor for EGF); the *ras* proteins[22], all of which may be peripheral membrane proteins with functions analogous to G proteins[20]; and diverse nuclear proteins[4], whose kinship remains largely conjectural and whose functions remain mysterious.

The mere fact that we can prepare a summary with such particulars is itself a wonder. A decade ago, none of this was known – not a single product of a retroviral oncogene or cellular proto-oncogene. Now dozens of these proteins are in hand, providing the first outlines of a biological 'road-map' to carcinogenesis.

Oncogenes and the control of growth

Oncogenes impinge on the chain of command that directs the response to polypeptide growth factors (Table 4). Several of the proteins encoded by oncogenes represent abnormal versions of cell surface receptors for growth factors. At least one of the proteins encodes a portion of a growth factor proper. Several of the proteins reside on the inner surface of the plasma membrane, well situated to transduce signals received from outside the cell, and others may be in the nuclear chain of command that directs a cell to divide in response to growth factors.

Table 4. Proto-oncogenes and the control of cellular replication

Oncogene	Biochemical activity	Possible function
erb-B	Tyrosine kinase	Cell surface receptor (EGF)
fms	Tyrosine kinase	Cell surface receptor (M-CSF/CSF-I)
neu	Tyrosine kinase	Cell surface receptor (presently unidentified)
ros	Tyrosine kinase	Cell surface receptor (presently unidentified)
sis	Growth factor	PDGF (B subunit)
src	Tyrosine kinase	? Transducer at inner surface of plasma membrane
abl	Tyrosine kinase	? Transducer at inner surface of plasma membrane
ras	?	? Transducer at inner surface of plasma membrane
fos	?	? Nuclear effector of mitogenesis
myc	?	? Nuclear effector of mitogenesis
myb	?	? Nuclear effector of mitogenesis

These findings no longer surprise, since we know that retroviral oncogenes are drawn from the genetic repertoire of the normal cell and might therefore represent functions that normally govern cellular replication. What does amaze is the fact that the natural selection of oncogenes by retroviruses has brought to view growth factors, receptors and biochemical pathways that we had encountered before in other experimental wanderings. Perhaps our grasp of cellular controls is more extensive than we had any right to expect, although I am dubious that this is so.

The tasks of proto-oncogenes

What role do proto-oncogenes play in the daily affairs of normal cells and organisms? Hypothetical answers to this question have generally taken two forms: the genes may govern the cell-division cycle; or they are part of the machinery that directs differentiation. No unitary view has yet emerged. Strains of yeast deficient in c-*ras* fail to execute the cell cycle normally[23,24]. By contrast, the expression of c-*src* in both chickens[25] and *Drosophila melanogaster*[36] is most pronounced in differentiated cells that are no longer dividing: the action of c-*src* may have no bearing on the cell cycle.

How are these matters to be pursued? For the moment, the future seems to lie mainly with the fruit fly. No other metazoan organism is more accessible to genetic manipulation, and *Drosophila melanogaster* possesses a substantial variety of proto-oncogenes, ripe for analysis[26]. *Saccharomyces cerevisiae* permits great virtuosity in genetic analysis, but c-*ras* is the only possible counterpart of a proto-oncogene as yet found in yeast, and a unicellular organism may not offer all the lessons we need to learn. In the longer view, there is hope that the formation of transgenic mice may permit the elucidation of how individual genes participate in development. First efforts to use this tactic with proto-oncogenes have fallen shy of the mark. For example, artificial implantation of c-*myc* into the mouse germ line produced carcinoma of the adult breast rather than abnormalities of development[27].

Proto-oncogenes and cancer

By one means or another, by circumstantial evidence of considerable variety, many of the known proto-oncogenes have been implicated in the genesis of tumors[2,3]. In some instances, the genes have been mutated to change the functions of the proteins they encode; in others, chromosomal translocations, mutagenesis, or gene amplification have altered expression of the offending genes.

Norman Mailer has reminded us that the genesis of cancer is not a simple matter. 'None of the doctors have a feel for cancer... The way I see the matter, it's a circuit of illness with two switches... Two terrible things have to happen before the crud can get its start. The first cocks the trigger. The other fires it'[28]. In no instance can we yet count and name the steps that lead to a given malignancy; we cannot speak of oncogenes as if their activity were alone responsible for tumorigenesis – we are not even certain that oncogenes are the key we hope they are; and it is possible that not all the steps to malignancy are genetic in nature. But it remains true that the emergence of proto-oncogenes has given new substance to various events in the genesis of a cancer cell: insertional mutagenesis by retroviruses[3] and point mutations within proto-oncogenes[29] may on occasion exemplify first steps in tumorigenesis; at least one gene has been isolated that confers the ability to metastasize[30]; amplification of several proto-oncogenes seems to correlate with the unruly growth of advanced malignancy[15,16]; at least one oncogene permits tumor cells to escape from dependence upon hormones[31]; and the manner in which two distinct genetic lesions might combine to produce malignant growth has been reconstructed in cell culture[32,33].

Some observers quarrel with these findings, faulting the fabric before it is fully woven[34]. But there are realities that cannot be easily dismissed: the same genetic lesions have been found repeatedly in the DNA of human tumors; with frequencies that seem beyond coincidence, these lesions have involved proto-oncogenes already known to us from the study of retroviral oncogenes; provocative correlations can be made between the occurrence of at least some genetic lesions and the biological behavior of the tumors in which the lesions are found; and several proto-oncogenes have returned to the stage repeatedly because they are affected by diverse forms of genetic damage – *myc* provides the most visible example because it has figured in mutagenesis by the integration of retroviral DNA, in chromosomal translocations, and in gene amplification. Where there is smoke, there is usually fire.

Where do we go from here? We must first confront the fact that genetic lesions have not been detected in most human tumors. We may have to invent new means of searching for these lesions, and remain open to the possibility that they will not always be there. We need to explore how recessive genetic damage might interact with proto-oncogenes[35]. And what of the inherited diathesis to cancer that first engendered the image of cancer genes? Can we find explanations for these through the study of proto-oncogenes? So far, we have not. In the end, we must learn how the products of oncogenes act before we can know the inner life of the cancer cell, before we can hope to parlay the explication of oncogenes into strategies for the treatment and prevention of cancer.

References

1 Norris, W. (1820) *Edinburgh Med. Surg. J.* 16, 562–565
2 Bishop, J. M. (1983) *Annu. Rev. Biochem.* 52, 301–354
3 Varmus, H. E. (1984) *Annu. Rev. Genet.* 18, 553–612
4 Bishop, J. M. (1985) *Cell* 42, 23–38
5 Land, H., Parada, L. F. and Weinberg, R. A. (1984) *Science* 222, 771–778
6 Yunis, J. J. (1983) *Science* 221, 227–235
7 Rowley, J. D. (1983) *Nature* 301, 290–291
8 Nowell, P. C. *et al.* (1984) *Cancer Surveys* 3, 531–542

9   Klein, G. and Klein, E. (1985) *Nature* 315, 190–195
10 Shtivelman, E. *et al.* (1985) *Nature* 315, 550–554
11 Konopka, J. B. *et al.* (1985) *Proc. Natl Acad. Sci. USA* 82, 1810–1815
12 George, D. (1984) *Cancer Surveys* 3, 497–513
13 Schwab, M. *et al.* (1983) *Nature* 305, 245–248
14 Kohl, N. E. *et al.* (1983) *Cell* 35, 359–367
15 Brodeur, G. M. *et al.* (1984) *Science* 224, 1121–1124
16 Nau, M. M. *et al.* (1984) in *Current Topics in Microbiology and Immunology,* Vol. 113, pp. 172–177, Springer-Verlag
17 Lee, W-H., Murphree, A. L. and Benedict, W. F. (1984) *Nature* 309, 458–460
18 Hunter, T. and Cooper, J. A. (1985) *Annu. Rev. Biochem.* 54, 897–930
19 Heldin, C-H. and Westermark, B. (1984) *Cell* 37, 9–20
20 Toda, T. *et al.* (1985) *Cell* 40, 27–36
21 Kingston, R. E., Baldwin, A. S., Jr and Sharp, P. A. (1985) *Cell* 41, 3–5
22 Ellis, R. W., Lowy, D. R. and Scolnick, E. M. (1982) in *Advances in Viral Oncology* (Klein, G., ed.), Vol. 1, pp. 107–126, Raven Press
23 Kataoka, T. *et al.* (1984) *Cell* 37, 437–445
24 Tatchell, K. *et al.* (1984) *Nature* 309, 523–528
25 Sorge, L. K., Levy, B. T. and Maness, P. F. (1984) *Cell* 36, 249–257
26 Shilo, B-Z. and Hoffmann, F. M. (1984) *Cancer Surveys* 3, 299–320
27 Stewart, R. A., Pattengale, P. K. and Leder, P. (1984) *Cell* 38, 627–637
28 Mailer, N. (1984) in *Tough Guys Don't Dance,* p. 158, Random House, New York
29 Zarbl, H. *et al.* (1985) *Nature* 315, 382–385
30 Bernstein, S. C. and Weinberg, R. A. (1985) *Proc. Natl Acad. Sci. USA* 82, 1726–1731
31 Kasid, A. *et al.* (1985) *Science* 228, 725–728
32 Land, H., Parada, L. F. and Weinberg, R. A. (1983) *Nature* 304, 596–601
33 Ruley, H. E. (1983) *Nature* 304, 602–606
34 Duesberg, P. H. (1985) *Science* 228, 669–677
35 Cavenee, W. K. *et al.* (1983) *Nature* 305, 779–784
36 Simon, M., Drees, B., Koinberg, T. and Bishop, J. M. (1985) *Cell* 42, 831–840

J. M. Bishop is at the Department of Microbiology and Immunology and the G. W. Hooper Foundation, University of California Medical Center, San Francisco, CA 94143, USA.

Cellular oncogenes

R. A. Weinberg

Of all areas of biochemistry, that which has probably seen the greatest change since the first issue of TIBS is oncogene research. We knew almost nothing about cellular oncogenes in 1976, and we know quite a bit now. In those days, we knew much about the gross, biological phenomena of cancer, but little about the underlying molecular mechanisms. Today, some of these central mechanisms are being revealed.

The cancer literature of 1976 provided demonstrations without end of the differences in phenotype between normal cells and their transformed counterparts. This catalog of cancer phenotypes, increasing to this day, derived from measurements of cellular morphology, metabolic priorities, surface antigenicities, growth rates, social behavior, growth factor requirements, and so forth. Such an endless list of cancer-specific phenotypes was most bewildering, since it was impossible to ferret out those phenotypes which were central and essential to the cancer state from the remainder, which seemed to represent distracting epiphenomena.

By 1976, two rather different types of work gave hope of some simplification. The first body of work, decades in the making, indicated that genetic damage was a frequent precursor to cellular transformation. This strengthened the hand of those who believed that the powerful tools of genetics could one day be brought to bear on the cancer problem. The other input came from virology, from the laboratories of those who studied DNA tumor viruses such as SV40 or polyoma, and transforming retroviruses such as Rous sarcoma virus. The tumor virologists established a simple point, which is deeply embedded in much of our present thinking. They found that a tumor virus with a small genome could transform a cultured cell from a normal into a tumorigenic state.

It was apparent that the process of tumorigenic conversion could be orchestrated by an extraordinarily small amount of genetic information. SV40 and Rous virus have genomes in the 5–10 kb range, almost a million times smaller than that of the cellular genome. Yet these minute amounts of genetic information were able to dramatically redirect the behavior of the host cells into which they had insinuated themselves. The viral transforming genes – oncogenes – were seen to act pleiotropically; an obviously small number of genes elicited a great number of phenotypic shifts. This suggested that the study of relatively simple genes would allow us to circumvent the endless complexity of the cancer phenotypes.

Unfortunately, most types of carcinogenic processes apparently involved no viruses or viral oncogenes. But in the year of the first *TIBS*, all this changed because of experiments performed on Rous sarcoma virus (RSV) and its oncogene, known as *src*. It had been clear that this single viral gene was sufficient for virus-induced transformation. What now emerged from an analysis of the pedigree of *src* was the startling finding that the *src* gene is of cellular origin, having been acquired from the chicken genome during the formation of RSV[1]. This showed that the cellular genome harbored, in apparently latent form, a gene which could assume malignant roles when properly activated. This paradigm was soon extended, in that we now know of at least 18 cellular genes, 'proto-oncogenes', each one of which has assumed an oncogenic configuration after associating with a transducing retrovirus[2]. These proto-oncogenes provided a vital element in the puzzle. They explained how cells could become transformed by genes residing within their own genomes. Intervention by exogenous genomes no longer seemed essential.

At the same time, the presence of these proto-oncogenes raised a provocative question that remains unanswered to this day: what are they doing within the normal cellular genome? That they subserve important cellular functions seems clear. Some of these proto-oncogenes have been found in homologous form in *Drosophila* and even in yeast[3,4]. Retention over a billion years and more of evolution implies indispensability, and the presence of some of these genes in yeast indicates important roles that preceded even the evolution of multicellularity. The popular truism has been that the proto-oncogenes must specify normal growth, since their oncogenic counterparts induce abnormal growth. This is probably correct, but still has only a minimum of experimental support, as we discuss later.

Proto-oncogenes and non-viral cancers

Another shift in the winds came in 1978 and 1979, when much of the earlier work on cellular proto-oncogenes acquired a relevance to chemically induced tumors and to human tumors of unknown etiology which apparently harbored no viruses. The use of gene transfer (transfection) allowed the transmission of the cancer state from one cell to another with DNA as the vehicle[5,6]. This work showed that distinct cellular determinants of transformation resided in tumor cell DNA. As we learned in the ensuing years, these determinants – oncogenes – followed the paradigm of the retrovirus-associated genes, in that normal cellular proto-oncogenes could serve as precursors to active oncogenes. What distinguished these two groups of oncogenes was the mechanism of activation, in one case viral transduction, in the other, some form of somatic mutation. Importantly, several of the oncogenes detected by transfection were soon found to be related to oncogenes transduced by retroviruses[7–10]. This meant that the same cellular proto-oncogene could become activated by a somatic mutation or by affiliation with a retrovirus.

All this was enormously satisfying for those interested in knowing the molecular basis of cancer. We now believe that the phenotypes of the cancer cell can be traced back to a few central regulator genes that have gone awry. We believe that the arrows and boxes that are often used to describe metabolic pathways or electronic circuitry will soon be used to interconnect the oncogenes with the plethora of cancer phenotypes. Lest this enthusiasm grow uncontrolled, we should keep in mind that the current progress on this front is very slow indeed. We are almost as puzzled now as we were in 1976 as to how an oncogene protein is able to transform a cell.

One relief from our otherwise total ignorance of the mechanism of oncogene action came from the discovery that the *src* protein[11] and some related proteins were tyrosine kinases. Such results suggested that a single protein could act pleiotropically on the cell by modifying a number of important intracellular targets. This line of work has been frustrated in recent years because no one has identified the targets whose modification by *src* is essential to the transformation process.

Moreover, many oncogenes do not encode protein kinases. The oncogenes found in human tumors by transfection have almost without exception been found to be members of the *ras* gene family[7-10,12,13], which has no structural homology with the *src*-like genes. These *ras* oncogenes were originally named because of their association with Kirsten and Harvey rat sarcoma viruses. Only later was it realized that they are well represented among the human oncogenes. Their encoded proteins (21 000 mol. wt) are certainly not tyrosine kinases. They bind GDP and GTP and are associated with the plasma membrane[14]. Their mode of action is obscure.

30 oncogenes equals 30 mechanisms?

We know of at least 18 cellular oncogenes and perhaps a dozen more carried by various DNA tumor viruses. If there are 30 oncogenes, are there also 30 different mechanisms of cellular transformation, or does this large number of oncogene-encoded proteins act upon a small number of critical targets? Another troubling question concerns the pleiotropy of oncogenes, the ability of each to elicit a large number of shifts in cellular phenotype. How pleiotropically acting is each of the well-known oncogenes? Can a single oncogene elicit all the phenotypes that are required for the complete progression from normality to fully competent tumorigenicity?

The beginnings of answers have emerged over the last several years in work with DNA tumor viruses, such as adenovirus and polyoma virus[15,16] and with cellular oncogenes[17-19]. For example, studies of the Ela and Elb oncogenes of adenovirus indicate that neither gene can induce tumorigenicity, but both acting in concert can achieve this state[15]. The middle T or the large T oncogenes of polyoma virus, each acting on its own, is unable to induce tumorigenic conversion, but acting together they are able to produce virtually all of the tumor cell phenotype[16]. An analogous description can be made about actions of the cellular *ras* and *myc* oncogenes. Neither the cellular *ras* nor *myc* genes can transform normal cells singly, but together they achieve full transformation[17].

In all these cases it appears that each oncogene, while eliciting several cellular responses, is nonetheless unable to elicit the full complement of traits required for tumorigenicity. Cooperation among several oncogenes seems to be required. These observations on the molecular level may explain the multistep process of natural carcinogenesis, each step reflecting perhaps the activation of another cellular gene. Moreover, the data show that two oncogenes may act in distinct, complementary ways.

The analogies among adenovirus, polyoma virus and the cellular oncogenes rest on more than the presence of a pair of cooperating genes in each set. In fact, it now appears that the middle T polyoma oncogene and the *ras* oncogene act very similarly, each able to cooperate with *myc* to induce tumorigenicity. Oncogenes of the other group, *myc*, polyoma large T, and adenovirus Ela, seem also able to mimic one another in their mode of action. Each seems able to immortalize cells in culture and to cooperate with *ras*.

Two 'complementation groups' of oncogenes

All this allows us to think that perhaps there are only a small number of central regulatory pathways governing cell proliferation. Each of the pathways may be acted upon by any one of a number of different oncogene-encoded proteins. The designation of as few as two regulatory pathways and associated oncogenes may seem premature and arbitrary, given the paucity of evidence. But interesting insights have already emerged from a scheme in which oncogenes are lumped into two 'complementation groups'.

The *myc*-like genes all appear to encode proteins found in the nucleus[17]. One member of this group, the adenovirus Ela gene, encodes a protein that is known to function as a *trans*-acting regulator of transcription. It appears able to enhance the transcription of a number of viral and cellular genes[20]. Recent work by R. Kingston and P. Sharp suggests similar properties may be exhibited by other gene products of the *myc* group. We are left with the most intriguing hypothesis that the *myc*-like proteins (including the *myc* protein itself) act to induce transcription of a bank of cellular genes that are critical for cellular proliferation. Because of their nuclear location, these proteins may regulate cell growth by interacting directly with the transcriptional apparatus or with the inducible target genes. It remains to be seen whether the cellular immortalization that is elicited by the *myc*-like proteins depends mechanistically on the power of these proteins to affect transcription.

The *ras*-like proteins behave differently. Those studied to date are localized to the cytoplasm, apparently to the inner surface of the plasma membrane. They seem involved in the issues of cell shape and anchorage independence, and their cytoplasmic localization may give a clue to their mechanism of action. Do they act on the tethers that connect the cytoarchitecture to the cell surface? Or do they stand astride a critical pathway for growth signals that are received from outside the cell and are passed on to intracellular targets? This latter model is suggested by analogy of the *ras* protein with another guanosine nucleotide-binding membrane protein, the G protein of the adenyl cyclase, which is known to act by transducing surface receptor signals to an intracellular target[21].

Extracellular signals and their transduction

These notions of extracellular signals and signal transduction are rapidly becoming central to our conceptualization of how oncogene proteins function. The reasons are obvious. Oncogene proteins can only elicit exaggerated versions of the phenotypes produced by their normal cellular counterparts. This forces confrontation, once again, with the roles of the proto-oncogenes and their encoded proteins. Perceptions on the role of the normal proteins in regulating cell growth ultimately touch on a single, obvious idea – that cells in metazoa grow in response to intercellular signals. Thus, the elements in the growth control pathways must either be the carriers of intercellular signals (e.g. growth factors) or their cell surface receptors, or the proteins that are responsible for further transducing growth signals from the receptors to critical intracellular targets.

In fact, work over the past year has begun to place elements into such a pathway. One finding of great interest was the finding of homology between the *sis* oncogene protein and the platelet-derived growth factor (PDGF)[22,23]. This implies that one mechanism for transformation may operate at the top of the pathway, causing a cell to become transformed because it synthesizes an excess of growth-stimulating factor. This factor may then act to overstimulate growth of the same cell that has just released it. Such an 'autocrine' mechanism has been discussed for some years by those who have noted that certain types of transformed cells may secrete growth factors which themselves are able to elicit transformed phenotypes[24].

The second elements in a growth-regulating pathway are the cell surface receptors. One might think that an altered growth factor receptor, that behaves as if it is constitutively binding its ligand, could also act as an oncogenic protein.

A recent report in *Nature* demonstrates homology between the erbB oncogene protein and the receptor for epidermal growth factor[25].

The subsequent elements in the pathway are the intracellular transducers of signal. Examples of this, such as the normal version of the *src-* or *ras*-encoded proteins, would seem to act by receiving growth-stimulatory signals and passing them on to downstream targets. The abnormal, oncogenic versions of these proteins would appear to act autonomously, stimulating downstream targets without receiving the normally required stimuli from an upstream source. The experimental justification of such a model, eagerly sought, is still lacking.

That such interacting pathways exist is clear. The most dramatic demonstration of this comes from recent work showing that extracellular PDGF can strongly stimulate the expression of the normal *myc* gene[26]. Thus, the homolog of the *sis* oncogene is able to regulate transcription of the normal homolog of a second oncogene. Quite possibly, other proto-oncogene-encoded proteins intervene to pass the signals down the pathway from PDGF to *myc*. The next years will see us working out these pathways. We shall soon fit many pieces of this puzzle together.

References

1 Stehelin, D., Varmus, H. E., Bishop, J. M. and Vogt, P. K. (1976) *Nature* 260, 170–173
2 Coffin, J. M., Varmus, H. E., Bishop, J. M., Essex, M., Hardy, W. D., Martin, G. S., Rosenberg, N. E., Scolnick, E. M., Weinberg, R. A. and Vogt, P. K. (1981) *J. Virol.* 40, 953–957
3 Shilo, B. Z. and Weinberg, R. A. (1981) *Proc. Natl Acad. Sci. USA* 78, 6789–6792
4 Gallwitz, D., Donath, C. and Sander, C. (1983) *Nature* 306, 704–706; DeFeo-Jones, D., Scolnick, E. M., Koller, R., Dhar, R. (1983) *Nature* 306, 706–709
5 Shih, C. *et al.* (1979) *Proc. Natl Acad. Sci. USA* 76, 5714–5718
6 Krontiris, T. G. and Cooper, G. M. (1981) *Proc. Natl Acad. Sci. USA* 78, 1181–1184
7 Der, C. J., Krontiris, T. and Cooper, G. M. (1982) *Proc. Natl Acad. Sci. USA* 79, 3637–3640
8 Parada, L. F., Tabin, C. J., Shih, C. and Weinberg, R. A. (1982) *Nature* 297, 474–478
9 Santos, E., Tronick, S., Aaronson, S. A., Pulciani, S. and Barbacid, M. (1982) *Nature* 298, 343–347
10 Goldfarb, M., Shimizu, K., Perucho, M. and Wigler, M. (1982) *Nature* 296, 404–409
11 Collett, M. S. and Erikson, R. L. (1978) *Proc. Natl Acad. Sci. USA* 75, 2021–2024
12 Cooper, G. M. (1982) *Science* 218, 801–806
13 Land, H., Parada, L. F. and Weinberg, R. A. (1983) *Science* 222, 771–778
14 Ellis, R. W., Lowy, D. R. and Scolnick, E. M. (1982) *Advances in Viral Oncology*, pp. 107–126, Raven Press
15 van den Elsen, P. J., de Pater, S., Houweling, A., vander Veer, A. and van der Eb, A. (1982) *Gene* 18, 175–185
16 Rassoulzadegan, M. *et al.* (1982) *Nature* 300, 713–718
17 Land, H., Parada, L. F. and Weinberg, R. A. (1983) *Nature* 304, 596–602
18 Newbold, R. F. and Overell, R. W. (1983) *Nature* 304, 648–651
19 Ruley, H. E. (1983) *Nature* 304, 602–606
20 Berk, A. J. *et al.* (1979) *Cell* 17, 935–944; Jones, N. and Shenk, T. (1979) *Cell* 17, 683–689; Jones, N. and Shenk, T. (1979) *Proc. Natl Acad. Sci. USA* 76, 3665–3669
21 Ross, E. M. and Gilman, A. G. (1980) *Annu. Rev. Biochem.* 49. 533–564
22 Doolittle, R. F., Hunkapiller, M., Hood, L., Devare, S., Robbins, K. C., Aaronson, S. A., Antoniades, H. N. (1983) *Science* 221, 275–276
23 Waterfield, M., Scrace, G., Whittle, N., Stroobant, P., Johnsson, A., Wasteson, A.,

Westermaker, B., Heldin, C.-H., Huang, J. and Deuel, T. (1983) *Nature* 304, 35–39
24   DeFalco, J. and Todaro, G. J. (1978) *Proc. Natl Acad. Sci. USA* 75, 4001–4005
25   Downward, J. *et al.* (1984) *Nature* 307, 521–527
26   Kelly, K., Cochran, B. H., Stiles, C. D. and Leder, P. (1983) *Cell* 35, 603–610

R. A. Weinberg is at the Center for Cancer Research, Massachusetts Institute of Technology, and Whitehead Institute for Biomedical Research, Cambridge, MA 02142, USA.

Amplification of cellular oncogenes in cancer cells

Kari Alitalo

Amplification of certain oncogenes is common in some tumors and also occurs as a rare sporadic event associated with various types of cancer. Amplified oncogenes are also expressed at elevated levels in some cells where they are normally silent and may or may not be associated with chromosomal abnormalities that signify DNA amplification. The increased dosage of an oncogene following amplification may contribute to the multistep progression of at least some forms of cancer.

Regulatory or structural alterations of cellular oncogenes have been implicated in various forms of cancer[1]. Point mutations in oncogenes can result in protein products with strongly enhanced tumorigenic potential. Aberrant expression of cellular oncogenes may result from tumor-specific chromosomal translocations that dysregulate the normal function of a proto-oncogene. The amplification of cellular oncogenes can enhance their expression by increasing the amount of DNA template available for the production of mRNA.

Chromosomal abnormalities and oncogene amplification

Somatic amplification of specific genes has been implicated in a variety of adaptive responses of cells to environmental stresses[2]. Two cytogenetic abnormalities, double minute chromosomes (dmins) and homogeneously staining chromosomal regions (HSR) associated with DNA amplification were originally discovered in tumor cells and in cells selected for drug-resistance[3-5]. In metaphase spreads, dmins appear as small, spherical, usually paired chromosome-like structures that lack a centromere[3]. HSRs stain with uniform intermediate intensity rather than with the normal alternating dark and light bands in trypsin-Giemsa stained chromosome preparations[3,4].

The dmins and HSRs are apparently rare in tumor cells *in vivo*, although frequency data are difficult to obtain since these abnormalities are easily missed in routine cytogenetic analysis. They frequently occur in cultured malignant cells, notably in neuroblastoma cell lines[6]. Culture conditions apparently select for tumor cells that contain either dmins or HSRs. Moreover, during growth in culture, dmins often disappear with the appearance of clonal populations of cells that have developed an HSR, suggesting that the two cytogenetic abnormalities are alternative forms of gene amplification. It has been assumed that HSRs can break down to form dmins and that dmins can integrate into chromosomes to generate HSRs[2,3].

Work on drug-resistant cells has shown that in the absence of a selection pressure (drug), dmins and the amplified genes that they contain are lost, whereas amplified DNA in the form of HSRs is retained in the cells[2]. This is explained by the fact that dmins segregate unevenly in mitosis and are frequently lost from the nucleus because they lack centromeres. HSR chromosomes carry centromeres and are therefore divided evenly at mitosis.

Although dmins and HSRs have been predominantly detected in tumor cells selected for resistance to cytotoxic drugs, they are sometimes present in cancer cells before therapy[3,6]. It was in this context that we and others first explored the possible amplification of cellular oncogenes.

The somatic amplifications of cellular oncogenes reported to date in tumor cells are summarized in Table 1. Amplification which can range from a few-fold to many hundred-fold affects at least five out of 20 or so known cellular oncogenes. The first oncogene amplification reported involved the c-*myc* oncogene (see Table 1) in a promyelocytic leukemia cell line HL-60[7,8]. This gene was amplified 8–32 times both in the HL-60 cells and in primary leukemic cells from the patient[7,8]. Original clonal lines of HL-60 were later found to contain some dmins in culture but not sufficient to establish any clear correlation with amplified c-*myc*. However, such a correlation was discovered for c-*myc* amplification in a neuroendocrine cell line from a colon carcinoma, COLO 320[9]. In these cells, about 30 copies of c-*myc* (Fig. 1) were mapped either to HSRs of a marker chromosome by *in situ* hybridization or to isolated dmins, depending on the particular subline studied (Fig. 2). Similarly, amplified copies of the c-Ki-*ras* oncogene were mapped to dmins and HSRs of a mouse adrenocortical tumor Y1[10]. An extensive search for changes in other oncogenes and tumor cells has since revealed amplifications that do not show up as dmins or HSRs. For example, the c-*myb* oncogene is amplified in a characteristic marker chromosome of a colon carcinoma without evidence of HSRs[11,12]. This suggests that (onco) gene amplification may be more common than the structural alterations revealed by chromosome banding and microscopy. Furthermore, somatic amplifications of oncogenes have also been found in fresh tumor cells from patients (Table 1).

Translocations and DNA rearrangements

The evolution and progression of the karyotype of tumor cells is a complex process. Concomitant with amplification, DNA sequences acquire an increased

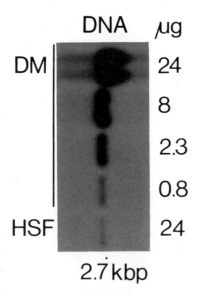

Fig. 1. Estimation of the copy number of c-myc in COLO 320 DM cells. DNA was cleaved with SstI, diluted as indicated, electrophoresed, blotted and hybridized with a cloned radioactive 320 bp DNA fragment from the 3' exon of c-myc. The intensity of the signal from the 2.7 kbp fragment in the autoradiogram is similar in 24 µg of DNA from human skin fibroblasts (HSF) and 0.8 µg of DNA from COLO 320 DM cells. Thus, c-myc is amplified about 30 times.

Table 1. Sporadic and tumor-specific amplification of cellular oncogenes

Tumor cells	Oncogene	Amplification	Chromosomal location of amplified gene	Remarks	Refs
Sporadic					
HL-60 (acute promyelocytic leukemia)	c-*myc*	20×	8q(ABR)	Amplification present in primary leukemic cells	7, 8, 13
COLO 320 (colon carcinoma)	c-*myc*	30×	dmin, HSR	Part of the amplified c-*myc* sequences rearranged	9
Y1 (adrenocortical tumor)	c-Ki-*ras*	50×	dmin, HSR	Levels of p21 (c-Ki-*ras*) elevated	10
COLO 201/205 (colon carcinoma)	c-*myb*	10×	mar1	Patient treated with 5-fluorouracil before culturing of tumor cells	11, 12
K562 (chronic myelogenous leukemia)	c-*abl*	10×	mar(ABR)	CA coamplified in the marker that may be derived from chromosome 22. c-*abl* protein-associated tyrosine kinase activated	15, 34
A-431 (epidermoid carcinoma)	c-*erbB*	15–20×	nd	Amplification associated with chromosome 7 translocation and sequence rearrangements	14
ML1-3 (acute myelogenous leukemia)	c-*myb*	5–10×	nd	Abnormalities of chromosome 6q22–24, where c-*myb* is normally located	39
SK BR-3 (breast carcinoma)	c-*myc*	10×	nd		17
Tumor-specific					
small-cell lung cancer	c-*myc* N-*myc* L-*myc*	up to 80×	nd	Most amplifications in the variant phenotype of SCLC	24
neuroblastomas	N-*myc*	up to 250×	dmin, HSR	N-*myc* also amplified in primary tumors of advanced grade	25
glioblastomas	c-*erbB*	up to 50×	nd	Some amplifications associated with sequence rearrangements	26

nd, not determined; mar, marker chromosome

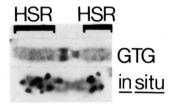

Fig. 2. *Trypsin-Giemsa banding (GTG) and* in situ *hybridization for c-myc in a long marker chromosome of COLO 320 HSR cells. The marker has evolved from the X chromosome by replacement and extension of both chromosomal arms with homogeneously staining regions (HSR)*[9].

mobility in the genome with extrachromosomal intermediates visualized as dmins, transpositions and translocations to other chromosomal segments, etc.[3,6]. There may not be preferred chromosomal sites for the apparent reintegration of dmins as HSRs[6]. However, in one case, an amplified oncogene has been observed *in situ* in its resident chromosomal site which had an abnormal banding region[13]. At least three examples of oncogene amplification accompanied by oncogene rearrangement have been reported. In the colon carcinoma COLO 320, both damaged and normal versions of the c-*myc* gene are amplified[9]. Part of the amplified copies of the c-*erb*B oncogene in A431 epidermoid carcinoma cells are also rearranged and produce a truncated EGF receptor protein[14]. In the chronic myeloid leukemia (erythroleukemia) cell line K562, an amplified DNA segment consists of portions of both the c-*abl* oncogene, the *bcr*-1 gene and the immunoglobulin C_λ locus[15]. In all three cases, abnormal transcripts are produced from the rearranged amplified oncogenes[9,14,16]. In K562 cells, the protein product of the abnormal c-*abl* oncogene has also been activated as a tyrosine kinase[17]. It is not known whether structural alterations of the genes preceded their amplification or whether they were acquired during amplification. However, most reported cases of amplified oncogenes are apparently normal on the basis of restriction endonuclease mapping (see Table 1). Therefore, mutation does not seem to be a necessary companion of oncogene amplification.

Gene amplification mechanisms
   The mechanisms of gene amplification and the structure of the amplified DNA have been worked out mainly in experimental settings involving selection for drug-resistance in cell culture[2]. Although they are still incompletely resolved and may vary in different cases, some general features have emerged. Spontaneous illegitimate DNA replication seems to occur in normal cells so that various segments of DNA replicate more than once during a single cell cycle[2,5]. In nonselective conditions this DNA is probably lost because the newly synthesized extra copies of DNA are not covalently linked to chromosomal DNA of mitotic cells. However, if there is selection for increased gene dosage, progressive gene multiplication occurs. The incidence of cells bearing amplified genes under conditions of cytotoxic selection can vary by two orders of magnitude and is greatly increased by presence of mitogenic substances (hormones or tumor promotors) during selection or of certain carcinogenic or cytotoxic agents before selection[18,19]. Mariani and Schimke[19] point out that most of the cytotoxic agents which enhance gene amplification are inhibitors of DNA synthesis. Aberrant replication takes place after transient inhibition of DNA synthesis and this response can lead to gene amplification[2]. Mitogenic hormones probably increase

disproportionate DNA replication but also enhance the colony-forming efficiency of drug-resistant cells in selective conditions[2,18].

The chromosomal site of integration of transfected genes significantly affects the frequency and cytogenetic result of their experimentally-induced amplification[20]. Amplification in some transformants has been found to be 100 times that of the others[20]. This suggests that there are preferred chromosomal positions for amplification of cellular genes and that chromosomal rearrangements may facilitate gene amplification by positioning crucial DNA sequences in a favorable array. DNA rearrangements involving variation in gene copy number have been found in the human genome between clusters of short repetitive interspersed DNA sequences called *Alu* family sequences[21]. It is not known if these kinds of repetitive sequences are involved in generating amplified oncogene sequences in tumors.

Amplification, enhanced expression and clonal selection of cancer cells

The rapid induction of gene amplification which apparently occurs frequently through extrachromosomal intermediates may provide tumor cells with genetic material for subsequent selective pressures operating in harmful conditions[2]. This may promote the emergence and evolution of clonal populations of cells with increasingly malignant properties. Such genetic instability is clearly enhanced in cancer cells. An important question is whether drug-resistance in treated patients also selects for cells that have an enhanced ability to amplify (onco)genes[18]. It is also possible that some mutagenic insults are only carcinogenic as a result of subsequent amplification events facilitated by tumor promotors or by hormones[2].

The persistence of dmins in some tumors suggests that there is selection for them. Amplified DNA in dmins must contain an origin for DNA replication and must be selected for in daughter cell populations, where it is unevenly segregated. In at least one study, the length of an HSR was found to increase during selection of malignant cells for enhanced tumorigenicity[22]. A naive supposition is that the amplified sequences in dmins (and possibly in HSRs) of tumors contain growth-promoting genes. This fits in well with recent findings on amplified oncogenes, though in many cases amplified oncogenes are still being sought. Even positive findings do not confirm a role for amplified cellular oncogenes, however, because the domain of amplified DNA is inevitably much larger than a single genetic locus[23].

All the amplified oncogenes studied are abundantly expressed at the RNA level, roughly in proportion to the amount of DNA amplification (see Table 1). Examples of enhanced gene dosage include abnormal RNA and ectopic expression[11]. In several cases, this enhancement is not limited to synthesis of RNA (see Table 1). For example, the Y1 cells that have amplified c-Ki-*ras* contain exceptionally high concentrations of its protein product on their plasma membrane[10]. High concentrations of the c-*myc* encoded protein are also found in COLO 320 cells that have amplified the gene. In general, enhanced expression of an oncogene seems to be a prerequisite for the growth advantage of cells having extra copies of the gene. This effect could also be the principal contribution of amplification to tumorigenesis.

Tumor cell and stage specificity of amplified oncogenes

In at least some tumor cells, amplified oncogenes may complement mutationally activated oncogenes[27,28]. The N-*myc* gene is consistently amplified in most neuroblastoma cell lines and in about 40% of neuroblastoma tumors (Table 1). Also, some retinoblastoma and small-cell lung cancer cell lines contain multiple copies of N-*myc*[29,30]. The size of the amplicon in neuroblastomas may be of the order of 200–2000 kbp and is complex in structure, containing distinct segments from chromosomal arm 2p[31]. About 50% of advanced stages (III–IV) of neuroblastoma tumors contain amplified N-*myc*[32]. The amplifications of N-*myc* in neuroblastomas and c-*myc* in small-cell lung cancer are correlated with a poor prognosis, independent of the stage of the tumor (Ref. 33 and J. Minna, pers. commun.). The N-*myc* and L-*myc* genes can also be found amplified in small-cell lung cancer[34]. These three *myc* genes show similar structures and encode related nuclear phosphoproteins. The c-*erb*B-1 gene has been found amplified in some glioblastomas and several squamous-cell carcinomas[26,35]. The related c-*erb*B-2 (*neu*) gene is amplified in some adenocarcinomas[36].

When does oncogene amplification come into play during tumorigenesis? Gene amplification may not be an initiating event in carcinogenesis. Amplification and enhanced expression of c-*myc* and N-*myc* apparently occur during malignant progression of human carcinoma of the lung and neuroblastoma cells[24,25]. However, there may not be a mandatory sequence of oncogene amplifications for the genesis of any particular tumor. Perhaps amplification of an oncogene affects the malignant progression of already initiated cells. Moreover, even amplified oncogenes may become transcriptionally silent upon induction of tumor cell differentiation[37,38].

Acknowledgements

I thank Manfred Schwab, Gerard Evan, J. Michael Bishop, Harold Varmus, Robert Winqvist, Kalle Saksela, Tomi Mäkela, Lea Sistonen, Päivi Koskinen and Jorma Keski-Oja for their collaboration. Studies in my laboratory were supported by the Finnish Cancer Research Fund and by the Academy of Finland. Part of the studies were carried out under contract with the Finnish Life Insurance Companies.

References

1 Bishop, J. M. (1983) *Annu. Rev. Biochem.* 52, 301–354
2 Schimke, R. T. (1984) *Cell* 37, 705–713
3 Barker, P. E. (1982) *Cancer Genet. Cytogenet.* 5, 81–94
4 Cowell, J. K. (1982) *Annu. Rev. Genet.* 16, 21–52
5 Stark, G. R. and Wahl, G. M. (1984) *Annu. Rev. Biochem.* 53, 447–491
6 Biedler, J. L., Meyers, M. B. and Spengler, B. A. (1983) *Adv. Cell. Neurobiol.* 4, 268–301
7 Collins, S. and Groudine, M. (1982) *Nature* 298, 679–681
8 Dalla-Favera, R. D., Wong-Staal, F. and Gallo, R. C. (1982) *Nature* 299, 61–63
9 Alitalo, K., Schwab, M., Lin, C. C., Varmus, H. E. and Bishop, J. M. (1983) *Proc. Natl Acad. Sci. USA* 80, 1707–1711
10 Schwab, M., Alitalo, K., Varmus, H. E., Bishop, J. M. and George, D. (1983) *Nature* 303, 497–501
11 Alitalo, K., Winqvist, R., Lin, C. C., de la Chapelle, A., Schwab, M. and Bishop, J. M. (1984) *Proc. Natl Acad. Sci. USA* 81, 4534–4538
12 Winqvist, R., Kmuubila, S., Lepince, D., Stekelin, D. and Alitalo, K. *Cancer Genet. Cytogenet.* (in press)
13 Nowell, R., Finan, J., Favera, R. D., Gallo, R. C., Ar-Rushdi, A., Romanczu, K. G., Selden, J. R., Emanuel, B. S., Rovera, G. and Croce, C. M. (1983) *Nature* 306, 494–497
14 Ullrich, A., Coussens, L., Hayflick, J. S., Dull, T. J., Gray, A., Tam, A. W., Lee, J., Yarden, Y., Libermann, T. A., Schlessinger, J., Downward, J., Mayes,

E. L. V., Whittle, N., Waterfield, M. D. and Seeburg, P. H. (1984) *Nature* 209, 418–425

15 Collins, S. J. and Groudine, M. T. (1983) *Proc. Natl Acad. Sci. USA* 80, 4813–4817
16 Collins, S. J., Kubonishi, I., Miyoshi, I. and Groudine, M. T. (1984) *Science* 225, 72–74
17 Kozobor, D. and Croce, C. M. (1984) *Cancer Res.* 44, 438–441
18 Barsoum, J. and Varshavsky, A. (1983) *Proc. Natl Acad. Sci. USA* 80, 5330–5334
19 Mariani, B. D. and Schimke, R. T. (1984) *J. Biol. Chem.* 259, 1901–1910
20 Wahl, G. M., de Saint Vincent, B. R. and DeRose, M. L. (1984) *Nature* 307, 516–520
21 Shmookler Reis, R. J., Lumpkin, C. K., McGill, J. R., Riabowol, T. K. and Goldstein, S. (1983) *Nature* 201, 394–398
22 Gilbert, F., Balaban, G., Brangman, D., Herrman, N. and Lister, A. (1983) *Int. J. Cancer* 31, 765–768
23 Roberts, J. M., Buck, L. B. and Axel, R. (1983) *Cell* 33, 53–63
24 Little, C. D., Nau, M. M., Carney, D. N., Gazdar, A. F. and Minna, J. D. (1983) *Nature* 306, 194–196
25 Schwab, M., Alitalo, K., Klempnauer, K.-H., Varmus, H. E., Bishop, J. M., Gelbert, F., Brodeur, G., Goldstein, M. and Trent, J. (1983) *Nature* 305, 245–248
26 Libermann, T. A., Nusbaum, H. R., Razon, N., Kris, R., Lax, I., Soreq, H., Whittle, N., Waterfield, M. D., Ullrich, A. and Schlessinger, J. (1985) *Nature* 313, 143–147
27 Land, H., Parada, L. F. and Weinberg, R. A. (1983) *Science* 222, 771–778
28 Murray, M. J., Cunningham, J. M., Parada, L. F., Dautry, F., Lebowitz, P. and Weinberg, R. A. (1983) *Cell* 33, 749–757
29 Lee, W-H., Murphree, A. L., Benedict, W. F. (1984) *Nature* 309, 458–460
30 Nau, M. M., Carney, D. N., Battey, J., Johnson, B., Little, C., Gazdar, A. and Minna, J. D. (1984) *Curr. Top. Microbiol. Immunol.* 113, 172–177
31 Shiloh, Y., Shipley, J., Brodeur, G. M., Bruns, G., Korf, B., Donlon, T., Schreck, R. R., Seeger, T., Sakai, K. and Latt, S. A. (1985) *Proc. Natl Acad. Sci. USA* 82, 3761–3765
32 Brodeur, G. M., Seeger, R. C., Schwab, M., Varmus, H. E. and Bishop, J. M. (1984) *Science* 224, 1121–1124
33 Seeger, R. C., Brodeur, G. M., Sather, H., Dalton, A., Siegel, S. E., Wong, K. Y. and Hammond, D. (1985) *N. Engl. J. Med.* 313, 1111–1116
34 Nau, M. M., Brookds, B. J., Battey, J., Sausville, E., Gazdar, A. F., Kirsch, I. R., McBride, O. W., Bertness, V., Hollis, G. F. and Minna, J. D. (1985) *Nature* 318, 69–73
35 Yamamoto, T., Kamata, N., Kawano, H., Shimizu, S., Kuroki, T., Toyoshima, K., Rikimaru, K., Nomura, N., Ishizaki, R., Pastan, I., Gamou, S. and Shimizu, N. (1986) *Cancer Res.* 46, 414–416
36 Yokota, J., Yamamoto, T., Toyoshima, K., Terada, M., Sugimura, T., Baatifora, H. and Cline, M. J. (1986) *The Lancet* 765–766
37 Thiele, C. J., Reynolds, C. P. and Israel, M. A. (1985) *Nature* 313, 404–406
38 Westin, E. H., Wong-staal, F., Gelmann, E. P., Dalla-Favera, R., Papas, T. S., Lautenberger, J. A., Eva, A., Prekumar Reddy, E., Tronick, S. R., Aaronson, S. A. and Gallo, R. C. (1982) *Proc. Natl Acad. Sci. USA* 79, 2490–2494
39 Pelicci, P.-C., Lanfrancone, L., Brathwaite, M. D., Wolman, S. R. and Dalla-Favera, R. (1984) *Science* 224, 1117–1121

K. Alitalo is at the Department of Virology and Recombinant DNA Laboratory, University of Helsinki, Haartmaninkatu 3, 00290 Helsinki 29, Finland.

The *c-myc* proto-oncogene: involvement in chromosomal abnormalities

T. H. Rabbitts

The c-myc *proto-oncogene has been implicated in oncogenesis because of dramatic changes associated with the gene in the chromosomes of some tumours. The abnormalities include provirus insertion, chromosomal translocation and gene amplification. The changes are thought to involve an alteration in* c-myc *expression, which contributes to the aetiology of these tumours.*

Scepticism has been expressed about the real contribution of oncogenes to tumour formation. The c-*myc* oncogene is one of the most convincing examples of an oncogene with a positive role in tumour aetiology, since consistent, gross abnormalities within or near this gene occur in various tumour types. The most consistent abnormality is that observed in the human B-lymphocyte tumour called Burkitt's lymphoma. This tumour has a regularly occurring chromosomal translocation involving the c-*myc* gene. Other crucial observations of the involvement of the c-*myc* gene in tumours were the finding of provirus insertion adjacent to c-*myc* in chicken B-cell lymphomas and c-*myc* amplification in some human cancers. These three abnormalities, involving c-*myc,* lend considerable credence to the view that c-*myc* proto-oncogene has a role in tumour formation.

Definition of the c-*myc* gene and viral transduction of c-*myc*
   The *myc* oncogene was originally observed in the genomes of a group of acutely-transforming retroviruses which can induce a variety of neoplastic diseases in birds. The best characterized virus of this group is MC29 whose genome encodes a single polypeptide of 110 kDa. The aminoterminal half of this protein is specified by the retroviral *gag* gene. However, the 47 kDa carboxy-terminal moiety of this polypeptide is not of retroviral origin and has been designated 'viral *myc*' or v-*myc*.
   Cellular homologues of v-*myc* have been observed in chicken as well as mammalian genomes. Sequences of the cellular or c-*myc* gene which share homology with MC29 occur in two exons; an additional exon has been identified in c-*myc* which is not present in v-*myc* (see Fig. 1). The existence of a cellular homologue of the v-*myc* gene allows an explanation of the viral gene. A specialized form of viral transduction can occur in which a spliced transcript of the c-*myc* gene is incorporated into a retrovirus genome. The transforming activity of the viral *myc* gene may be explained by a number of mechanisms, such as high levels of transcription resulting from the potent activating elements in the viral long terminal repeat sequences.

The c-*myc* proto-oncogene is normally expressed in a variety of tissue types
   The first article in this book (J. M. Bishop, p. 1–10) explained that proto-oncogenes are genes used by cells as part of their normal activity. Operationally,

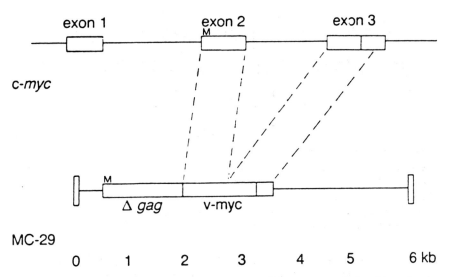

Fig. 1. The relationship of v-myc and c-myc genes. The sequence relationships of v-myc and c-myc genes are shown by the dotted lines. M refers to the methionine translational initiation codon.

they are termed oncogenes only after they are altered in some way by mutational events (for example, base changes as in the *ras* gene or gene amplification as in N-*myc*, a gene related to c-*myc*). The c-*myc* gene is an excellent example of a proto-oncogene; it is normally expressed in a variety of growing cell types, notably lymphoid cells. Transcription from the gene can be seen very soon after resting spleen cells are activated with polyclonal mitogens[2] and synthesis of c-*myc* mRNA and protein takes place throughout the cell cycle[3-5], transcription is shut off when the cells stop dividing[6]. The c-*myc* protein is usually located in the nucleus and is capable of binding strongly to DNA *in vitro*, albeit non-specifically[27]. The data support, but by no means prove, the idea that the c-*myc* gene product is a regulatory protein of some sort but we cannot be certain that this will ultimately prove an adequate description. These results indicate that c-*myc* activity is controlled by a delicate balance in the cell and that c-*myc* expression is finely coupled to the differentiation and/or division state of the cell. This view is supported by the fact that both c-*myc* mRNA[8] and protein normally have a rather short half-life *in vivo*. It is perhaps not surprising, therefore, that disruptions of the gene are frequently associated with cancer.

Provirus insertion

The c-*myc* gene became implicated in mammalian tumour formation when it was discovered that avian leukosis virus (ALV, a replication-competent retrovirus which does not carry a transforming gene or oncogene) can induce, with a high frequency, B-cell lymphomas in chickens, with a chromosomal insertion site nearly always near to c-*myc*[9,10]. The c-*myc* gene was already known as a genomic gene because of its homology to v-*myc*, the transforming gene present in the avian myelocytomatosis (AMV) retrovirus. The insertion of ALV near to c-*myc* was therefore a highly significant discovery. This led to the idea of promoter insertional activation of the c-*myc* gene whereby the ALV promoter takes over the transcriptional control of c-*myc*, causing deregulation (see below) which is probably (at least partly) responsible for ALV-induced B-cell lymphomas. The site and orientation of provirus insertion does not seem to be all that important since it can be found upstream or downstream of c-*myc*, in the opposite or the same transcriptional orientation, respectively. The important feature is proximity to c-*myc*, which can result in a large increase in the magnitude of c-*myc* mRNA expression. This is thought to be a crucial effect of provirus insertion into the genome of the prelymphomatous tissue and constitutes the tumorigenic activation of the c-*myc* gene which eventually leads to B-cell lymphoma.

Chromosomal translocation involving the c-*myc* gene

In the human B-cell tumour, Burkitt's lymphoma (BL), and the mouse plasmacytomas, specific chromosomal translocation involving c-*myc* occur. There is an absolute correlation between these types of tumour and the presence of the specific chromosomal translocation, making a causative correlation extremely likely. The single locus encoding human c-*myc* occurs at 8q24(q = chromosome long arm) and contains a single copy of c-*myc* consisting of three exons (Figs 1 and 2). The first exon (about 500 base pairs) is thought to be non-coding and the protein coding part (the only part with an equivalent in the v-*myc* gene of AMV) is encoded by exons two and three. Two main mRNA species are derived from the normal c-*myc* gene, since there are two RNA start sites and promoters (designated P1 and P2 in Fig. 2). The function of the long exon 1 is

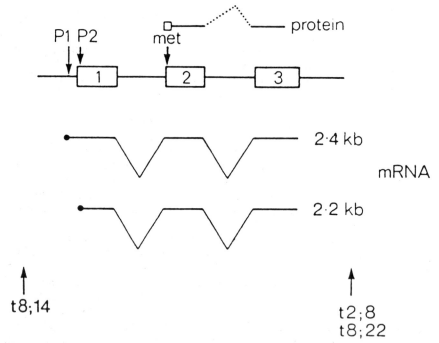

Fig. 2. The c-myc gene and products. The gene has three exons: the codon for protein synthesis initiation is at the start of exon 2; the protein is encoded by exons 2 and 3. Two major RNA species (2.4 kb and 2.2 kb mRNA, indicated with splice positions) are derived from two major promoters, P1 and P2. The translocation breakpoints in the Burkitt's lymphomas are indicated.

unknown. The possibilities put forward include the ideas that a transcriptional repressor molecule binds to it[11] or, that it is involved in the control of protein synthesis by the mRNA[12]. However, data which might validate these hypotheses have yet to be produced. In fact, recent studies on the stability of c-*myc* mRNA in cells expressing truncated c-*myc* genes show that truncated *myc* mRNA is more stable than the normal counterpart[13]. These observations argue that exon 1 plays a post-transcriptional role in the process of c-*myc* mRNA degradation *in vivo* and therefore that truncation of the c-*myc* gene (see below) may be a crucial tumorigenic event.

Three specific translocations are found in BL, each involving 8q24 with either 14q32 (in the majority of cases) or with 2p12 or 22q11 (the so-called variant BL translocations). The positions of breakpoints adjacent to c-*myc* are illustrated in Fig. 2. The genes located on chromosomes 14, 2 and 22 are for immunoglobulin (*Ig*) heavy (H) chains, kappa light (L) chains and lamba light chains respectively. Molecular cloning studies and *in situ* hybridizations have elucidated the reorganization events accompanying the cytogenetic changes associated with the translocations. The c-*myc* gene lies near to the tip of the chromosome long arm and the 5' end of the gene faces the centromere. In t(8;14), the breakpoint is proximal (i.e. on the centromeric side) to c-*myc* so that the piece of 8q translocated to chromosome 14 includes c-*myc*. This is not the case in the variant translocations where breakage on 8q is distal (i.e. on the telomeric side) to c-*myc* and the L-chain genes are included in the segment translocated to chromosome 8. Therefore, the translocation breakpoints occur upstream of c-*myc* in t(8;14) and downstream in the variant BL.

At the molecular level, DNA studies have shown that the BL t(8;14) translocations bring the c-*myc* and *Ig* H-chain genes very close together (as depicted in Fig. 3) in a head-to-head orientation. The breakage point on chromosome 14 is frequently, but not always, within the switch region (involved in the *Ig* switch recombination) but there seems to be no sequence specificity in the c-*myc* locus since the breakpoint on 8q is rather variable[13,15]. Indeed, this variability is so large that a new region of clustered breakpoints, called *pvt*, some distance from the mouse c-*myc* has been described in plasmacytomas which have variant translocations[16] analogous to those in BL. Occasionally, translocation of c-*myc* in BL t8;14 results in truncation of the gene, the breakpoint being within the intron between exons 1 and 2. In mouse plasmacytomas, this is the most frequent occurrence. Since exon 1 is non-coding, the c-*myc* protein, which would result from such a truncated transcript, is unaffected. When truncation does occur, transcription of the gene proceeds from previously cryptic promoters within the intron[17].

We are still rather uncertain about the consequences of translocation on the c-*myc* gene. It was expected that *Ig* gene controlling elements would affect translocated c-*myc*, causing c-*myc* to be expressed like *Ig* genes (i.e. essentially incapable of inactivity once switched on). It should be emphasized that chromosomal translocation can, but does not necessarily, result in elevated amounts of c-*myc* mRNA. However, the major transcriptional enhancer associated with *Ig* H-chains does not usually remain on 14q+ after translocation[18] (see Fig. 3) and therefore cannot exert its *cis* acting effect on c *myc*. Exceptions occur[19] in which the c-*myc* gene is controlled by the *Ig* enhancer. Other *Ig* controlling elements may come to light in future studies but, at present, our view of the mechanism of disruption of translocated c-*myc* activity is murky. Even though there may be no unifying hypothesis to account

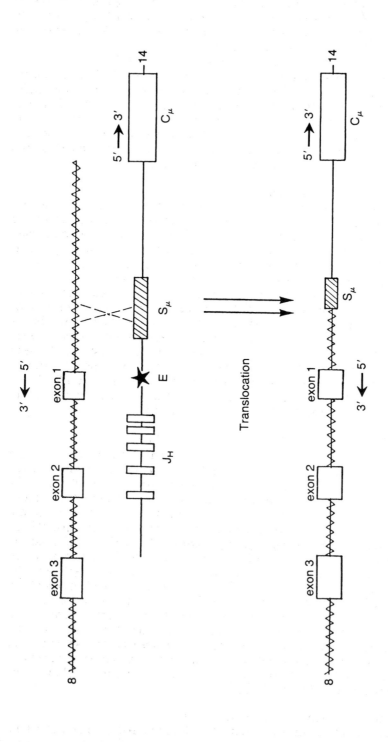

*Fig. 3. An 8;14 translocation in Burkitt's lymphoma. The c-*myc *gene from chromosome 8 is shown joining the* Ig *μ-chain gene from chromosome 14 through the* Ig *switch sequences. The resulting 14q$^+$ chromosome has c-*myc *and* Ig*μ head-to-head. The star depicts the major transcriptional enhancer of the* Igh *locus.*

for both the variety of translocation points and the apparently consistent activation of the c-*myc* gene, the common feature is probably deregulation of the translocated gene. Indeed, there may be several ways in which chromosomal translocation can achieve this deregulation.

One intriguing feature of many translocations in Burkitt's lymphoma is that extensive somatic mutations have occurred within exon 1[11,14]. These mutations are presumably introduced into the translocated c-*myc* gene during the joining event. The widespread occurrence of such mutations (which can be deletions or point mutations) suggests that they may affect the function of an element in or around the gene, not necessarily exon 1 but perhaps an upstream element. Furthermore, coding region changes have also been described[26] and these may well exert their influence on the progression of the tumour.

Amplification of the c-*myc* gene

Amplification of c-*myc*, and associated larger amounts of mRNA, has been found in a variety of tumour types (reviewed in Ref. 20). This amplification can be associated with gross cytogenetic abnormalities, described as double minute chromosomes (small spherical structures in metaphase chromosome preparations) and homogeneously staining regions (so-called because of the Giemsa staining characteristics of the amplified chromosomal regions).

Amplification of c-*myc* has been observed in colon carcinoma (seen as both double minute chromosomes and homogeneously staining regions), promyelocytic leukaemia, large and small lung cell carcinoma and breast carcinoma. It is not a phenomenon restricted to c-*myc*; a related gene, N-*myc*, was first discovered as an amplified gene in neuroblastomas[21]. Gene amplification need not result in increased amounts of the relevant mRNA; however, in most examples of amplified c-*myc* genes, there is more mRNA and presumably this has a crucial bearing on the origin of the tumour or on its progression, as in neuroblastomas with N-*myc* amplification[22].

Co-operative transforming effect of the c-*myc* oncogene

One very convincing piece of evidence that oncogenes can cause tumours is the *in vitro* transforming assay of NIH3T3 cells. For example, c-*ras* genes isolated from tumour cell DNA will cause morphological transformation (i.e. focus formation) of cells in culture and these cells will subsequently cause tumour formation in mice. Primary cultures of fibroblasts, on the other hand, are resistant to such induced transformation but can be transformed if transfected with tumour cell-derived c-*ras* plus a c-*myc* gene which is both truncated (i.e. the coding region only) and controlled by an SV40 promoter[23]. Such co-operative transformation can also be achieved with a combination of c-*ras* and the adenovirus gene *Ela*[24]. This experiment illustrates clearly two features of the generation of the tumour phenotype. Firstly, that it is a multi-step event (i.e. involving several proto-oncogene activations) and secondly, that there is more than one way to reach the neoplastic state. Elucidation of the function of the various oncogenes in this process is a major goal of molecular biology and offers some hope that we can define and understand the steps in tumour progression. Whether this knowledge will help to cure or prevent cancer remains to be seen but there is certainly an optimistic note.

'Pre-induced c-*myc* activation' of tumour cells

The processes of provirus insertion, translocation and gene amplification (which affect the c-*myc* gene in tumours) are superficially very different.

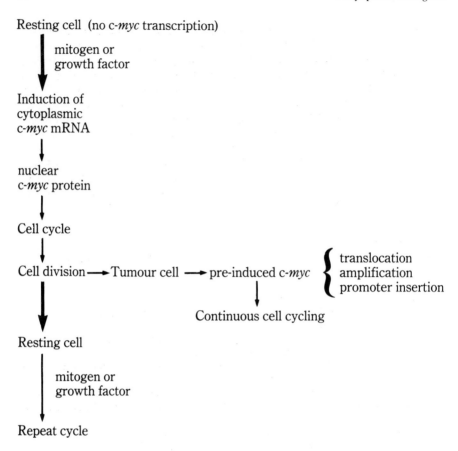

Fig. 4. Pre-induced c-myc *activity in tumour cells.*

However, the view of deregulation of c-*myc* may be a common feature in these aberrations with the possible exception of gene amplification, since amplified genes can exhibit apparently normal regulation[25]. A hypothesis which fits all these processes is that the end result of the abnormality is the availability of c-*myc* mRNA, in unusually and critically large amounts, throughout the life of the cell. This might be called 'pre-induced c-*myc* gene activation' and provides an explanation for continued progression of tumour cells through successive cell divisions. A diagrammatic representation is shown in Fig. 4. A normal resting cell rapidly becomes activated (at the early stage of the G_0–G_1 transition) by growth factors or polyclonal mitogens, as in, for example, activated spleen cells. The c-*myc* RNA and protein are synthesized throughout the cell cycle, culminating in cell division (a causative role for c-*myc* in replication is possible but not necessarily implied). After division, the progeny cells may become resting cells or they may progress through a further cycle of division. In the continued presence of mitogens or growth factors, the daughter cells will continue to divide, c-*myc* mRNA will continue to be made in response to these factors and no effective resting phase will occur in the population of cells. Tumour cells differ crucially from normal cells in that they do not return to a resting phase because they have an effective pre-induction of c-*myc* expression. In tumour cells, the continuance of the cyclical process does not require growth factor stimulation but is achieved in different ways; for example, in BL cells with chromosomal translocation, c-*myc* is deregulated by proximity to *Ig* genes; in tumours with provirus insertion, c-*myc* is deregulated by the presence of viral transcriptional control sequences; and in tumours with amplified c-*myc* the consequent high concentration of c-*myc* mRNA is equivalent to deregulation, resulting in c-*myc* mRNA availability for a greater time even though myc mRNA turns over rapidly after cessation of production.

The precise function of the c-*myc* protein remains to be determined. It seems to be important for many normal growing cells and so, like many aspects of cancer therapy, specific targeting into the c-*myc* gene of the tumour cell may prove difficult, to say the least.

Acknowledgement

I wish to thank Dr R. Baer for his suggestions concerning this article.

References

1   Klein, G. and Klein, E. (1985) Evolution of tumours and the impact of molecular oncology. *Nature* 315, 190–195

2   Kelly, K. *et al.* (1983) Cell-specific regulation of the c-*myc* gene by lymphocyte mitogens and platelet-derived growth factor. *Cell* 35, 603–610

3   Thompson, C. B. *et al.* (1985) Levels of c-*myc* oncogene mRNA are invariant throughout the cell cycle. *Nature* 314, 363–366

4   Hann, S. R., Thompson, C. B. and Eisenman, R. N. (1985) c-*myc* oncogene protein synthesis is independent of the cell cycle in human and avian cells. *Nature* 314, 366–369

5   Rabbitts, P. H. *et al.* (1985) Metabolism of c-*myc* gene products: c-*myc* mRNA and protein expression in the cell cycle. *EMBO J.* 4, 2009–2015

6   Campisi, J. *et al.* (1984) Cell cycle control of c-*myc* but not c-*ras* expression is lost following chemical transformation. *Cell* 36, 241–247

7   Persson, H. and Leder, P. (1984) Nuclear localisation and DNA binding properties of a protein expressed by human c-*myc* oncogene. *Science* 225, 718–720

8   Dani, K. *et al.* (1984) Extreme instability of c-*myc* mRNA in normal and transformed cells. *Proc. Natl Acad. Sci. USA.* 81, 7046–7050

9   Hayward, W. S., Neel, B. G. and Astrin, S. M. (1981) Activation of a cellular oncogene by promoter insertion in ALV-induced lymphoid leukosis. *Nature* 290, 475–479

10 Payne, G. S., Bishop, J. M. and Varmus, H. (1982) Multiple arrangements of viral DNA and inactivated host oncogene in bursal lymphomas. *Nature* 295, 209–217

11 Leder, P. *et al.* (1983) Translocations among antibody genes in human cancer. *Science* 222, 765–771

12 Saito, H. *et al.* (1983) Activation of the c-*myc* gene by translocation: a model for translational control. *Proc. Natl Acad. Sci. USA* 80, 7467–7480

13 Rabbitts, P. H. *et al.* Truncation of exon 1 from the c-*myc* gene results in prolonged c-*myc* mRNA stability (1985) *EMBO J.* 4, 3727–3733

14 Rabbitts, T. H. *et al.* (1984) Effect of somatic mutation within translocated c-*myc* genes in Burkitt's lymphoma. *Nature* 309, 592–597

15 Bernard, O. *et al.* (1983) Sequences of the murine and human cellular *myc* oncogenes and two modes of *myc* transcription resulting from chromosome translocation in B lymphoid tumours. *EMBO J.* 2, 2375–2383

16 Cory, S. *et al.* (1985) Variant (6;15) translocations in murine plasmacytomas involve a chromosome 15 locus at least 72 kb from the c-*myc* oncogene. *EMBO J.* 4, 675–681

17 Stanton, L. W., Watt, R. and Marcu, K. B. (1983) Translocation, breakage and truncated transcripts of c-*myc* oncogene in murine plasmacytomas. *Nature* 303, 401–404

18 Rabbitts, T. H. *et al.* (1983) Transcription enhancer identified near the human $C\mu$ immunoglobulin heavy-chain gene is unavailable to the translocated c-*myc* gene in a Burkitt lymphoma. *Nature* 306, 806–809

19 Hayday, A. C. *et al.* (1984) Activation of a translocated human c-*myc* gene by an enhancer in the immunoglobulin heavy-chain locus. *Nature* 307, 334–340

20 Alitalo, K. (1984) Amplification of cellular oncogene in cancer cells. *Med. Biol.* 62, 304–317

21 Schwab, M. *et al.* (1983) Amplified DNA with limited homology to *myc* cellular oncogene is shared by human neuroblastoma cell lines and a neuroblastoma tumour. *Nature* 305, 245–248

22 Brodeur, G. M. *et al.* (1984) Amplification of N-*myc* in untreated human neuroblastomas correlates with advanced disease stages. *Science* 224, 1121–1124

23 Land, H., Parada, L. F. and Weinberg, R. A. (1983) Tumorigenic conversion of primary embryo fibroblasts requires at least two co-operating oncogenes. *Nature* 304, 596–602

24 Ruley, H. E. (1983) Adenovirus early region IA enables viral and cellular transforming genes to transform primary cells in culture. *Nature* 304, 602–605

25 Westin, E. M. *et al.* (1982) Expression of cellular homologues of retroviral *onc* genes in human hematopoietic cells. *Proc. Natl Acad. Sci. USA.* 73, 2490–2494

26 Rabbitts, T. H., Hamlyn, P. H. and Baer, R. (1983) Altered nucleotide sequences of a translocated c-*myc* gene in Burkitt lymphona. *Nature* 306, 760–765

T. H. Rabbitts is at the MRC Laboratory of Molecular Biology, Hills Road, Cambridge, CB2 2QH, UK.

Myc/Ig juxtaposition by chromosomal translocations: some new insights, puzzles and paradoxes

George Klein and Eva Klein

Human Burkitt's lymphoma and murine plasmacytoma cells contain characteristic chromosomal translocations[1] that show the following common features: juxtaposition of the c-myc oncogene to one of the three immunoglobulin loci[2-4]; wide variability of the translocation breakpoint in and outside the oncogene, but with rigorous avoidance of any damage to the two coding exons[5-21]; high expression of the Ig-juxtaposed c-myc gene with concomitant shutdown of the normal, non-translocated allele[4,7,11,14,15,18]. The latter fact suggests that the translocation has removed the oncogene from its normal regulatory circuit and placed it under the constitutively activating influence of an Ig-locus. This is believed to play an essential role in the malignant transformation[23]. Numerous papers have dealt with the possible role of the translocations in tumorigenesis. Less attention has been given to their implications with regard to the normal DNA rearrangement process that takes place during B-cell differentiation. In this article both areas and their interrelations are considered.

It is reasonable to assume that the translocations occur during the normal re-arrangement of the Ig-genes which create vulnerable sites and increase the risk of illegitimate recombination. In the typical, i.e. most common, translocations, the transposed *myc*-gene joins one of the IgH switch sites, suggesting that the switch recombination enzymes participate in the event. Exceptions where the IgH cluster breaks elsewhere, e.g. in the neighborhood of a J sequence or within the V_H region, do occur, but are rare[24,25]. The less frequent variant translocations[19,20] involve one of the light chain loci. The switch regions can therefore be regarded as favored hot spots, but they are not exclusive translocation sites.

There are no similar hot spots within or in the vicinity of the c-*myc* gene: the variability of the breakpoints is much too great. In the majority of the 12 ; 15 translocations in murine plasmacytomas (MPCs) and in a substantial fraction of the 8 ; 14 translocations in Burkitt's lymphomas (BLs), the break occurs within exon 1 or intron 1 of the gene, however. The break can also occur outside the gene; this happens more frequently in BL than in MPC. In the typical (IgH) translocations the breaks are always upstream of the gene in both species. They can be located between the 5'-end of c-*myc* and the nearest *Eco*RI restriction site (10 kb in the mouse, 17 kb in man) or further upstream, outside the restriction site. The maximum distance that is compatible with the tumor phenotype is not known, but it is likely that the *cis*-activating effect of the IgH locus can act on the *myc*-gene over considerable distances[16].

The variant translocations that involve one of the light chain loci[26,27] differ from the IgH translocations in two ways, at least in the more extensively investigated BL system. The first difference is that chromosome 8 breaks downstream of the c-*myc* gene and the C_{kappa} or C_{lambda} sequences are transposed to it telomerically, carried by the terminal fragments of chromosome 2 or chromosome 22[18-20]. The second important difference concerns the relative orientation of c-*myc* and the juxtaposed Ig-region. The IgH sequences face c-*myc* head to head in the typical translocations. In the variant translocations the 5'-end of the transposed light chain sequences face the tail end of c-*myc*.

These differences may be trivial and merely reflect the orientation of the participating genes or may have some important biological reason. The orientation of c-*myc* and of the Ig loci in relation to the centromere is well established in man but is still ambiguous in the mouse. The 5'-end of c-*myc* points towards the centromere on human chromosome 8. The IgH locus on H14 is in the opposite orienta-

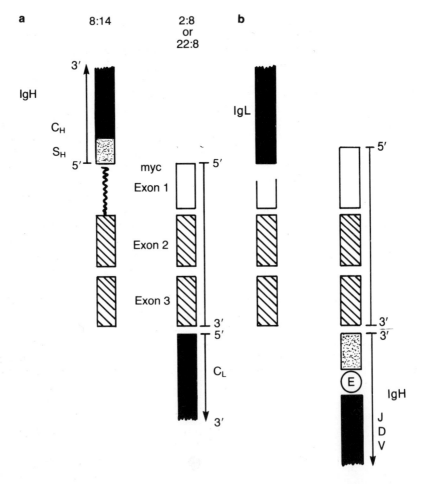

Fig. 1. (a) Consistent features of the myc/Ig juxtapositions associated with the tumorigenic phenotype in BL and MPC. The typical (IgH) and the variant (IgL) translocations differ in breaking the chromosome upstream and downstream of the c-myc gene, respectively. Invariable requirement: intact coding exons (2 and 3) of myc. Favored IgH breakpoint: a switch region (S_H), flanked by C_H sequences. (b) Presumably lethal or nontumorigenic combinations with reverse joining patterns, that have not been found.

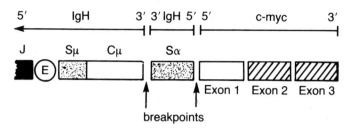

Fig. 2. *Schematic map of the rearranged c-*myc *gene in the ABPC 45 mouse plasmacytoma that has no cytogenetically visible translocation (after Ref. 28).*

tion, with its 5'-end towards the telomere. Reciprocal translocations led to the exchange of terminal chromosome fragments, as a rule. If the *myc*-carrying chromosome breaks at random, while the Ig-loci provide vulnerable, translocation-prone regions, and if tumor development depends on the constitutional activation of the *myc* gene, the regularities of the structural pattern may either reflect the localization of recombinational hot spots within the Ig loci or, and perhaps more probably, the localization of the strongest activators. The evidence suggests that the *myc*-juxtaposed IgH switch region needs to be flanked by IgH-constant region sequences in the 3'-direction in order to permit tumorigenic activation (Fig. 1). If the *myc*-gene stayed on chromosome 8 and the breakage occurred 3' of the gene as in the variant translocations, a switch site would be transposed from chromosome 14, joining the oncogene tail to tail, flanked by upstream IgH sequences, including the enhancer region. This configuration has not been found, however, but some unusual and more complex rearrangements have been identified that may be pertinent. In a recent study, performed in collaboration by K. Marcu's and our group[28], we have examined a mouse plasmacytoma, ABPC45, that carries an interstitial deletion on chromosome 15 but has no detectable translocation[29]. We found that a 5'–3' oriented C_{mu}–S_{mu}– enhancer–J sequence was positioned tail to tail to an S_{alpha} sequence which in turn faced an intact c-*myc* gene, head to head (Fig. 2). This extraordinary structure must have arisen by at least three cytogenetic events, two translocations and one inversion. It stresses the likely importance of head-to-head confrontation between a switch site and the c-*myc* gene, as in the typical translocations. Moreover, in spite of the fact that the IgH enhancer is usually removed by the typical translocation breaks, this finding suggests that the presence of the enhancer may nevertheless contribute to the tumorigenic activation of c-*myc* in exceptional cases. Other exceptions where the IgH enhancer was in a position to activate the coding exons of c-*myc* have been found by others, both in MPC[30] and in some BLs[31,32].

The tail-to-head *myc*-C_{kappa} or C_{lambda} orientation in the variant translocations can be seen as a consequence of the parallel centromeric 5'–telomeric 3' orientation of both light chain genes. The regularity of this finding suggests that the regions immediately upstream of the constant regions are prone to break and/or that the resulting translocation configuration is particularly suitable for the downstream activation of the *myc*-gene. It also suggests that the mirror configuration where chromosome 8 would break 5' of *myc* as in the typical translocations and the oncogene would be transposed to face the light chain sequences in a head-to-tail configuration does not provide the proper conditions for tumorigenic activation.

In the mouse, the centromere–telomere orientation of the *myc* and IgH loci has not been decisively established. The analysis is difficult due to the relative morphological uniformity of the mouse chromosomes. Some suggestions were made but they are not conclusive. Meo *et al.*[33] have firmly established that the IgH, Pre 1 and the T31H breakpoint (BP) markers are linked on chromosome 12. They have also shown that IgH maps between the centromere and the T31H BP. The order centromere–IgH– Pre-1–T31H–telomere was proposed by these authors on the basis of a single recombinant mouse, however. This would only be compelling if a double crossover could have been excluded, but such an exclusion was admittedly not possible. To determine the orientation of IgH, Owen *et al.*[34] studied the expression of the Tsu[d] locus, a T-cell antigen controlled by an IgH linked gene. Several RI strains were typed for Tsu[d] and IgH. The recombination frequencies were interpreted to suggest that the Tsu[d] locus was located in the close neighborhood of the IgH-C region, on the same side of the Pre-1 gene. Their conclusion was based on the localization of the Pre-1 locus between IgH and T31H BP as proposed by Meo *et al.*[33]. If the latter conclusion is wrong and the order is centromere–Pre-1–IgH–telomere, the conclusion of Owen *et al.* about the relative positions of IgH-C and IgH-V would also have to be reversed.

The uncertainty of the gene orientation in the mouse inhibits the precise coordination of the cytogenetic and the molecular findings. This question will have to be addressed by direct methods, e.g. *in-situ* hybridization, in order to decide whether the MPC translocations resemble the BL translocations as a direct or a mirror image.

Some of the main features of the MPC and the BL associated translocations are shown comparatively in Table 1.

Pseudofunctional correlations

It is paradoxical that while the BL/MPC associated translocations affect the non-functional (allelically excluded) Ig-locus, there is nevertheless a certain relationship between the affected sequences and the Ig-product. This pseudofunctional correlation is interesting because it may elucidate some aspects of the normal rearrangement process and can provide clues for the mechanism of the *myc*-translocation. One set of relationships applies to the typical (*myc*/heavy chain) and another to the variant (*myc*/light chain) juxtapositions.

In MPC, the S_{alpha} region is the common *myc* acceptor site, while in BL it is S_{mu}. This gives the appearance of a functional correlation, because most BLs produce mu and most MPCs produce alpha chains. This is merely a statistical difference, however, since numerous exceptions are known where the tumors produce a noncorresponding heavy chain[4,5,13,40,41].

For MPC, a clue may be sought in the fact that this tumor usually originates from the B-cells of the omentum and the mesentery that are largely IgA producers. These lymphocytes are believed to switch to alpha chain production at an early stage of the maturation, after having received a signal from a specialized T-cell subset. If it is assumed that the translocation of c-*myc* to the S_{alpha} region of the functionally excluded IgH locus occurs as an accident *of the $S_{mu}S_{alpha}$ switch recombination*, it would follow that the switch occurs in both homologous chromosomes. This makes sense, since it is hard to see how the mechanism that executes the T signal could distinguish between a functionally and a non-functionally rearranged IgH gene. Alternatively, the switch recombination enzymes that operate in the functional rearrangement may favor the illegitimate recombination of c-*myc* to the S_{alpha} region on the homologous chromosome while this is still in the germ line

Table 1. *Many, but not all, features of the human Burkitt lymphoma (BL) and the mouse plasmacytoma (MPC)-associated translocations are identical*

Only BL	Common for BL and MPC	Only MPC
Most frequent IgH breakpoint 5′ of S_{mu}	Typical (myc/IgH) translocations are more frequent than variant (myc/light chain locus) juxtapositions	Most frequent IgH breakpoint 5′ of S_{alpha}
Breakpoints in myc carrying chromosome highly variable, 60% or more outside the gene	Coding exons (no 2 and 3) of c-myc are always intact	Myc-breakpoints are spread in a narrower area, frequently in first intron, only rarely outside the gene
Variant translocations are of two types, involving the kappa or the lambda gene	Pseudofunctional correlation between the chromosome affected by the variant translocation and the light chain product	There is only one variant translocation involving the kappa gene
Variant translocations break chromosome 8 downstream of the myc gene	Typical translocations break the myc-carrying chromosome 5′ of the gene. Myc may or may not be rearranged	Unknown
Association between the tumour and one of the translocations		
100%		85%. Translocation-negative tumors may carry interstitial deletions on chromosome 15, accompanied by myc-rearrangement and activation[29]
Additional contributory factors in tumor development and/or progression		
EBV, chronic malaria, immunosuppression		Oil granuloma. Secondary changes: IAP-activation of c-mos[35,36], 10 ; 6[37] or (12 ; 14) translocation[38], synergistic effect of v-abl in ABPC[39]

configuration. This possibility is supported by the finding[40] that the IgH sequences on the 5' side of the S_{alpha} associated breakpoint are in the germ line configuration in some exceptional MPCs, as shown by the analysis of the reciprocal recombination fragment.

The BL precursor must be a pre-B or early B-cell that has not yet started to switch its heavy chain genes. The participation of switch recombination enzymes in the myc/S_{mu} juxtaposition event is therefore unlikely. The mu region is hypomethylated in normal IgM producing lymphocytes, indicating selective activation[42,43]. In conjunction with class switching, other heavy chain regions become hypomethylated as well. Therefore, in the non-switched cell, the $S_{mu}-C_{mu}$ area appears to represent a more active chromatin region than other heavy chain genes. If so, the tumorigenic activation of the translocated *myc* gene may be restricted to this area in the non-switched cell. This argument also postulates that the regulatory processes that activate the heavy chain constant regions act on both homologous chromosomes.

The pseudofunctional correlation in the variant translocations is more regular and precise. A correlation between the light chain product and the translocation chromosome was first noted in MPC. Tumors with the typical 12 ; 15 translocation produce either kappa or lambda. In contrast, all examined tumors with the 6 ; 15 translocation produced kappa[26,39]. Similarly, all BL lines that carried the variant (2 ; 8) translocation and made a functional light chain were found to produce kappa[44,45]. Likewise, all light chain-producing BLs that carried the 8 ; 22 translocation were found to make lambda chains, with the exception of one that produced kappa[46].

In the limited number of lines with variant translocations that were analysed at the molecular level, the *myc*-juxtaposed light chain locus was broken, precluding the production of a functional chain[47]. The very strong correlation between the translocated locus and the light chain product is therefore in need of an explanation. It may be the consequence of the sequential rearrangement of kappa and lambda genes during B-cell maturation[48-51]. When a functional kappa rearrangement has been achieved, lambda genes do not rearrange, as a rule. The *myc*-translocation can be regarded as a special type of non-functional rearrangement. Therefore, it would be expected that some of the 8 ; 2 translocation carrying BLs have succeeded in rearranging the kappa locus on the normal chromosome 2 functionally, while others failed. This is indeed the case: BLs with 8 ; 2 variant translocations make either kappa or produce no functional light chain[44]. One would also expect, however, that some of the kappa non-producers proceed to rearrange their lambda genes and become lambda producers. So far, no 8 ; 2 carrying lambda producers have been found, however. Conceivably, the *myc*-translocation may have interfered with the orderly continuation of the normal rearrangement process. Alternatively, the mechanism that excises the majority of the non-functionally rearranged kappa genes in lambda producing B-cells may damage the *myc*/kappa translocation complex, preventing the malignant development of the corresponding clone. This possibility is also supported by the fact that BLs with the (8 ; 22) are about twice as frequent, compared to the 2 ; 8 variants[44,45]. If the *myc* translocation is equally likely to occur during the rearrangement of the kappa and the lambda locus, the opposite would be expected, since the kappa rearrangement precedes and, if successful, precludes lambda rearrangement.

The good correlation between the (8 ; 22) translocation and lambda chain production is not surprising, since kappa producers do not rearrange their lambda genes, as a rule. Some of the (8 ; 22) translocation carriers are expected to contain a second non-functionally rearranged and some a functionally rearranged lambda gene. Both types were found to exist[44]. No explanation can be provided for the single exceptional (8 ; 22) translocation carrying BL line that produces kappa chains[46].

The 'heavy chain paradox' in Burkitt's lymphoma

All BLs so far studied carry one of the three *myc*/Ig translocations[23,52]. Moreover, all tested BL biopsies and derived lines were found to produce a heavy chain, while light chain production is more variable. Since the likelihood of functional and non-functional rearrangements is equally high, a substantial proportion of the 8 ; 14 translocation carrying BLs would be expected to have two non-functionally rearranged IgH loci. Such tumors would produce no heavy chains. The lack of such BLs suggests that the production of a functional heavy chain may be essential for the survival of the translocation-carrying cell and/or its development into a malignant tumor. Conceivably, the same mechanism that removes normal B cells with two non-functionally rearranged IgH loci may also eliminate them if one of the IgH loci is attached to a *myc* gene. Alternatively, a translocation carrying BL-precursor cell that cannot make a functional heavy chain may not possess the proliferative capacity required during a critical period of tumor development.

Why are the Ig-loci favored as recipients of the *myc*-translocation?

This question is often raised. There are many other genes that are equally or more active than the Ig-loci in B-cells, but have not been found to participate in oncogene translocations. This would suggest that high gene expression is not sufficient *per se*. DNA rearrangement during differentiation may be required in addition, to provide vulnerable, illegitimate recombination prone sites.

Only the genes of the immune system are presently known to rearrange during normal differentiation. Apart from the virtually unknown nervous system, the immune system is unique in its ability to generate a wide diversity of proteins. DNA rearrangements arc at least partly responsible for this diversity.

The human T-cell receptor beta chain locus has been localized to chromosome 7[53]. Screening a computer-based registry[54] did not reveal any chromosome 7 associated specific breaks or translocations in human leukemia. While the T-cell receptor gene also rearranges during differentiation, it is transcribed at a lower level than the immunoglobulin genes in B-cells. Recently, the T-cell receptor alpha chain gene has been localized to band 14q11[55], a frequent breakpoint in the fragile T-cell chromosomes of ataxia telangiectasia (AT) patients that was recently also shown to be involved in translocations associated with chronic T-cell leukemias[56]. While such translocations are not equally regular as their IgH region (14q32) localized counterparts in B-cell malignancies, they may play a primary or secondary role in the natural history of their carrier tumors.

Why is *myc* regularly favored in BL and MPC, to the exclusion of other oncogenes?

In spite of the large number of BLs and MPCs that have been studied, no exception has been found to the exclusive role of c-*myc* (or the corresponding chromosome region) as the regularly Ig-juxtaposed oncogene in these two tumors. As already discussed, this cannot be ascribed to any favored hot spot or Ig-homologous sequence on the *myc*-carrying chromosome, because the breakage can occur in many different sites and since no switch or other Ig-homologous sequences have been found. Known breakpoints have affected a variety of non-coding regions of the c-*myc* gene within exon 1 or intron 1 and also flanking regions, both upstream and downstream of the gene. The various combinations that have emerged may merely reflect the end result of random breakage of the *myc*-carrying chromosome, followed by the juxtaposition of the coding exons to an activating Ig-region, and selection for the tumorigenic phenotype.

If this scenario is correct, there is no reason why other oncogenes than c-*myc* might not be transposed to the Ig-'hot spots' occasionally as well. This is actually the case in some other human B-cell leukemias and lymphomas, as discussed below, but not in BL and MPC. It would therefore appear that *only* the constitutive activation of c-*myc*, but *not* of other oncogenes, may induce tumorigenic behavior in B-cells at the maturation stages characteristic for the BL and MPC precursor cell. Alternatively, the *myc*/Ig juxtaposition may *ipso facto* position the affected cell in the BL or MPC 'differentiation window'. Croce's somatic hybrid studies[57] have shown that stage specific restrictions may influence the expression of translocated *myc* and probably other oncogenes as well. Another striking example for a competitive interaction between an activated oncogene and differentiation inducing signals is provided by the HL60 myeloid leukemia cell that carries amplified and highly transcribed c-*myc* sequences. The induction of terminal differentiation leads to an early switch-off of *myc* transcription.

The phenotypic (tumorigenic) expression of an oncogene can also be regulated at the post-transcriptional level. The constellation of receptors for growth vs. differentiation inducing factors and other maturation dependent programs may be decisive. There are many precedents in the field of viral oncology that show the profound influence of cell differentiation or maturation on the phenotypic consequences of oncogene activation[59]. For the B-cell series, an interesting recent example is provided by the spectrum of tumors that appear in Balb/c mice after exposure to Abelson virus, with or without concomitant intraperitoneal injection of mineral oil[60-62]. Three types of tumors were seen. One type, designated ABLS, corresponded to the usual AbLV induced pre B-cell leukemias and transcribed the virally transduced v-*abl* oncogene at a high rate, as expected. It was previously known that such leukemias are stably diploid and carry no cytogenetic markers[63]. The second type, designated ABPC, corresponded to the plasmacytomas induced in Balb/c by mineral oil alone, but appeared after much shorter latency periods[64]. They carried the usual MPC-associated (12 ; 15) or (6 ; 15) translocations, and transcribed both c-*myc* and v-*abl* at a high rate[39], suggesting that the combined action of the two oncogenes may have increased the frequency of the tumorigenic change, as reflected by the shortened latency period. A third type of tumor was designated as plasmacytoid lymphosarcoma (ABPL). Initially, this was regarded as a B-cell derived tumor, at a somewhat earlier stage of maturation than the plasmacytomas. Recently, their B-cell origin has been questioned, however, and it has been suggested that they may belong to the monocytic series (Mushinski and Shen-Ong, unpublished data). Molecular analysis brought the unexpected information that the ABPLs have no v-*abl* transcripts but contain abundant c-*myb* RNA of an unusually large size, not seen in either ABLS or ABPC[60]. Moreover, c-*myb* but not c-*myc* was rearranged. There was no evidence for any v-*abl* expression. The rearrangement of c-*myb* could be attributed to the insertion of a retroviral LTR region 5' of the gene, probably derived from the Moloney helper virus.

The main characteristics of three histologically different tumors, induced by the same experimental strategy, are summarized in Table 2. The ABPCs illustrate how the interaction of a virally carried and a resident cellular oncogene can enhance the malignant transformation. A comparison of all three tumor forms

Table 2. Different oncogenes are activated in three histologically different tumors arising after the combined administration of Abelson virus and mineral oil (after Mushinski et al. Refs 39, 60–62)

Tumor	Histology	Cell type	Activated oncogene	Activation mechanism
ABLS	Lymphosarcoma	Pre-B	v-*abl*	Transducing virus
ABPL	Plasmacytoid lymphoma	B?	c-*myb* No v-*abl* transcription	Retroviral insertion
ABPC	Plasmacytoma	Mature B	c-*myc*	Chromosomal translocation
			v-*abl*	Transducing virus

shows major differences in the relative contribution of several oncogene activation mechanisms, such as retroviral transduction (v-*abl* in ABLS and ABPC), activation of a cellular oncogene by retroviral insertion in its proximity (c-*myb* in ABPL) or by translocation to a highly active chromatin region (c-*myc* in ABPC). These differences enforce the view that the occurrence and/or the phenotypic expression of each event is strongly dependent on the maturation stage of the target cell.

Can other chromosomal translocations identify further tumorigenic mechanisms?

This question occupies a central position in current discussions concerned the implications of non-random chromosomal changes associated with human tumors[65]. A very interesting case is unfolding in relation to the Ph_1 chromosome in CGL. It shares some features with the *myc*/Ig juxtaposition in BL and MPC but is markedly different in other respects. In the typical (9 ; 22) translocation, the c-*abl* oncogene, localized on the distal tip of chromosome 9, moves to the Ph_1 breakpoint on chromosome 22[66–68]. Initially, this finding was not compelling, due to the large diversity of the variant Ph_1 translocations where the distal fragment of chromosome 22 moves to other autosomes than chromsome 9. However, recent *in-situ* hybridization experiments revealed that the cytogenetically invisible c-*abl*-containing telomeric fragment of chromosome 9 moves regularly to the Ph_1 breakpoint on chromsome 22 in these cases as well[69]. The transposed c-*abl* gene is activated to produce an abnormally long mRNA[70], that codes for a 210K protein, a combined product of chromosome 22 and chromosome 9-derived sequences, instead of the normal 145 K c-*abl* protein[71]. The 210 K protein has an abnormal tyrosine kinase activity like the product of the virally carried (v-*abl*) gene. In contrast to the behavior of the c-*myc* in the BL/MPC where the translocated c-*myc* is expressed but the normal allele is switched off, Ph_1 positive CGL cells express both the translocated gene and the normal c-*abl*. This may reflect an important difference in the mechanism by which the *myc* vs. the *abl* translocation contributes to the tumorigenic process. The Ig-juxtaposition of the normal c-*myc* gene induces a regulatory change in the production of the normal protein whereas the Ph_1 translocation acts by generating an abnormal fusion protein with an altered function.

Other interesting chromosomal translocations that may act by oncogene activation are found among the non-BL lymphomas and leukemias of B-cell origin that carry 14q + markers with a breakpoint at 14q32, corresponding to the IgH locus, and a transposed distal segment derived from chromosomes other than chromosome 8[72,73]. Croce's group has recently identified the sequences transposed from chromosome 11 in 11 ; 14 translocation-carrying B-CLL and diffuse large cell lymphoma (designated bcl-1) and the chromosome 18-derived sequence in 14 ; 18 translocation-carrying follicular small cell lymphomas (designated bcl-2)[74,75]. The association of these presumptive new oncogenes with specific B-cell lymphoma subtypes is in line with the hypothesis that the constitutive activation of a given oncogene may trigger a tumorigenic step only in cells at certain specific stages of maturation.

Conclusions

Ig/c-myc juxtaposition by chromosomal translocation is an essential step in the genesis of human Burkitt's lymphoma and murine plasmacytoma. This conclusion is based on the extraordinary regularity of the event and its occurrence even under cytogenetically complicated circumstances. The coding exons of the oncogene are always intact, indicating that the expression of the normal myc-protein is essential for the tumorigenic step. Occasional point mutations show no consistency and have only been detected in some long-passaged BL lines. The tumorigenic effect of the Ig-juxtaposed myc-gene may be due to dysregulation. The cis-acting influence of a constitutively expressed immunoglobulin gene, may permit c-myc to escape its normal, presumably finely poised regulation. The strong contrast between the expression of the translocated myc and the repression of its normal homologue is in line with this explanation. It is known that the normal c-myc gene is switched off when cells proceed towards terminal differentiation[58,76]. This inability of the translocated gene to follow this instruction may keep the cells permanently in cycle. Switch recombination sites appear as the hot spots of the typical IgH/myc translocations. This is not invariable, however, and breakpoints have also been found near a J sequence or in the V_H region. In the variant translocations, the light chain genes break between the V and C regions. It is thus clear that a variety of Ig-associated sequences can cis-activate the transposed oncogene, sometimes over considerable distances. Therefore, no single enhancer can bear the total responsibility for myc activation. Probably, there are multiple alternative sites that can assume this role. Perhaps the activated state of the chromatin bears the main responsibility.

The wide variability of the breakpoints on the myc-carrying chromosome indicates that there is no hot spot in or around the oncogene. The chromosome appears to break at random. The range of the breakage sites that have been identified may merely reflect the restrictions posed by the selection for tumorigenicity. It follows from this reasoning that other parts of the genome should be equally prone to Ig-juxtaposition during the long preneoplastic history of BL and MPC. If so, the exclusive role of c-myc requires an explanation. It appears most likely that the activation of a certain oncogene is only tumorigenic if it occurs at a narrowly restricted stage of maturation. This is supported by the different oncogene activation patterns within the tumor spectrum arising after the combined administration of Abelson virus and mineral oil to Balb/c mice, and by the transposition of new (non-myc) presumptive oncogenes to the IgH region in specific non-BL lymphomas of B-cell origin that carry a 14q + marker.

The myc/Ig juxtapositions in BL and MPC have a number of unexpected features that reflect both on the oncogene translocation and on the normal DNA rearrangement in Ig-producing cells.

Most MPCs are IgA producers. In the majority, c-myc has been transposed to face the S_{alpha} region of the IgH complex. Most BLs are IgM producers and S_{mu} is the most frequent rearrangement site in the typical translocations. In the variant translocations, the affected light chain locus usually corresponds to the light chain product of the tumor cell. These are not true functional correlations, however, since the translocation affects the non-functional allele.

It is puzzling that all BLs that have been tested were found to produce a heavy chain, in spite of the high likelihood of double non-functional rearrangements in 8 ; 14 translocation allele.

The following explanations may be considered for these paradoxical phenomena:

(i) The mechanism that induces the S_{mu}/S_{alpha} 'deletion switch' during the differentiation of normal peritoneal B-lymphocytes affects the functionally and non-functionally rearranged IgH loci indiscriminately;

(ii) Translocation-carrying pre-BL cells may have to produce a functional heavy chain in order to emerge as an autonomous lymphoma clone. Alternatively, translocation-carrying cells that fail to produce a normal heavy chain may be eliminated by the surveillance mechanism that removes non-functionally rearranged normal B-lymphocytes;

(iii) The correlation between the chromosome affected by the variant translocations and the functional light chain product suggests that the translocations occur as accidents of the normal DNA rearrangement, follow similar time sequences, and are subject to some of the corresponding feedback regulations;

(iv) The higher frequency of BL variants with 8 ; 22 compared to 8 ; 2 translocations carriers suggests that cells that proceed to rearrange their lambda genes may occasionally remove translocated kappa/*myc* complexes, similarly to the excision of normal non-functionally rearranged kappa genes in normal lambda producing B-cells.

Finally, we may ask the question why the Ig/*myc* juxtapositions are so strictly confined to BL and MPC, and why they do not occur in their histological counterparts in the opposite species, such as in human multiple myelomas or plasmacytomas and murine B-cell lymphomas. Recently, we have found that c-*myc* was amplified in the most malignant form of human plasma cell tumor, plasma cell leukemia (PLC), in contrast to ordinary plasmacytomas or multiple myelomas that showed neither *myc*-rearrangement nor *myc*-amplification (Sümegi et al. unpublished observations). Murine B-cell leukemias may have 15 trisomy, but no translocations[77]. We have previously proposed that chronic preneoplastic stimulation of the target cell is the common factor in the natural history of BL and MPC that makes both of them translocation prone[52]. The mineral oil granuloma is essential for the development of MPC; if it is prevented by, e.g. cortisone treatment, no tumor develops[64]. In African BL, chronic malaria and EBV appear to be the most frequent cofactors. In the more recently identified AIDS-related BLs HTLV-3, EBV and the typical combination of chronic infections may play an analogous role[78]. Chronic malaria and the AIDS-associated infections share the double impact of B-cell activation and T-cell suppression. EBV is an immortalizing agent for B-cells *in vitro* and it is likely to increase the life span of B-cells *in vivo*, and to block their terminal differentiation fully or in part. Under the impact of chronic activation, such B-cells may undergo a large number of cell divisions. The recently demonstrated BCGF-production of EBV activated B-cells may add an autocrine component as well[79].

The risk of all cytogenetic aberrations is proportional to the number of cell divisions in a given cell lineage. The *myc*/Ig translocation can be regarded as a rare genetic accident in the chronically stimulated B-cell population. Unlike other genetic accidents, it conveys a major tumorigenic advantage on its host cell, provided that it occurs at a narrowly restricted stage of maturation.

References

1   Klein, G. (1981) *Nature (London)* 294, 313–318
2   Klein, G. (1983) *Cell* 32, 311–315
3   Cory, S. (1983) *Immunol. Today* 4, 205–207
4   Leder, P., Battey, J., Lenoir, G., Moulding, C., Murphy, W., Potter, H., Steward, T. and Taub, R. (1983) *Science* 222, 765–771
5   Shen-Ong, G. L., Keath, E. J., Piccoli, S. P. and Cole, M. D. (1982) *Cell* 31, 443–452
6   Adams, J. M., Gerondakis, S., Webb, E., Mitchell, J., Bernard, O. and Cory, S. (1982) *Proc. Natl Acad. Sci. USA* 79, 6966–6970
7   Adams, J. M., Gerondakis, S., Webb, E., Corcoran, L. M. and Cory, S. (1983). *Proc. Natl Acad. Sci. USA* 80, 1982–1986
8   Cory, S., Adams, J. M., Steven, D., Gerondakis, S. D., Miller, J. F. A. P., Gamble, J., Wiener, F., Spira, J. and Francke, U. (1983) *EMBO J.* 2, 213–216
9   Cory, S., Gerondakis, S. and Adams, J. M. (1983) *Science* 219, 963–967
10 Dalla-Favera, R., Martinotti, S. and Gallo, R. C. (1983) *Science* 291, 963–967
11 Erikson, J., Ar-Rushdi, A., Drwinga, H. L., Nowell, P. C. and Croce, C. M. (1983) *Proc. Natl Acad. Sci. USA* 80, 820–824
12 Taub, R., Kirsch, I., Morton, C., Lenoir, G., Swan, D., Tronick, S., Aaronson, S. and Leder, P. (1982) *Proc. Natl Acad. Sci. USA* 79, 7837–7841
13 Calame, K., Kim, S., Lalley, P., Hill, R., Davis, M. and Hood, L. (1982) *Proc. Natl Acad. Sci. USA* 79, 6994–6998
14 Harris, L. J., Lang, R. B. J. and Marcu, K. B. (1982) *Proc. Natl Acad. Sci. USA* 79, 4175–4179
15 Stanton, L. W., Watt, R. and Marcu, K. B. (1983) *Nature (London)* 303, 401–406
16 Perry, R. P. (1983) *Cell* 33, 647–649
17 Bernhard, O., Cory, S., Gerondakis, S., Webb, E. and Adams, J. M. (1983) *EMBO J.* 2, 2375–2383
18 Croce, C. M. and Klein, G. (1985) *Sci. Am.* 252, 54–60
19 Erikson, J., Nishikura, K., Ar-Rushdi, A., Finan, J., Emanuel, B., Lenoir, G., Rabbitts, T., Nowell, P. C. and Croce, C. M. (1983) *Proc. Natl Acad. Sci. USA* 80, 7581–7585
20 Croce, C. M., Thierfelder, W., Erikson, J., Nishikura, K., Finan, J., Lenoir, G. M. and Nowell, P. (1983) *Proc. Natl Acad. Sci. USA* 80, 6922–6926
21 Emanuel, B. S., Selden, J. R., Chaganti, R. S. K., Suresh, J., Nowell, P. C. and Croce, C. M. (1984) *Proc. Natl Acad. Sci. USA* 82, 2444–2446
22 Harris, L. J., Lang, R. B. and Marcu, K. B. (1982) *Proc. Natl Acad. Sci. USA* 79, 4175–4179
23 Klein, G. and Klein E. (1984) *Carcinogenesis* 5, 429–435
24 Hayday, A., Gillies, S. D., Saito, H., Wood, C., Wiman, K., Hayward, W. S. and Tonegawa, S. (1984) *Nature (London)* 307, 334–340
25 Pegoraro, L., Palumbo, A., Erikson, J., Falda, M., Giovanazzo, B., Emanuel, B. S. J., Rovera, G., Nowell, P. C. and Croce, C. M. (1984) *Proc. Natl Acad. Sci. USA* 82, 7166–7170
26 Ohno, S., Babonits, M., Wiener, F., Spira, J., Klein, G. and Potter, M. (1979) *Cell* 18, 1001–1007
27 Bernheim, A., Berger, R. and Lenoir, G. (1981) *Cancer Genet. Cytogenet.* 3, 307–315
28 Fahrlander, P. D. J., Sümegi, J., Yang, Jian-qing, Wiener, F., Marcu, K. B. and Klein, G. (1985) *Proc. Natl Acad. Sci. USA* 82, 3746–3750
29 Wiener, F., Ohno, S., Babonits, M., Sümegi, J., Wirschubsky, Z., Klein, G., Mushinski, J. F. and Potter, M. (1984) *Proc. Natl Acad. Sci. USA* 83, 1159–1163
30 Corcoran, L. M. N., Cory, S. and Adams, J. M. (1985) *Cell* 40, 71–79

31 Siebenlist, U., Hennighausen, L., Battey, J. and Leder, P. (1984) *Cell* 3, 381–391
32 Hayday, A. C., Gillies, S. D., Saito, H., Wood, C., Wiman, K., Hayward, W. S. and Tonegawa, S. (1984) *Nature (London)* 307, 334–340
33 Meo, T., Johnson, J., Beechey, C. V., Andrews, S. J., Peters, J. and Searle, A. G. (1980) *Proc. Natl Acad. Sci. USA* 77, 550–553
34 Owen, F. L., Riblet, R. and Taylor, B. A. (1981) *J. Exp. Med.* 153, 801–810
35 Rechavi, G., Givoli, D. and Canaani, E. (1982) *Nature (London)* 300, 607–611
36 Canaani, E., Dreazen, O., Klar, A., Rechavi, G., Ram, D., Cohen, J. B. and Givol, D. (1983) *Proc. Natl Acad. Sci. USA* 80, 7118–7122
37 Perlmutter, R. M., Klotz, J. L., Pravtacheva, D., Ruddle, F. and Hood, L. (1984) *Nature (London)* 307, 473–476
38 Wiener, F., Babonits, M., Bregula, U., Klein, G., Leonard, A., Wax, J. S. and Potter, M. (1984) *J. Exp. Med.* 159, 276–291
39 Ohno, S., Migita, S., Wiener, F., Babonits, M., Klein, G., Mushinski, F. and Potter, M. (1984) *J. Exp. Med.* 159, 1762–1777
40 Cory, S., Gerondakis, S. and Adams, K. M. (1983) *EMBO J.* 2, 697–703
41 Harris, L. J., D'Estachio, P., Ruddle, F. H. and Marcu, K. B. (1982) *Proc. Natl Acad. Sci. USA* 79, 6622–6626
42 Yagi, M. and Koshland, M. E. (1981) *Proc. Natl Acad. Sci. USA* 78, 4907–4911
43 Rogers, J. and Wall, R. (1981) *Proc. Natl Acad. Sci. USA* 78, 7497–7501
44 Lenoir, G. M., Preud'Homme, J. L., Bernheim, A. and Berger, R. (1982) *Nature (London)* 298, 474–476
45 Klein, G. and Lenoir, G. (1982) *Adv. Cancer Res.* 37, 381–387
46 Hollis, G. F., Mitchell, K. F., Battery, J., Potter, H., Taub, R., Lenoir, G. M. and Leder, P. (1984) *Nature (London)* 307, 752–755
47 Croce, C. M., Erikson, J., Nishikura, K., Ar-Rushdi, A., Giallongo, Y., Rovera, G., Finan, J. and Nowell, P. C. (1984) in *Cancer Cells* (Vande Woide, G. F. *et al.* eds), pp. 235–242, Cold Spring Harbor Laboratory
48 Alt, F., Rosenberg, N., Lewis, S., Thomas, E. and Baltimore, D. (1981) *Cell* 27, 381–390
49 Coffman, R. L. and Weissman, I. L. (1983) *J. Mol. Cell Immunol.* 1, 31–38
50 Maki, R., Kearney, J., Paige, C. and Tonegawa, S. (1980) *Science* 209, 1366–1370
51 Alt, F. W., Yancopoulos, G. D., Blackwell, T. K., Wood, C., Thomas, E., Boss, M., Coffman, R., Rosenberg, N., Tonegawa, S. and Baltimore, D. (1984) *EMBO J.* 3, 1209–1214
52 Klein, G. and Klein E. (1984) *Prog. Med. Virol.* 30, 87–106
53 Caccia, N., Kronenberg, M., Saxe, D., Haars, R., Bruns, G. A. P., Goverman, J., Malissen, M., Willard, H., Yoshikai, Y., Simon, M., Hood, C. and Mak, T. W. (1984) *Cell* 37, 1091–1099
54 Mitelman, F. (1983) *Cytogenet. Cell Genet.* 36, 1–515
55 Croce, C. M., Isobe, M., Palumbo, A., Puck, J., Ming, J. J., Tweardy, D., Erikson, J., Davis, M. and Rovera, G. (1985) *Science* 227, 1044–1047
56 Zech, L., Gahrton, G., Hammarström, L., Juliusson, G., Mellstedt, H., Robert, K. H. and Smith, C. I. E. (1984) *Nature (London)* 308, 858–860
57 Croce, C. M., Erikson, J., Ar-Rushdi, A., Aden, D. and Nishikura, K. (1984) *Proc. Natl Acad. Sci. USA* 81, 3170–3174
58 Reitsma, P. H., Rothburg, P. G., Astrin, S. M., Trial, J., Bar-Shavit, Z., Hall, A., Teitelbaum, S. L. and Kahn, A. J. (1983) *Nature (London)* 306, 492–494
59 Graf, T., Beng, H. and Hayman, M. J. (1980) *Proc. Natl Acad. Sci. USA* 67, 389–393
60 Mushinski, J. F., Potter, M., Bauer, S. R. and Reddy, E. P. (1983) *Science* 200, 795–798
61 Lavu, S., Mushinski, J. F., Shen-Ong, G. L. C., Potter, M. and Reddy, P. (1984) *Curr. Top. Microbiol. Immunol.* 113, 37–40
62 Shen-Ong, G. L. C., Reddy, E. P., Potter, M. and Mushinski, J. F. (1984) *Curr. Top. Microbiol. Immunol.* 113, 41–46

63 Klein, G., Ohno, S., Rosenberg, N., Wiener, F., Spira, J. and Baltimore, D. (1980) *Int. J. Cancer* 25, 805–811

64 Potter, M., Wiener, F. and Mushinski, J. F. (1984) *Adv. in Viral Oncol.* 4, 139–162

65 Rowley, J. D. (1983) *Nature (London)* 301, 290–291

66 Heisterkamp, N., Groffen, J., Stephenson, J. R., Spurr, N. K., Goodfellow, P. N., Solomon, E., Carritt, B. and Bodmer, W. F. (1982) *Nature (London)* 299, 747–750

67 de Klein, A., van Kessel, A. G., Grosveld, G., Bartram, C. R., Hagemeijer, A., Bootsma, D., Spurr, N. K., Heisterkamp, N., Groffen, J. and Stephenson, J. R. (1982) *Nature (London)* 300, 765–767

68 Groffen, J., Stephenson, J. R., Heisterkamp, N., de Klein, A., Bartram, C. R. and Grosveld, G. (1984) *Cell* 36, 93–99

69 Bartram, C. R., de Klein, A., Hagemeijer, A., van Agthoven, T., van Kessel, A. G., Bootsma, D., Grosveld, G., Gerguson-Smith, M. A., Davies, M., Stone, M., Heisterkamp, N., Stephenson, J. R. and Groffen, J. (1983) *Nature (London)* 277, 277–280

70 Canaani, E., Gale, R. P., Steiner-Saltz, D., Berrebi, A., Aghai, E. and Januszewics, E. (1984) *Lancet* i, 593–595

71 Witte, O. N. and Konopka, J. (1985) *Oncogene in B-cell Neoplasia* (Melchers, F. ed.) *Current Topics Microbiol.* (in press)

72 Fukuhara, S. and Rowley, J. D. (1978) *Int. J. Cancer* 22, 14–21

73 Fukuhara, S. and Uchino, H. (1983) *New Engl. J. Med.* 308, 1603–1604

74 Tsujimoto, Y., Uynis, J., Onorator-Showe, L., Erikson, J., Nowell, P. C. and Croce, C. M. (1984) *Science* 224, 1403–1406

75 Pegoraro, L., Palumbo, A., Erikson, J., Falda, M., Giovanazzo, B., Emanuel, B. S., Rovera, G., Nowell, P. C. and Croce, C. M. (1984) *Proc. Natl Acad. Sci. USA* 81, 7166–7170

76 Gonda, T. J. and Metcalf, O. (1984) *Nature (London)* 310, 249–251

77 Wiener, F., Babonits, M., Spira, J., Bregula, U., Klein, G., Merwin, R. M., Asofsky, R., Lynes, M. and Haughton, G. (1981) *Int. J. Cancer* 27, 51–58

78 Klein, E. (1985) in *Immunity to Cancer.* (Reif, A. E. and Mitchell, M. S. eds) Academic Press, New York and London

79 Gordon, J., Aman, P., Rosen, A., Ernberg, I., Ehlin-Henriksson, B. and Klein, G. (1985) *Int. J. Cancer* 35, 251–256

G. Klein and E. Klein are at the Department of Tumour Biology, Karolinska Institute, Box 60 400, S-104 01 Stockholm, Sweden.

Chromosomal translocations and the c-*myc* gene: paradigm lost?

Nick Gough

Specific chromosomal translocations appear to play an important role in the genesis of certain tumours. In particular, two malignancies of the B lymphoid lineage, murine plasmacytomas and human Burkitt lymphomas, display specific chromosomal translocations involving bands bearing immunoglobulin (Ig) genes[1]. In most murine plasmacytomas the distal portion of chromosome 15 is translocated either to chromosome 12, which carries the Ig heavy-chain locus, or less frequently to chromosome 6, which carries the Ig kappa genes. Similarly, in human Burkitt lymphomas, the terminal part of chromosome 8 is usually translocated to chromosome 14, which carries the Ig heavy-chain locus, or occasionally to chromosomes 2 or 22, which carry the kappa and lambda genes respectively. Klein's suggestion[2] that an oncogene on chromosome 15 (in the mouse) or 8 (in the human) might be activated as a result of its accidental transposition to a functionally active Ig gene region was amply supported by two pieces of evidence. First, the relevant bands on murine chromosome 15 and human chromosome 8 carry the cellular proto-oncogene c-*myc*. Second, and more strikingly, most of the murine 15;12 (and human 8;14) translocations involve recombination events within or immediately upstream of the c-*myc* gene on the one hand, and close to an Ig heavy-chain gene on the other[3]. The major consequence of this translocation is that the rearranged c-*myc* allele is constitutively, and thus inappropriately, expressed. Whilst it is not clear why or how the expression of the c-*myc* gene is altered, it is fairly easy to be persuaded that regulatory elements adjacent to the promoters of the c-*myc* gene might be removed by translocation, or that the Ig locus plays a more active role, bringing its own regulatory elements to bear on the c-*myc* gene.

Translocation variants

Since the chromosome 15 breakpoint in a 15;6 translocation is cytogenetically indistinguishable from that in a t15;12 and given the consistency at the molecular level of the recombination event in 15;12 translocations, one could have been forgiven for assuming that the 'variant' 15;6 translocations would follow much the same pattern as their 15;12 counterparts: not so. Recent work from Suzanne Cory and Jerry Adams' laboratory[4,5] has revealed a new locus on chromosome 15 at which many of the breakpoints in the variant (15;6) murine translocations occur. Since this locus is distant from c-*myc*, it perhaps challenges the uniquely pivotal role of the c-*myc* gene in lymphocyte transformation.

Recently Webb *et al.*[4] cloned the t15;6 junction from a tumour in which both alleles of the c-*myc* gene were shown by Southern blotting experiments to be unaltered. Pursuing the hypothesis that the t15;6 involved a breakpoint close to the C_x gene (albeit distinct from c-*myc*) they cloned both C_x alleles from this tumour: one of the alleles represents a conventionally rearranged and activated Ig gene, while the other proved to have undergone recombination with a region of chromosome 15. They then used molecular probes derived from this chromosome 15 locus to examine its status in other variant t(15;6) tumours[5]. Nine t15;6 tumours were examined; in none is the chromosome 15 breakpoint within the immediate vicinity of the c-*myc* gene (27 kb 5' or 23 kb 3'). This is in striking contrast with the vast majority of 15;12 translocations which are clustered very close to or within the 5' exon of c-*myc*. However, in five of the nine tumours the breakpoints on chromosome 15 are clustered within 4.5 kb of each other, around the previously identified breakpoint; this region has therefore been denoted the *pvt*-1 locus (plasmacytoma variant translocation) (see Fig. 1). Four of the 15;6 translocation breakpoints were unaccounted for, appearing to map close to neither c-*myc* nor *pvt*-1[5]. This raises the possibility of other *pvt* loci within this band on chromosome 15.

In an attempt to determine the distance between, and the relative orientations of, the *pvt*-1 and c-*myc* loci, Cory *et al.*[5] cloned a 108 kb region spanning the *pvt*-1 locus. This region does not, however, overlap with a region of 58 kb encompassing the c-*myc* gene that they also cloned. While the relative location and orientation of *pvt*-1 and c-*myc* are still not known (although, by analogy with the variant human 8;2 and 8;22 translocations, *pvt*-1 might be 3' to the c-*myc* gene), the distance between the two loci must be *at least* 72 kb.

More recently the same group[6] have also demonstrated that some murine T lymphomas have retroviral inserts within the *pvt*-1 locus. Of the seven retroviral inserts identified within the 108 kb region spanning *pvt*-1, four lie within the same cluster as the translocation breakpoints, while three lie some distance away (see Fig. 1).

This raises a number of intriguing questions. Foremost, of course, is the nature of the *pvt*-1 locus. Since most thinking has hitherto focused on the involvement of c-*myc* in the genesis of plasmacytomas, it is natural to attempt to relate *pvt*-1 to c-*myc*. Certainly, in all tumours examined, the levels of c-*myc* mRNA are similar to that in t15;12 plasmacytomas and therefore it is assumed that somehow the c-*myc* gene has indeed been deregulated, but it is unclear how translocations at the *pvt*-1 locus might deregulate *myc* expression. Given the distance between the two loci, it is difficult to see how a derangement at *pvt*-1 could disrupt the regulation of c-*myc*, although Cory *et al.*[5] point out that if *pvt*-1 and c-*myc* were brought into proximity in the chromatin superstructure then perturbation of the *pvt*-1 locus might well affect c-*myc*. The more obvious possibility, however, is that *pvt*-1 is another structural gene whose product is implicated (directly or indirectly) in the transformation of lymphoid cells. Such a gene product might be a *trans*-acting regulator of c-*myc* or may act independently. If *pvt*-1 is a structural gene, the fact that the translocations and insertions are spread over a 70–80 kb range (although most are clustered, see Fig. 1) favours the notion that they alter the gene's expression by interrupting its transcriptional unit, rather than by influencing its regulatory elements or promoters.

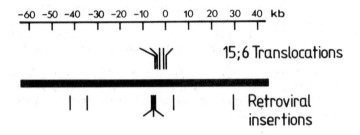

Fig. 1. Location of translocation breakpoints (top) and retroviral inserts (bottom) in the pvt-*1 locus (adapted from Refs. 5 and 6).*

Gene rearranagement

It is also intriguing that most 15;12 translocations involve the c-*myc* locus (but not *pvt*-1), whereas many 15;6 translocations involve *pvt*-1 (but none c-*myc*). Since light- and heavy-chain Ig genes undergo rearrangement at different stages of B lymphoid maturation, it is conceivable that *pvt*-1 might be 'available' for translocation (in the correct chromatin configuration perhaps) only at the time of kappa gene rearrangement and c-*myc* only at the time of heavy-chain rearrangement. This, however, seems a little implausible, particularly since the c-*myc* gene is probably expressed at every cell division and would presumably be in the same configuration at the time of both heavy and kappa rearrangement. One is left to speculate, therefore, that structural constraints favour recombination of C_x with *pvt*-1 rather than c-*myc,* and the converse for the heavy-chain locus.

Finally, it is unclear *how* the 15;6 translocations occur. Since the t15;12 normally map within regions of the Ig heavy-chain locus involved in 'switch recombination'[1,3], it has been assumed that the enzymatic machinery involved in class switching plays a role in the translocation. This is unlikely to be the case for the t15;6, since light-chain genes do not undergo switch recombination and do not contain switch sites. However, since the chromosome 6 breakpoints map reasonably close to the kappa joining gene segments[5] (a locus with a propensity for rearrangement, both normal and aberrant), Cory *et al.*[5] suggest that, at the time of Ig gene rearrangement or activation, this locus may participate in fairly nonspecific recombination events; transformation then selects those which have occurred at *pvt*-1.

Note added in proof

The relative locations and orientations of the c-*myc* and *pvt*-1 loci on chromosome 15 have since been determined by Banerjee *et al.*[7]

References

1   Klein, G. (1983) Specific chromosomal translocations and the genesis of B-cell-derived tumors in mice and men. *Cell* 32, 311–315
2   Klein, G. (1981) The role of gene dosage and genetic transpositions in carcinogenesis. *Nature* 294, 313–318
3   Perry, R. P. (1983) Consequences of *myc* invasion of immunoglobulin loci: facts and speculation. *Cell* 33, 647–649
4   Webb, E., Adams, J. M. and Cory, S. (1984) Variant (6;15) translocation in a murine plasmacytoma occurs near an immunoglobulin kappa gene but far from the *myc* oncogene. *Nature* 312, 777–779
5   Cory, S., Graham, M., Webb, E., Corcoran, L. and Adams, J. M. (1985) Variant (6;15) translocations in murine plasmacytomas involve a chromosome 15 locus at least 72 kb from the c-*myc* oncogene. *EMBO J.* 4, 58–59
6   Graham, M., Adams, J. M. and Cory, S. (1985) Murine T lymphomas with retroviral inserts in the chromosomal 15 locus for plasmacytoma variant translocations. *Nature* 314, 740–743
7   Banerjee, M., Wiener, F., Spira, J., Babonits, M., Nilsson, M-G., Sumeji, J. and Klein, G. (1985) Mapping of the c-*myc, pvt*-1 and immunoglobulin kappa genes in relation to the mouse plasmacytoma-associated variant (6;15) translocation breakpoint. *EMBO J.* 4, 3183–3188

N. Gough is at the Ludwig Institute for Cancer Research, Royal Melbourne Hospital, Victoria 3050, Australia.

Amplification of N-*myc* in human neuroblastomas

Manfred Schwab

Enhanced expression consequent to amplification of the N-myc *gene may contribute to malignant progression of human neuroblastomas. Cytogenetic analyses of human neuroblastomas provide evidence for specific chromosomal abnormalities and have presented an opening for the study of the molecular biology of various forms of human cancer including neuroblastoma, small-cell lung cancer and retinoblastoma. A previously unknown human gene,* N-myc, *seems to contribute to the growth control of cells and according to contemporary definition can be regarded as a cellular oncogene. A prominent feature is its abnormally high expression due to amplification in numerous human neuroblastomas, several cases of small-cell lung cancer and some retinoblastomas.*

Amplification of cellular genes is one of the adaptive genetic mechanisms cells have for acquiring the capacity to synthesize large amounts of specific cellular products. Unscheduled amplification involving extensive DNA domains is a frequent mechanism by which cells gain resistance against selective drugs (for review see Ref. 1), while scheduled amplification of genes can occur during certain phases of normal development (for instance in the ovarian follicle cells of the fruitfly[2]). Cytogenetic studies of human and animal tumor cells have repeatedly provided evidence for mysterious chromosomal manifestations of amplified cellular DNA: 'double minutes' (DMs; Fig. 1a)[3], 'C-bandless chromosomes' (CMs; Fig. 1b)[4] and homogeneously-staining chromosomal regions' (HSRs; Fig. 1c)[5], but their origin, genetic information and possible significance have long been enigmatic[6,7]. Surveys of mRNA expression of cellular oncogenes in tumor cell lines known to contain DMs, CMs or HSRs uncovered unusually large amounts of c-*myc* mRNA in the human APUDOma cell line COLO 320 (Ref. 8) and in the murine SEWA tumor cell lines[9], and of c-Ki-*ras* mRNA in the murine adrenocortical tumor cell line Y1 (Ref. 10). Subsequent analyses of the genomic DNA revealed multiple copies of the cellular oncogenes c-*myc* in COLO 320 and SEWA cells, and of c-Ki-*ras* in Y1 cells[8–10] which could be localized to DMs, CMs and HSRs[8–10] (for review see Ref. 11).

The N-*myc* gene
To find out if amplification of cellular oncogenes is not only a feature of established cell lines but can also be found in tumor specimens derived directly from patients, we turned to human neuroblastoma because cells of this tumor frequently carry DMs or HSR. When total genomic DNA from neuroblastoma cell lines carrying DMs or HSRs was analysed with different oncogene probes, amplification of a domain was detected with viral *myc* probe[12]. Analyses of the topography, and especially of the nucleotide sequence ruled out the possibility that the amplified DNA is part of the c-*myc* gene, the cellular homolog of v-*myc*[12]. The new DNA sequence soon assumed a distinctive name: N-*myc*.

The strongest similarity between c-*myc* and N-*myc* is within the first coding exon of c-*myc*[12] (Fig. 2). Nucleotide sequence analyses identified similarities

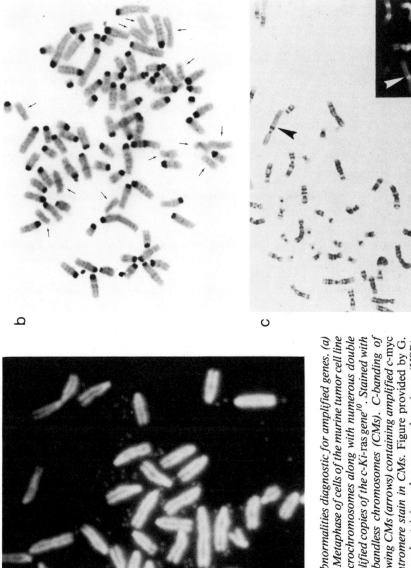

Fig. 1. *Chromosomal abnormalities diagnostic for amplified genes. (a) Double minutes (DMs). Metaphase of cells of the murine tumor cell line Y1 showing normal macrochromosomes along with numerous double minutes containing amplified copies of the c-Ki-ras gene[10]. Stained with Hoechst 33258. (b) C-bandless chromosomes (CMs). C-banding of murine SEWA cells showing CMs (arrows) containing amplified c-myc gene[9]. Note lack of centromere stain in CMs. Figure provided by G. Levan. (c) Homogeneously-staining chromosomal regions (HSR). G-banding of COLO 320-HSR metaphase spread. Arrow indicates HSR marker-chromosome containing amplified c-myc. Inset: Q-banded preparation. Figure provided by C. C. Lin; from Ref. 8.*

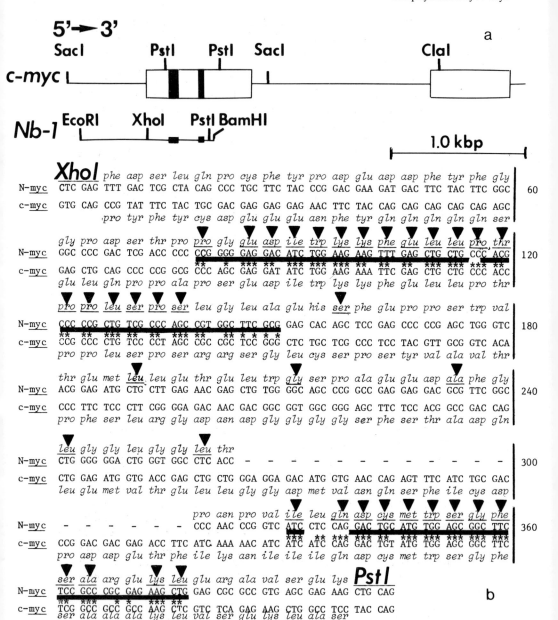

Fig. 2. *Similarities between c-myc and N-myc. (a) Localization of regions of similarity between N-myc and c-myc (myc-boxes). The two myc-boxes are localized in c-myc within the first coding exon, as indicated by solid black bars. Nb-1 represents a portion derived from the 5'-end of N-myc. (b) Nucleotide sequence analyses of DNA encompassing the myc-boxes. Sequence spans the region between the XhoI and PstI restriction endonuclease sites of N-myc as indicated in (a). Black bars under N-myc sequence indicate myc boxes I and II. Asterisks indicate bases, filled triangles amino acids identical between N-myc and c-myc. Relative to the c-myc gene, box I starts at nucleotide position 133, box II at position 385 (Ref. 31). Sequence analysis by K. H. Klempnauer, from Ref. 12.*

between N-*myc* and c-*myc* in two major domains (here referred to as *myc*-boxes), separated by a heterologous sequence. Box I (72 nucleotides) shows 78% similarity between N-*myc* and c-*myc* and box II (48 nucleotides) shows 83% similarity.

The similarities are even more significant at the level of the amino acid sequences of the proteins. The deduced amino acid sequence of N-*myc* reveals in box I 19 out of 24 amino acids identical to those of the c-*myc* proteins, and in box II 13 out of 16 amino acids are identical. Of these, in box I 18 form contiguous stretches and in box II 10 do so. Interestingly, differences in the nucleotide sequences between N-*myc* and c-*myc* within the *myc*-boxes are mostly in the third position of the codons resulting in conservation of the amino acid sequences. This suggests that the protein domains encoded by the *myc*-boxes serve a conserved function common to c-*myc* and N-*myc*. Additional but less extensive regions of similarity between c-*myc* and N-*myc* have been discovered in a 3'-coding exon of N-*myc*[13].

It is possible that N-*myc* is a member of a family of *myc*-related genes (*myc*-box genes) present in vertebrates from man to fish (Ref. 14; and author unpublished). At least one *myc*-box gene additional to N-*myc*, L-*myc*, has been implicated in human cancer (M. Nau, pers. commun.).

Amplification of N-*myc* in neuroblastomas

Among the 26 neuroblastoma cell lines tested to date, 22 have amplification of N-*myc* ranging from about 10- to 700-fold (Table 1)[12,13,15]. Four lines lack amplification. In all cases, amplification of N-*myc* was localized to DMs and HSRs[12,15,17].

Given the frequency of DMs reported in direct preparations of cells from patients it came as no surprise to find N-*myc* amplification in DNA directly prepared from a neuroblastoma tumor[12]. These tumors are usually classified into four stages (Evans stages I–IV), depending on the degree of progression and the prognosis. Stage I defines a locally confined tumor with good prognosis and stage IV a metastatic tumor with poor prognosis. A study involving 64 tumors of patients not subjected to therapy revealed (without exception) that amplification of N-*myc* was limited to stage III and IV tumors[18]. Amplification was discovered in approximately 50% of all stage III and IV tumors. This implies that amplification of N-*myc* is a late event in the development of neuroblastomas. It should be interesting to see now whether stage I and II tumors which have been surgically treated but later went into relapse with higher malignancy (equivalent to stages III or IV) now have developed amplification. Also, is amplification present in the metastases of stage III and IV tumors which themselves did not carry amplified N-*myc*?

The normal position of N-*myc* is on the short arm of chromosome 2 (2p23–24)[15,17], but HSRs in neuroblastoma cells have been reported on numerous different chromosomes (Table 1). It is not clear whether N-*myc* is translocated before being amplified, or whether the emergence of an HSR in different chromosomal positions is the result of prior amplification. Neuroblastoma cell line IMR-32 has amplified N-*myc* within an HSR on chromosome 1. DNA flanking amplified N-*myc* has been also found in this cell line on the short arm of chromosome 2 as what appears to be single copy[19], and it is likely that N-*myc* is also present as single copy on chromosome 2. If further analyses confirm that sequences present in HSRs on different chromosomes are still retained as a single copy at their germ-line position, then relocation of N-*myc* is, in general,

Table 1. N-myc *amplification in human neuroblastoma cell lines*

Cell line	Fold amplification	DMs	HSR[a]	Ref.
Kelly	100-120	−	+ (4,12)	12
NGP	120-140	−	+ (9)	12
NFL	20- 25	−	+ (9)	12
CHP-134	20- 25; 700	−	+ (6,7)	12,15
CHP-126	100-120	+	+ (5)	12,15
IMR-32	15- 20; 25	−	+ (1)	12,15
NMB	100-120	−	+ (13)	12
MCN-1	5- 10	+	−	12
LA-N-1	100	−	+	15
LA-N-5	50	+	−	15
NB-9	300	+	−	15
NB-16	300	+	−	16
NB-19	600	−	+ (13)	16
BE(2)-C	150	+	−	16
NAP(H)	100[b]	−	+	16
SK-N-BE(1)	50	+	−	16
NAP(D)	100[b]	+	−	16
CHP-234	100[b]	+	−	16
SMS-KAN	100[b]	+	−	16
SMS-KCN	100[b]	+	−	16
SMS-MSN	100[b]	+	−	16
SMS-KANR	100[b]	−	− (ABR)[d]	16
SH-SY5Y	0	−	−	16
SK-N-SH	0	−	−	12,15
CHP-100	0[c]	?		15
NB-69	0	−		16

[a] numbers in parentheses indicate chromosome.
[b] estimates on the basis of data presented in Ref. 16.
[c] three-fold amplification of c-*myc*.
[d] abnormally staining chromosomal region.

probably the result of amplification. This relocation mechanism might involve mobile genetic elements (possibly DMs) and it is supported by cytogenetic data showing a tendency in human neuroblastoma for HSRs to evolve from DMs[20].

N-*myc* may regulate cellular differentiation

N-*myc* is expressed as a major mRNA of 3.0–4.0 kb[13,21]. Low expression of N-*myc* is detectable in neuroblastoma cells lacking amplification such as the human neuroblastoma line SK-N-SH or the murine neuroblastoma line Neuro-2a (Ref. 21), while approximately 40–60-fold elevated expression is found in other neuroblastoma cell lines or in tumors carrying amplification of N-*myc*[21].

Human neuroblastomas often consist of heterogeneous cell populations ranging from primitive neuroblasts to cells displaying features of ganglion differentiation. Hybridization *in situ* to tissue sections has been used to identify primitive neuroblasts as primary sites for enhanced expression of N-*myc*, while more differentiated cells tend to have small amounts of N-*myc* mRNA[21]. High expression of N-*myc*, as detected by hybridization *in situ*, appears to be correlated with a fatal outcome[22]. Whether high expression of N-*myc* turns out to be a useful marker for the diagnosis and evaluation of the prognosis of neuroblastomas as well as for devising therapies has yet to be addressed in prospective and retrospective clinical studies. The *in situ* hydridization results showing low expression of N-*myc* in more differentiated cells are corroborated by studies using neuroblastoma cell lines. Visible morphologic differentiation (neurite formation) induced by retinoic acid is preceded by drastic reductions in the amount of N-*myc* mRNA[23].

A survey of numerous cell lines established from various types of tumor including carcinomas, melanomas and leukaemias has shown that N-*myc* expression is restricted to cells derived from a set of related neuroectodermal tumors including neuroblastomas, small-cell lung cancer and retinoblastomas[21,24].

Analyses of mRNA isolated from various developmental stages of embryo in the mouse have revealed high concentrations of N-*myc* mRNA during mid-gestation[25]. Studies of sections of mouse embryos *in situ* should soon provide clues about the types of cells that produce N-*myc* mRNA. Even without gene amplification, surprisingly large amounts of N-*myc* mRNA were discovered in cells of different murine embryonal carcinoma lines[25].

Together, these results suggest that N-*myc* is a highly regulated gene and its product may be involved in the regulation of cellular differentiation.

Oncogenic activity of N-*myc*

Consistent amplification of N-*myc* alone does not prove that N-*myc* has a role in tumorigenesis. The amplified domain of DNA is presumably much larger than the N-*myc* gene, and has been estimated, for instance, to encompass as much as 3000 kb in the line IMR-32 (Ref. 19). This DNA domain could contain several genes and therefore the possible role of N-*myc* in control of cellular growth has been investigated. After defining the boundaries of the N-*myc* gene, a transcriptional enhancer derived from the U3 region of a long terminal repeat (LTR) of murine Moloney leukaemia virus was covalently linked to the 5′-end of N-*myc* derived from a human neuroblastoma cell line and from a normal individual to generate suitable expression vectors[26]. When these N-*myc* expression vectors are introduced into early passage rat embryo cells the host cells can survive for more than 200 generations in culture, but the cells cannot elicit tumors in suitable host animals (author unpublished). Previous experiments had shown that the viral *myc* gene, or cellular *myc* derived from a murine plasmacytoma line, can assist the mutated c-Ha-*ras* gene derived from the human bladder carcinoma cell line EJ in tumorigenic conversion of early passage rat embryo cells[27]. Cotransfection of c-Ha-*ras*(EJ) together with either one of the N-*myc* expression vectors resulted in formation of two types of foci (type I and II). Foci formation occurred whether N-*myc* was derived from a neuroblastoma or from normal cells, indicating that activation of the oncogenic potential of N-*myc* requires only alterations augmenting expression. Type I foci consisted of a loose array of highly refractile, small, round cells that were fairly independent of the substrate, grew in a three-dimensional pattern and elicited malignant tumors when injected into isogenic rats or athymic mice. In contrast, type II foci consisted of densely layered, elongated, fibroblast-like cells that were highly substrate dependent, formed a flat monolayer but have not been found to form tumors in suitable hosts. The relevance of these results to human neuroblasts is yet to be determined as is the exact function of N-*myc* in normal cells and in tumor cells. Answers will be facilitated by the identification and study of the N-*myc* product. Apart from this, the question still remains whether genes other than N-*myc* (which are presumably present within the amplified DNA domain) may also contribute to neoplastic transformation.

N-*myc* in retinoblastoma and small-cell lung cancer

Amplification of N-*myc* also occurs in retinoblastomas[28] and in small-cell lung cancer[29]. The data for small-cell lung cancer suggest that amplification of N-*myc* is associated with more malignant forms of this tumor as well as with classical forms, in contrast to neuroblastomas where amplification has so far been found exclusively in the more advanced stages. For retinoblastomas the situation appears to be different. Amplification has been discovered so far in three of 38 tumors[28] and, as in neuroblastomas, is accompanied by high expression of N-*myc*[21,28]. In contrast to neuroblastomas – where there is only low expression of N-*myc* in the absence of amplification – in both retinoblastomas cell lines and tumors (Ref. 28 and author unpublished), abundant expression of mRNA has been found in the absence of amplification. The significance and molecular basis for this high expression are unknown. It is possible, though, that the high levels of N-*myc* expression in retinoblastoma cells without amplification result from an arrest of the differentiation of the tumor cells in an embryonal stage at which high expression of N-*myc* is normal.

How does amplification of N-*myc* relate to tumorigenesis?

Gene amplification is an unstable genetic condition that can only be maintained by strong selective pressure. Drug-resistant cells carrying amplified genes quickly dispose of their genetic burden when grown under non-selective conditions. Nothing is known about the selective pressure maintaining amplified cellular oncogenes but it is fair to assume their existence. One experimental system substantiates this. Certain clones of murine SEWA tumor cells generate DMs when grown in a suitable host; after *in vitro* transfers the DMs rapidly disappear from these cells, as if the genetic information is no longer required under these growth conditions[30]. It is probably not a coincidence that DMs in SEWA cells are the sites of amplified c-*myc*[9], supporting the conclusion that amplified cellular oncogenes are needed for their contribution to the transformed phenotype.

Assuming that amplification of N-*myc* does have a role in neuroblastomas, the restriction of amplification to advanced metastatic tumors and the predominance of enhanced N-*myc* expression in primitive neuroblasts seem to indicate a connection with malignant progression. In line with this, is the positive correlation between presence of N-*myc* amplification and the capacity of cells of neuroblastomas to become established in culture: all known neuroblastoma cell lines are derived from stage IV tumors which usually do not produce significant amounts of differentiated nerve cells. Lack of N-*myc* amplification in about 50% of advanced neuroblastomas does not necessarily contradict this concept since neuroblastomas belong to a class of neuroectodermal tumors that often cannot be distinguished easily from each other. It is possible, therefore, that while one type of neuroectodermal tumor (such as typical childhood neuroblastoma) progresses as a consequence of N-*myc* amplification, another type (such as peripheral neuroectodermal tumor) progresses as a result of a different molecular alteration.

Conclusion

The apparent restriction of amplification to malignant, metastatic forms of neuroblastoma could turn out to be a useful diagnostic marker for assessing the prognosis and possibly for devising appropriate therapies. Beyond this, the study of neuroblastomas has allowed us to uncover a new human gene that may have a specific but unknown function during a defined phase in mammalian embryo development and, furthermore, it has brought to our attention the existence of a family of *myc*-related genes present in the genome of vertebrates.

Acknowledgements

I am indebted to the many colleagues I collaborated with on the project discussed here, especially Kari Alitalo, Harold Varmus and Michael Bishop. Most of my original work was done while a Heisenberg-Fellow of the Deutsche Forschungsgemeinschaft.

References

1 Schimke, R. T. (1984) Gene amplification in cultured animal cells. *Cell* 37, 705–713
2 Spradling, A. C. and Mahowald, A. P. (1980) Amplification of genes for chorion proteins during oogenesis in *Drosophila melanogaster*. *Proc. Natl Acad. Sci. USA* 77, 1096–1100
3 Cox, D., Yuncken, C. and Spriggs, A. (1965) Minute chromatin bodies in malignant tumours of childhood. *Lancet* ii, 55–58
4 Levan, A., Levan, G. and Mitelman, F. (1977) Chromosomes and cancer. *Hereditas* 86, 15–30
5 Biedler, J. L., Helson, L. and Spengler, B. S. (1973) *Cancer Res.* 33, 2543–2652
6 Cowell, J. K. (1982) Double minutes and homogeneously staining chromosomal regions: gene amplification in mammalian cells. *Annu. Rev. Genet.* 16, 21–59
7 Barker, P. E. (1982) Double minutes in human tumor cells. *Cancer Genet. Cytogenet.* 5, 81–94
8 Alitalo, K. *et al.* (1983) Homogeneously staining chromosomal regions contain amplified copies of an abundantly expressed cellular oncogene (c-*myc*) in malignant neuroendocrine cells from a human colon carcinoma. *Proc. Natl Acad. Sci. USA* 80, 1707–1711
9 Schwab, M. (1985) Amplification and enhanced expression of the c-*myc* oncogene in mouse SEWA tumor cells. *Nature* 315, 345–347
10 Schwab, M. *et al.* (1983) A cellular oncogene (c-Ki-*ras*) is amplified, overexpressed, and located within karyotypic abnormalities in mouse adrenocortical tumor cells. *Nature* 303, 497–501
11 Alitalo, K. and Schwab, M. (1986) Oncogene amplification in tumor cells. *Adv. Cancer Res.* 47 (in press)
12 Schwab, M. *et al.* (1983) Amplified DNA with limited homology to *myc* cellular oncogene is shared by human neuroblastoma cell lines and a neuroblastoma tumor. *Nature* 305, 245–248
13 Michitsch, R. W. and Melera, P. (1985) Nucleotide sequence of the 3′-exon of the human N-*myc* gene. *Nucleic Acids Res.* 13, 2545–2558
14 Dalla-Favera, R. *et al.* (1982) Cloning and characterization of different human sequences related to the onc gene (v-*myc*) of avian myelocytomatosis virus (MC29). *Proc. Natl Acad. Sci. USA* 79, 6497–6501
15 Kohl, N. *et al.* (1983) Transposition and amplification of oncogene related sequence in human neuroblastomas. *Cell* 35, 359–367
16 Michitsch, R. W., Montgomery, K. T. and Melera, P. W. (1984) Expression of the amplified domain in human neuroblastoma cells. *Mol. Cell. Biol.* 4, 2370–2380
17 Schwab, M. *et al.* (1984) Chromosome localization in normal human cells and neuroblastomas of a gene related to c-*myc*. *Nature* 308, 288–291
18 Brodeur, G. M. *et al.* (1984) Amplification of N-*myc* in untreated human neuroblastomas correlates with advanced disease stage. *Science* 224, 1121–1124
19 Kanda, N. *et al.* (1983) Isolation of amplified DNA sequences from IMR-32 human neuroblastoma cells: facilitation by fluorescence-activated flow sorting of metaphase chromosomes. *Proc. Natl Acad. Sci. USA* 80, 4069–4073

20 Biedler, J. *et al.* (1985) Growth stage-related synthesis and secretion of proteins by human neuroblastoma cells and their variants. In *Advances in Neuroblastoma Research* (Evans, A. E., A'Angio, G. J. and Seeger, R. C. eds), pp. 209–221, Alan R. Liss

21 Schwab, M. *et al.* (1984) Enhanced expression of the gene N-*myc* consequent to amplification of DNA may contribute to malignant progression of neuroblastoma. *Proc. Natl. Acad. Sci. USA* 81, 4940–4944

22 Grady-Leopardi, E. *et al.* (1986) Expression of N-*myc* oncogene in neuroblastoma by *in situ* hybridization and blot analysis: relationship to clinical outcome. *Cancer Res.* 46, 3196–3199

23 Thiele, C. J., Reynolds, C. P. and Israel, M. A. (1985) Decreased expression of N-*myc* precedes retinoic acid-induced morphological differentiation of human neuroblastoma. *Nature* 313, 404–406

24 Kohl, N., Gee, C. E. and Alt, F. (1984) Activated expression of the N-*myc* gene in human neuroblastomas and related tumors. *Science* 226, 1335–1337

25 Jacobovits, A. *et al.* (1985) Expression of N-*myc* in teratocarcinoma stem cells and mouse embryos *Nature* 318, 188–191

26 Schwab, M., Varmus, H. E. and Bishop, J. M. (1985) The human N-*myc* gene contributes to tumorigenic conversion of mammalian cells in culture. *Nature* 316, 160–162

27 Land, H., Parada, L. and Weinberg, R. (1983) Tumorigenic conversion of primary embryo fibroblasts requires at least two cooperating oncogenes. *Nature* 304, 596–602

28 Lee, W-H., Murphee, A. C. and Benedict, W. F. (1984) Expression and amplification of the N-*myc* gene in primary retinoblastoma. *Nature* 309, 458–460

29 Nau, M. M. *et al.* (1984) Amplification, expression and rearrangement of c-*myc* and N-*myc* oncogenes in human lung cancer. In *Current Topics in Microbiology and Immunology* (Potter, M., Melchers, F. and Weigert, M., eds), pp. 173-177, Springer-Verlag

30 Levan, A., Levan, G. and Mandahl, N. (1981) Double minutes and C-bandless chromosomes in a mouse tumor. In *Genes, Chromosomes and Neoplasia* (Arrighi, F. E., Rao, P. N. and Stubblefield, E. eds), pp. 223–251, Raven Press

31 Watt, R. *et al.* (1983) Nucleotide sequence of cloned cDNA of human c-*myc* oncogene. *Nature* 303, 725–728

M. Schwab is at the Hooper Foundation, School of Medicine, University of California, San Francisco, CA 94143, USA.

The activation of cellular oncogenes by retroviral insertion

Roel Nusse

Replication-competent retroviruses can induce a variety of tumors by insertional activation of cellular oncogenes. Transposon tagging techniques have uncovered many novel cellular genes implicated in tumorigenesis. Activation of these genes can occur by insertion of viral promoters, transcriptional enhancement over large distances, or the generation of novel chimeric proteins.

Retroviruses can induce tumors in several different ways. Transforming viruses have transduced host cell proto-oncogenes and express these genes in a modified form, such that target cells swiftly become tumorigenic[1,2]. Generally, transforming viruses have sacrificed some viral information in the process of transduction of cellular sequences, and are hence dependent on replication-competent helper viruses for propagation. Most replicating retroviruses are unable to transform cells directly, but they are not completely innocuous; many of them can cause tumors in susceptible animals, albeit after long incubation periods compared with their oncogene-carrying derivatives.

In recent years, the mechanism underlying oncogenesis by slowly oncogenic viruses has been elucidated to a large extent. The implications of these findings have been wide-ranging: from the first demonstration that cellular proto-oncogenes could actually contribute to tumorigenesis, to the discovery of a whole series of novel oncogenes that had not been encountered before in viral form.

Early indications and the activation of c-*myc*

A first glimpse of the mechanism of viral oncogenesis without viral oncogenes was obtained when restriction enzyme analysis of tumor DNA showed that proviral DNA was integrated in a clonal fashion, i.e. tumors were descendants of a single infected cell. It was realized that proviral insertions could cause mutations in the host cell DNA, not only recessive mutations due to disruption of a gene, but also integrations resulting in dominant mutations, as a consequence of *cis*-activation of cellular sequences. The strategy for identifying the relevant cellular genes was straightforward and analogous to transposon tagging techniques used by *Drosophila* geneticists: proviral DNA was used as a probe to isolate flanking DNA from tumor cell libraries[3]. This approach proved to be successful (see below), but the first discovery of a gene activated by an inserted provirus was actually made when Hayward, Neel and Astrin conjectured that cellular proto-oncogenes could be among the targets for proviral insertion. They simply tested their hypothesis by screening virus-induced tumors for disruption of restriction fragments of known oncogenes, and found that a large majority of avian leukosis virus (ALV)-induced bursal lymphomas contained a provirus just upstream from the c-*myc* gene[4].

Their discovery was a key event in the history of oncogenetics. Not only did the mechanism of oncogenesis by ALV become understandable, but the stage was set for the subsequent unmasking of the c-*myc* and c-*abl* genes at chromosomal breakpoints in non-viral tumors. Another rewarding highlight for tumor virologists was the identification of the *ras* oncogenes, again originally found in retroviruses, as the culprits in cellular transformation after transfection of tumor DNA into NIH/3T3 cells. These and other findings showed that the search for genes implicated in viral oncogenesis could also lead us to the genetic events underlying non-viral forms of cancer[1,2].

Other genes activated by proviral insertion

Meanwhile, the large variety of animal tumors induced by slowly oncogenic retroviruses was explored to find novel insertion sites and genes. Established cell lines from tumors provided additional sources of material. Retroviruses can induce many different tumors, ranging from lymphoid proliferative diseases to mammary carcinomas and nephroblastomas. In most of these tumors, integrated proviral DNA can be found, and used as a tag to identify the integration domain by molecular cloning of viral DNA–host cell DNA junction fragments. The presence of proviruses in the same region of the cellular genome in multiple, independent tumors is then taken as evidence for the presence of a cellular gene whose activation has given the cell a growth advantage. The argument is based on the widely held but formally unproven assumption that proviruses integrate at numerous, if not random sites in the cellular DNA[5]. A common integration site therefore indicates selection of one particular cell on its way to tumorigenicity out of a large population of infected but otherwise normal cells. The prediction that a relevant cellular oncogene is present in the integration domain can be tested by searching for transcriptional activity, structural analysis of the gene and biological assays.

By following this strategy, many different integration domains have been identified, and in some of them, novel putative oncogenes have been found. The mouse mammary tumor (MMTV) and murine leukemia (MLV) viruses proved to be particularly useful in this approach (Tables 1 and 2). In murine mammary tumors, MMTV insertions are frequently found near either of two genes, called *int*-1 and *int*-2 (Refs 6 and 7). The structure of these genes is known; they encode proteins not related to each other or to other oncogenes, and are both conserved in evolution, allowing the isolation of homologous genes from the human genome. Both *int*-1 and *int*-2 are transiently expressed

Table 1. Cellular genes activated by proviral insertion: known genes

Gene	Virus	Animal	Disease
c-*myc*	ALV, CSV, REV	Chicken	Bursal lymphoma
	MLV	Mouse	T-cell lymphoma
	FeLV	Cat	T-cell lymphoma
c-*erb*-B	ALV	Chicken	Erythroleukemia
c-*myb*	MLV	Mouse	Lymphosarcoma
c-*mos*	IAP	Mouse	Plasmacytoma line
c-Ki-*ras*	F-MLV	Mouse	Myeloid cell line
c-Ha-*ras*	MAV	Chicken	Nephroblastoma[a]
IL-2	GaLV	Ape	T-cell lymphoma cell line
IL-3	IAP	Mouse	Myelomonocytic leukemia

[a]The evidence for *cis*-activation of c-Ha-*ras* by MAV comes from analysis of the RNA, but physical linkage of the provirus and the gene has not been demonstrated[34].

Table 2. Cellular genes activated by proviral insertion: genes or integration domains identified by transposon tagging

Gene	Virus	Animal	Disease
int-1	MMTV	Mouse	Mammary carcinoma
int-2			
int-41			Mammary and kidney carcinoma
Mlvi-1	M-MLV	Rat	T-cell lymphoma
Mlvi-2			
Mlvi-3			
Pim-1	M-MLV	Mouse	T-cell lymphoma
Gin-1	G-MLV	Mouse	T-cell lymphoma
pvt(=Mis-1)	M-MLV	Mouse/rat	T or B cell lymphoma
Fis-1	F-MLV	Mouse	Lymphoma, myeloid leukemia
tck(=lskT)	M-MLV	Mouse	Thymoma cell line

during embryogenesis of the mouse, but during different periods and at different sites[6]. Additional *int* genes, still to be analysed in more detail, are found in other mammary tumors.

In T-cell leukemias and lymphomas induced by MLV in mice or rats, many different genes are implicated[9–12]. The characterization of *Pim*-1 and *tck* (also called *lskT*) is most well advanced; both genes encode proteins with significant homology to the protein kinase family of the oncogenes[11–13]. In other common integration domains of MLV proviruses in T-cell leukemias, there is no evidence yet for a transcriptionally active gene. One of these regions, called *pvt* and also *Mis*-1, was independently isolated from both retroviral integration mapping and by molecular cloning of junction fragments of chromosomal fusions in mouse plasmacytomas[14].

Some known genes were also encountered among those with proviral insertions, in addition to the already mentioned c-*myc* gene (Table 1). In erythroleukemias induced by ALV, the c-*erb*-B gene is often interrupted by an incoming provirus[15], in such a manner that entirely novel *erb*-B transcripts and proteins are synthesized (see below), and similar insertions are found in c-*myb* in MLV-induced lymphosarcomas[16]. Some factor-independent T-cell lines were found to make their own growth factors as a consequence of proviral insertions near the IL-2 or the IL-3 gene[17,18]. The latter two examples nicely illustrate the principle that oncogenes are actually normal genes; one would not normally put IL-2 on the list of oncogenes, but if the gene had been discovered first by transposon tagging we might now know it as T-cell induction gene (tig)!

Hepatitis B virus (HBV) is a DNA-containing virus that nevertheless replicates, like RNA retroviruses, through a round of reverse transcription. HBV is associated with the etiology of human hepatocellular carcinoma, and integrated viral DNA can be found in most of these tumors. Recently, HBV viral DNA has been identified within a gene homologous to steroid hormone receptors and to the *erb*-A oncogene[19]. This finding suggests that insertional mutagenesis plays a role in the oncogenicity of this virus, although the evidence rests on a single case, and many other attempts to show common integration domains have not met with success.

It was initially disappointing that no common integration domains were found for bovine leukosis virus (BLV)[20] and human T-cell leukemia virus (HTLV). We are now aware of other properties shared by these two retroviruses, namely their capacity to *trans*-activate their own transcription through synthesis of a viral protein, pX, also called *tat*[21]. Presumably, these viral products can also *trans*-activate the expression of cellular genes, and thereby carry out their role in tumorigenesis. In this respect, BLV and HTLV resemble transforming retroviruses with viral oncogenes since their mode of action is independent of the integration site; they differ from the classical transforming viruses in having oncogenes with no readily detectable cellular precursors.

The mechanism of activation of cellular genes

The mode of gene activation by inserted proviruses is rather diverse, but it always hinges on the property of retroviruses that they carry their own transcription signals. Present in the long terminal repeats (LTRs) of an integrated provirus are enhancers, promoters and polyadenylation signals at

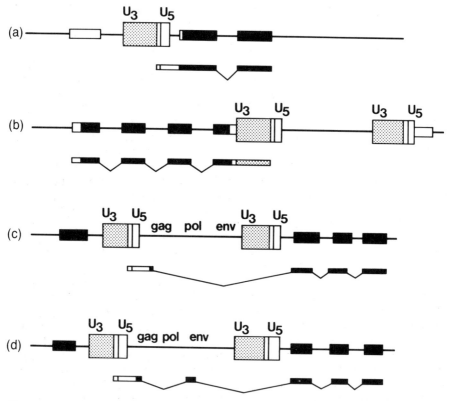

Fig. 1. *Generalized diagrams of four different configurations of inserted proviral DNA, an activated cellular gene and the resulting transcript. Protein-coding domains are in black boxes. (a) Insertion of the LTR of a deleted provirus in the promoter region of a gene, upstream from the first coding exon, such as occurs frequently near c-myc. (b) Enhancement activation of genes like int and Pim by a downstream intact provirus. In this example, the provirus is integrated in the untranslated trailer of the gene, leading to a hybrid RNA but to an unaltered protein. (c) Insertion of an intact MLV provirus within c-myb. The protein-encoding domain is disrupted and transcription starting from the 5' viral LTR joins viral gag sequences to the remainder of c-myb. (d). ALV insertions near c-erb-B, with similar disruptions to those in (c), but with a transcript containing viral env sequences as well. The remaining exons of c-erb-B correspond to the intracellular domain of the EGF receptor.*

both sides of the structural viral genes *gag, pol* and *env*[5]. Originally, it was proposed that the right LTR of an integrated provirus could directly serve as a transcriptional promoter of a gene downstream from the proviral element (Fig. 1a). This promoter-insertion model holds for many of the ALV-induced bursal lymphomas, but there were some important exceptions and variations. First, many, if not all proviruses near c-*myc* have sustained deletions of the viral genome, sometimes leaving little more than a solitary LTR intact (Fig. 1a). A mechanistic explanation of the requirement for these deletions was given by Cullen *et al.*[22], who showed that transcription starting in the right LTR of an intact provirus is quenched by transcription driven by the left LTR. By artificial termination of transcription within the provirus, or by deletions as found in the tumors, the activity of the right LTR becomes sufficient to act as a strong promoter[21].

Second, it was noticed by Payne *et al.* that ALV proviruses in tumors could also occur downstream of c-*myc*, or upstream in the opposite orientation[23]. This indirect form of transcriptional activation indicated the presence of transcriptional enhancers in retroviral LTRs, which has been widely documented subsequently. The importance of this type of activation lies in its less stringent requirements for the actual site of proviral insertion with respect to the gene. Moreover, the deletions apparently necessary for promoter insertions are not seen in proviruses activating at a distance.

Transcriptional enhancement is generally seen in the activation of the *int* genes by MMTV. Proviruses can be found at both sides of these genes[24], sometimes at large distances (more than 10 kbp from the promoter) but also within the transcriptional unit itself. The protein-encoding domains of the *int* genes nevertheless always remain intact[24,25], and tumorigenesis seems to be caused by inappropriate expression of an unaltered gene product. Insertions of MLV near *Pim*-1 follow the same principle, but are most frequently found within the 3' untranslated domain of the gene, indicating that perhaps stabilization of the *Pim*-1 mRNA contributes to gene expression as well[13]. Generalized diagrams of the configurations of insertions near the *int* and the *Pim* genes are shown in Fig. 1b.

More bizarre forms of proviral insertions are found at the c-*erb*-B gene in chicken erythroleukemias and near c-*myb* in mouse lymphosarcomas[15,16] (Fig. 1c and d). In both cases the protein-encoding domain of the cellular gene is disrupted as a consequence of insertion of a complete provirus within an intron. Novel hybrid proteins are generated by transcription starting in the left LTR of the provirus, readthrough into the *gag* domain and a splice onto the nearest 3' exon of the cellular oncogene. In the case of ALV insertion at c-*erb*-B, the splice also involves a short domain of the viral *env* gene[15]. Activation of c-*myb* can also occur by insertion within the 3' end of the gene with truncation of carboxy-terminal sequences of the protein[16]. These types of insertional mutations are highly interesting from the point of view of the requirements for converting a normal proto-oncogene protein into a transforming product, and suggest that truncation and a novel cellular location, guided by the newly acquired viral leader, are mandatory.

Proviral insertions near oncogenes herald transduction

The erythroleukemias induced by ALV show another interesting feature: quite often one can isolate new recombinant viruses that have transduced the cellular *erb*-B gene to become rapidly transforming viruses[26]. This observation is in line with the most tenable model for transduction of cellular oncogenes by retroviruses. In this scheme, a provirus integrates upstream from the oncogene, leading to a hybrid transcript containing viral and cellular sequences. By virtue of the presence of the viral packaging signal, the hybrid RNA ends up in a virion particle, is reverse transcribed upon reinfection and, by template switching of the reverse transcriptase and/or some other form of recombination, the oncogene becomes part of a new recombinant viral genome[5]. The hybrid transcript arising from the ALV inserts near c-*erb*-B fulfils the requirement of the first step, and is apparently frequently packaged and reverse transcribed. Less often, new *myc* viruses arise from either ALV-induced chicken tumors or feline leukemia virus (FeLV)-induced cat diseases[27]. One would expect that the MLV insertions near c-*myb* will also lead to new transforming MLV variants with a v-*myb* oncogene, but oddly, to date not even one murine *myb* virus has been isolated and only chicken *myb* viruses have been found.

The early clonal expansion of tumor cells containing a proviral insertion near an oncogene will undoubtedly favor the chance that the subsequent steps in transduction will take place. It is therefore likely that each transduction of a cellular oncogene has been initiated in a tumor resulting from insertional mutagenesis. Accordingly, this would predict that all of the cellular oncogenes that we know from transforming retroviruses are among the targets for slowly oncogenic viruses in tumors. Yet, the list in Table 1 does not comprise most of the known oncogenes, so we may have to look harder.

Conversely, many of the genes that are insertionally activated (Table 2) have never been transduced in the hitherto isolated transforming viruses. Perhaps their effects on cell growth are subtle and viruses acquiring these genes will not display conspicuous transforming abilities. One must keep in mind that oncogenesis by insertional mutagenesis probably involves more than one genetic event, quite unlike the rapid one step transformation by v-*onc*-carrying viruses. Additional mutations may occur elsewhere in the genome, as illustrated by the observations that tumors can have proviral insertions near two different genes[28,29].

Prospects

Proviral insertions are a rich source of mutations in tumor cells: mutations at known genes, showing how these genes are activated to become oncogenes, and mutations at unknown genes which can be uncovered because the provirus provides an easy starting point for molecular cloning.

The genes known to be activated by proviruses in tumors all act in a dominant way; undoubtedly a consequence of selection by investigators. Yet, there is growing evidence that many mutations in tumor cells are actually recessive. Finding recessive oncogenes is not an easy task; quite often they are mutated by large deletions in chromosomes and their precise location is unknown. Here, insertional mutagenesis by retroviruses may offer a valid approach to cloning. For example, one could attempt to culture cells from patients or experimental animals heterozygous for the gene of interest. Infection by an efficiently integrating retrovirus may cause the desired inactivation of the other allele of such a gene[30,31], and the emergence of the tumorigenic phenotype. This approach is complicated by the multitude of integrated viruses usually seen in virus-infected cells, but can nevertheless become feasible if adapted viruses are used that can easily be recovered as recombinant DNA[32].

A point that has to be considered in all of these experiments is the possibility that retroviral integration has a certain specificity for cellular sequences or chromatin structures. There are indications that insertion occurs more frequently in DNase hypersensitive sites[33], but there is clearly a need to examine this issue in more detail.

Acknowledgements

I thank David Greaves, Betsy Matthews and Anton Berns for comments on the manuscript, and Erica Spronk for secretarial assistance.

References

1 Varmus, H. E. (1984) *Annu. Rev. Genet.* 18, 553–612
2 Bishop, J. M. (1985) *Trends Genet.* 1, 245–249 (and this book, pp. 1–10)
3 Bingham, P. M., Levis, R. and Rubin, G. M. (1981) *Cell* 25, 693–704
4 Hayward, W. G., Neel, B. E. and Astrin, S. M. (1981) *Nature* 290, 475–480
5 Varmus, H. E. (1983) in *Mobile Genetic Elements* (Shapiro, J. A., ed.), pp. 411–503, Academic Press
6 Nusse, R. and Varmus, H. E. (1982) *Cell* 31, 99–109
7 Peters, G., Brookes, S., Smith, R. and Dickson, C. (1983) *Cell* 33, 369–377
8 Jakobowitz, A., Shackleford, G. M., Varmus, H. E. and Martin, G. R. *Proc. Natl Acad. Sci. USA* (in press)
9 Tsichlis, P. N., Strauss, P. G. and Hu, L. F. (1983) *Nature* 302, 445–449
10 Cuypers, H. T., Selten, G., Quint, W., Zijlstra, M., Maandag, E. R., Boelens, W., van Wezenbeek, P., Melief, C. and Berns, A. (1984) *Cell* 37, 141–150
11 Marth, J. D., Peet, R., Krebs, E. G. and Perlmutter, R. M. (1985) *Cell* 43, 393–404
12 Voronova, A. F. and Sefton, B. M. (1986) *Nature* 319, 682–685
13 Selten, G., Cuypers, H.Th., Boelens, W., Robanus-Maandag, E., Verbeek, J., Domen, J., Van Beveren, C. and Berns, A. *Cell* (in press)
14 Villeneuve, L., Rassart, E., Jolicoeur, P., Graham, M. and Adams, J. M. (1986) *Mol. Cell. Biol.* 6, 1834–1837
15 Nilsen, T. W., Maroney, P. A., Goodwin, R. G., Rottman, F., Crittenden, L., Raines, M. and Kung, H-J. (1985) *Cell* 41, 719–726
16 Sheng-Ong, G. L., Morse, H. C., Potter, M. and Mushinski, J. F. (1986) *Mol. Cell. Biol.* 6, 380–382
17 Chen, S. J., Holbrook, N. J., Mitchell, K. F., Vallone, C. A., Freengard, J. S., Crabtree, G. and Lin, Y. (1985) *Proc. Natl Acad. Sci. USA* 82, 7284–7288
18 Ymer, S., Tucker, W. Q. J., Sanderson, C. J., Hapel, A. J., Campbell, H. D. and Young, I. G. (1985) *Nature* 317, 255–258
19 Dejean, A., Bougueleret, L., Grzeschik, K-H. and Tiollais, P. (1986) *Nature* 322, 70–72
20 Kettmann, R., Deschamps, J., Couez, D., Claustriaux, J. J., Palm, R. and Burny, A. (1983) *J. Virol.* 47, 146–150
21 Fujisawa, J-I., Seiki, M., Kiyokawa, T. and Yoshida, M. (1985) *Proc. Natl Acad. Sci. USA* 82, 2277–2281
22 Cullen, B. R., Lomedico, P. T. and Ju, G. (1984) *Nature* 307, 241–254
23 Payne, G. S., Bishop, J. M. and Varmus, H. E. (1982) *Nature* 295, 209–213
24 Van Ooyen, A. and Nusse, R. (1984) *Cell* 39, 233–240
25 Moore, R., Casey, G., Brookes, S., Dixon, M., Peters, G. and Dickson, C. (1986) *EMBO J.* 5, 919–924
26 Miles, B. D. and Robinson, H. L. (1985) *J. Virol.* 54, 295–303
27 Neil, J. C., Hughes, D., McFarlane, R., Wilkie, N. M., Onions, D. E., Lees, G. and Jarrett, O. (1984) *Nature* 308, 814–820

28 Peters, G., Lee, A. E. and Dickson, C. (1986) *Nature* 309, 273–275
29 Cuypers, H.Th., Selten, G. C., Zijlstra, M., De Goede, R., Melief, C. and Berns, A. *J. Virol.* (in press)
30 Varmus, H. E., Quintrell, N. and Ortiz, S. (1981) *Cell* 25, 23–26
31 Jaenisch, R., Harbers, K., Schienke, A., Löhler, J., Chumakov, I., Jähner, D., Grotkopp, D. and Hoffmann, B. (1983) *Cell* 32, 209–216
32 Reik, W., Weiner, H. and Jaenisch, R. (1985) *Proc. Natl Acad. Sci. USA* 82, 1141–1145
33 Schubach, W. and Groudine, M. (1984) *Nature* 307, 702–708
34 Westaway, D., Papkoff, J., Mascovici, C. and Varmus, H. E. (1986) *EMBO J.* 5, 301–309

R. Nusse is at the Department of Molecular Biology, Netherlands Cancer Institute, Plesmanlaan 121, 1066 CX Amsterdam, The Netherlands.

Proto-oncogene *fos:* a multifaceted gene

Inder M. Verma

*Both v-*fos *and c-*fos *proteins, despite their altered carboxyl terminus, are nuclear and can transform fibroblasts in vitro. The c-*fos *gene is highly inducible and is expressed during development, differentiation and growth. Expression of c-*fos *protein exhibits complex regulation involving interaction with 3' non-coding sequences of c-*fos *RNA.*

A turning point in cancer research has been the realization that normal cellular genes have the potential to induce neoplasia. Such genes are now collectively called proto-oncogenes, a term rapidly gaining wide acceptance among cancer biologists[1,2]. Oncogenes were first discovered through the agency of retroviruses, which by far are the richest source of potent carcinogens[3], and over the last few years it has been firmly established that the transforming genes of retroviruses have been acquired from the genomes of normal cells[4,5]. The search for proto-oncogenes has widened with the very successful approach of using DNA transfection[6,7]; to date, nearly two dozen proto-oncogenes have been identified and the list is growing[3]. It seems a miracle that a cell remains normal in the face of such potential adversity. Why has the cell in its evolutionary wisdom not lost such potentially-lethal genes? The answer to these contradictions lies in delineating the role of proto-oncogenes in normal cellular metabolic processes.

In this review, I describe the salient features of the multifaceted proto-oncogene c-*fos*, which is expressed during cell growth, cell differentiation and development[8]. The viral homologue, v-*fos*, was identified as the resident transforming gene of FBJ-murine osteosarcoma virus which induces bone tumors in mice[14].

Molecular architecture of the *fos* gene

Elucidation of the complete molecular structure of the *fos* gene preceded knowledge of its expression in a variety of cell types. This was propitious because it is essential to know its detailed genomic organization in order to grasp the subtle and complex regulation of its expression. To date, two retroviruses containing the *fos* oncogene have been identified, namely FBJ-murine sarcoma virus (FBJ-MSV) and FBR-MSV (Refs 9 and 10). The complete nucleotide sequences of their proviral DNAs have been deduced[11]. In addition, the nucleotide sequence of the cellular progenitor of the *fos* gene from mouse and human cells has also been determined[11,12]. Figure 1 illustrates the organization of viral and cellular *fos* genes and their deduced products. The major features can be summarized as follows.

FBJ-MSV

(1) FBJ-MSV proviral DNA contains 4026 nucleotides, including two long terminal repeats (LTRs) of 617 nucleotides each, 1639 nucleotides of acquired cellular sequences (v-*fos*), and a portion of the envelope (*env*) gene. (2) Both

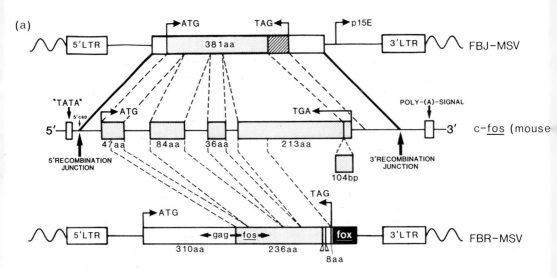

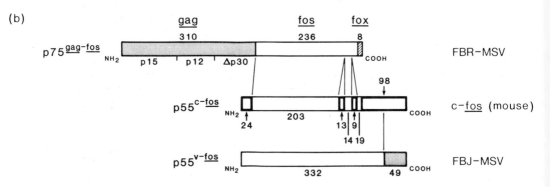

Fig. 1. *(a) Molecular architecture of FBJ-MSV (top) and FBR-MSV (bottom) proviral DNAs and the c-fos gene (middle). Top: the large open box indicates the acquired cellular sequences; solid, vertical bars indicate the initiation and termination codons of v-fos proteins; the stippled region indicates the carboxy-terminal 49 amino acids of the v-fos protein encoded in a different reading frame due to deletion of 104 bp of the c-fos sequence. Middle: the stippled boxes are the exons; the number of amino acids encoded by each exon is given; the 104 bp sequence that has been deleted in the v-fos sequence is indicated with a box below line; unlike the v-fos protein, the c-fos protein terminates at a TGA codon. Bottom: broken lines indicate the portions of the exon acquired from the c-fos gene; small, open triangles indicate deletion from FBR-MSV as compared with the c-fos gene; details of the structure of FBR-MSV proviral DNA have previously been described[16]. (b) A schematic comparison of p75^{gag-fos} (top), p55^{c-fos} (middle) and p55^{v-fos} (bottom) proteins. In p75 the gag- encoded portion is indicated with a stippled box, and that encoded by v-fos is shown by the hatched box. The region of p55^{c-fos} indicated by thickened boxes and vertical arrows are those portions deleted in p75^{gag-fos}. The hatched region in p55^{v-fos} is the carboxyl-terminal portion, which differs from that of p55^{c-fos}. The numbers refer to the number of amino acids encoded by each region.*

the initiation and termination codons of the v-*fos* protein are within the acquired sequences that encode a protein of 381 amino acids, having a molecular weight of 49 601. (3) In cells transformed by FBJ-MSV, a phosphoprotein with an apparent M_r of 55 000 (p55) on SDS polyacrylamide gel electrophoresis (SDS-PAGE) has been identified as the transforming protein. The discrepancy between the observed size and the size predicted by sequence analysis is probably due to the unusual amino acid composition of the *fos* protein (10% proline), since the v-*fos* protein expressed in bacteria has a similar mobility on SDS-PAGE[13].

Proto-oncogene fos

(1) The sequences in the c-*fos* gene that are homologous to those in the v-*fos* gene are interrupted by four regions of non-homology, three of which represent bona fide introns. (2) The fourth region (104 nucleotides), which is present in both mouse and human c-*fos* genes, represents sequences that have been deleted during the biogenesis of the v-*fos* gene. (3) The c-*fos* protein has 380 amino acids, which is remarkably similar to the size of the v-*fos* protein (381 amino acids) (the additional 104 nucleotides in the c-*fos* gene transcripts do not increase the predicted size of the c-*fos* proteins, because of a switch to a different reading frame). (4) In the first 332 amino acids, the v-*fos* and mouse c-*fos* proteins differ at only five residues, while the remaining 48 amino acids of the c-*fos* protein are encoded in a different reading frame from that in the v-*fos* protein. Thus the v-*fos* and c-*fos* proteins, though largely similar, have different carboxyl termini (Fig. 1b). (5) Despite their different carboxyl termini, both the v-*fos* and c-*fos* proteins are located in the nucleus. The c-*fos* protein undergoes more extensive post-translational modifications than the v-*fos* protein[14]. (6) The mouse and human c-*fos* genes share greater than 90% sequence homology, differing only in 24 residues out of a total of 380.

FBR-MSV

(1) The proviral DNA of FBR-MSV contains 3791 nucleotides (specifying a genome of 3284 bases) and encodes a single *gag–fos* fusion product of 554 amino acids[15,16]. (2) The *fos* portion of the gene lacks sequences that encode the first 24 and the last 98 amino acids of the 380 amino acid mouse c-*fos* gene product (Fig. 1b). In addition, the coding region has sustained three small in-frame deletions, one in the p30*gag* portion and two in the *fos* region. (3) The gene product terminates in sequences termed *fox* (Fig. 1a), which are present in normal mouse DNA at loci unrelated to the c-*fos* gene. The c-*fox* gene(s) is expressed as an abundant class of poly(A) RNA in mouse tissue[16].

Transformation by *fos* proteins

Both the viral and cellular *fos* proteins, despite their different carboxyl termini, can transform fibroblasts *in vitro*[17]. However, c-*fos*, upon transfection, can induce transformation only after undergoing two manipulations: (1) addition of viral LTR sequences, presumably to enhance transcription; and (2) more importantly, removal of sequences from the 3' noncoding region of the c-*fos* gene[17]. A stretch of 67 nucleotides, located 627–693 base pairs downstream of the coding domain and 123–189 base pairs upstream from the putative poly(A) addition site has been identified, removal of which confers transforming activity[18]. Alternatively, transformation by the c-*fos* gene can be accomplished if the carboxyl terminus of the coding domain is altered. Cells transfected with the c-*fos* gene actively transcribe *fos*-specific mRNA but little or no c-*fos* protein is detectable[17]. When the transcription of the c-*fos* gene is induced in a variety of cell types with a variety of agents, the c-*fos* protein is synthesized transiently[19]. For cellular transformation, a sustained synthesis of the c-*fos* protein is obligatory. We suggest that that c-*fos* protein may regulate its synthesis, perhaps by interaction with the 67 base pair region and/or the carboxy-terminal coding sequences. Because of the 104 base pair in-frame deletion during the biogenesis of the v-*fos* gene, the v-*fos* protein has an altered carboxyl terminus and thus escapes interaction with the *fos* protein. Consequently v-*fos* protein is synthesized constitutively and hence induces transformation.

Though both the p55^{fos} of FBJ-MSV and the p75$^{gag-fos}$ of FBR-MSV can induce morphological transformation, the latter has more pronounced transforming potential (Ref. 20 and R. Graham, pers. commun.). Although the p75$^{gag-fos}$ is a fusion protein the *gag* moiety does not appear to have any influence on its transforming ability[21]. The *fos* moiety has several alterations, as compared to p55^{v-fos} protein, which may be responsible for its enhanced transforming potential. Unfortunately, no transformation-defective mutants of *fos* genes are as yet available to allow complete analysis of the contribution of the various domains of the *fos* protein toward cellular transformation.

fos is a highly inducible gene

A remarkable property of the *fos* gene is its rapid induction in response to mitogens or differentiation-specific agents. Within minutes of the addition of an inducer, c-*fos* specific transcripts can be observed. Often the induction is transient and generally precedes the induction of proto-oncogene *myc*, another nuclear protein. Table 1 summarizes a number of biological systems where the induction of the c-*fos* gene has been reported. I would like to discuss the induction of c-*fos* gene during differentiation of monomyelocytic cells to mature macrophages, because it is the only system where the c-*fos* gene is constitutively turned on[22-24]. Furthermore, no c-*fos* gene is induced when the monomyelocytic cells differentiate to granulocytes, thus indicating a lineage specificity of the *fos* induction[23,24]. Upon addition of either TPA or vitamin D_3 to either U937 (a promonocytic cell line) or HL-60 (monomyelocytic cell line), the c-*fos* gene is expressed within 1–3 minutes with maximal levels of induction observed by 30 minutes. The levels of c-*fos* transcription decline to 20– 25% where they remain essentially unchanged for at least 10 days, by which time over 99% of the viable cells in the culture are fully adherent. Detection of c-*fos* transcripts cannot be due solely to their enhanced stability because the c-*fos* gene is actively transcribed. In contrast, c-*fos* protein is expressed for only 120 minutes, with maximal levels by around 60 minutes[23]. This observation lends further credence to the notion that *fos* protein may regulate its own synthesis.

Is *fos* protein required for myeloid differentiation? Direct evidence is lacking, but two sets of experiments indicate expression of the *fos* gene is neither sufficient nor essential for macrophage differentiation: serum stimulated U-937 cells exhibit *fos* expression without differentiation to macrophages; and variants of HL-60 which are resistant to TPA can be induced to differentiate with vitamin D_3 without expression of the *fos* gene (R. Mitchell and E. Huberman, pers. commun.). A definitive answer to the question of c-*fos* protein involvement in myeloid differentiation will have to await experiments where the synthesis of c-*fos* is selectively blocked or can be

Table 1. Induction of proto-oncogene fos

---

c-*fos* Induction

(1) Promonocyte/monomyelocyte $\xrightarrow[\text{Vitamin D}_3]{\text{TPA}}$ Macrophages

(2) PC12 $\xrightarrow[\text{cAMP, K}^+]{\text{NGF}}$ Neurites

(3) Partial hepatectomy
(4) Spleen cells stimulated with ConA or LPS
(5) Resting BALB/c or NIH 3T3 cells stimulated with PDGF, serum or TPA
(6) Hepatocytes stimulated with growth factors
(7) A431 + EGF

No c-*fos* induction

(1) Monomyelocyte $\xrightarrow{\text{DMSO}}$ granulocytes

(2) PC12 $\xrightarrow{\text{DEX}}$ chromaffin cells

---

constitutively turned on without the addition of inducing agents.

When most quiescent fibroblasts are treated with serum or growth factors like PDGF, EGF or TPA, c-*fos* is induced within 2–3 minutes[25–28]. Maximal levels of induction (over 20-fold) occur within 20 minutes, and decline by 60 minutes with no c-*fos* transcripts detected by 240 minutes. Addition of cycloheximide resulted not only in a 50-fold induction but the c-*fos* transcripts could be detected for considerably longer periods. Since no *de novo* transcription of c-*fos* could be detected, we presume this phenomenon to be largely due to stabilization of c-*fos* mRNA transcripts. Similar observations and conclusions have previously been proposed for proto-oncogene *myc* (Ref. 29). Several modified forms of c-*fos* protein were identified and maximal synthesis was observed with PDGF concentrations that saturate PDGF binding sites at 37°C (1 mM). Despite the similarities of rapid and transient c-*fos* induction, there is one major distinction in the *fos* gene expression in resting cells and differentiating monomyelocytic cells. No c-*fos* transcripts are observed by 240 minutes in stimulated fibroblasts while the c-*fos* RNA can be observed for 10 days during monocytic differentiation. It would thus appear that the transcriptional unit of the c-*fos* gene has different regulation in the two systems.

Regulation of c-*fos* transcription

Recent analysis of the c-*fos* promoter has identified the nature of the transcriptional enhancer and the inducible sequences[30,31]. An element essential for transcriptional activation and inducibility in response to serum is located between nucleotides −332 and −276, relative to the 5′ cap site I. However, when this sequence is linked to an heterologous promoter, the extent of induction with either serum or TPA is only 3- to 5-fold. Furthermore, the transcripts are more stable with increased constitutive levels. By making fusion genes between human c-*fos* and β-globin it has been shown that in addition to the 5′ activating element, transient accumulation of c-*fos* RNA following induction with serum also requires sequences at the 3′ end of the c-*fos* gene[30]. The precise nature of these sequences remains unknown but they are located downstream of the 3′ coding domain and include the interacting 67-nucleotide sequence discussed above. Two other points are worth noting:

(1) the 5' upstream sequences essential for transcriptional activation are conserved between human and mouse c-*fos* genes; these sequences also contain one of the two DNase I hypersensitive sites, and (2) the variety of cell types where *fos* gene expression can be induced show that, as expected, the *fos* enhancer is not tissue-specific[31].

Regulation of *fos* expression

The gene is versatile; the gene product may play a role during development, cellular differentiation and cell growth. Since the c-*fos* protein can induce transformation of at least fibroblasts *in vitro*, it is puzzling that cells expressing *fos* genes in response to inducers do not succumb to transformation[19]. It is possible that some cell types, such as peritoneal macrophages or macrophages in culture, are refractory to transformation by *fos* proteins. Perhaps fibroblasts and other cells susceptible to transformation by c-*fos* protein are not transformed because the expression of the *fos* protein is transient[21]. The synthesis of the *fos* gene product may be regulated post-transcriptionally or even more likely, at the translational level. As mentioned before, c-*fos* can induce cellular transformation if an AT-rich stretch of 67 base pairs located downstream of the termination codon is removed. We have no firm idea of the manner in which the 67 base pair sequences influence the synthesis of the c-*fos* protein, but it could either affect the stability of the mRNA or alter the translational efficiency of the c-*fos* mRNA. Little or no c-*fos* protein is detected in cells transfected with *fos* recombinant DNA constructs containing the 67 base pairs. Promonocytic or monomyelocytic cell lines induced to differentiate into macrophages continue to express *fos* mRNA for at least 10 days, but the *fos* protein is detected only for up to 120 minutes following induction. It is possible that the *fos* antiserum is unable to detect *fos* proteins because they are extensively modified. It is also difficult to comprehend how a protein found exclusively in the nucleus can influence translation. Apparently post-transcriptional or translational control of the expression of *fos* gene product is abrogated in mouse amnion cells where both the RNA and protein can be detected during prenatal development[8,14]. Regardless of the molecular mechanism influencing *fos* expression, we believe that the natural expression of the c-*fos* protein does not transform cells because it is synthesized only transiently. In contrast, the v-*fos* gene escapes this regulation, due to an altered carboxyl terminus, and its sustained synthesis leads to cellular transformation.

Delineation of the function of the *fos* protein is a top priority for researchers in the field and elucidation of the molecular mechanism by which non-coding sequences influence the transforming potential of the c-*fos* gene remains a challenge. Why does *fos* protein cause only bone tumors? Are rearrangements or chromosomal translocation of the *fos* gene involved in any human tumors? With such marvellous prospects, no wonder *fos* gene will continue to generate excitement.

References
1 Bishop, J. M. (1983) *Annu. Rev. Biochem.* 52, 301–54
2 Hunter, T. (1984) *Sci. Am.* 251, 70–79
3 Bishop, J. M. (1985) *Trends Genet.* 1, 245–249 (and this book, pp. 1–10)
4 Bishop, J. M. (1985) *Cell* 42, 22–38
5 Van Beveren, C. and Verma, I. M. (1985) *Curr. Top. Microbiol. Immunol.* 123, 73–98
6 Cooper, G. M. (1982) *Science* 217, 801–806

7   Weinberg, R. A. (1983) *Sci. Am.* 249, 126–142
8   Müller, R. and Verma, I. M. (1984) *Curr. Top. Microbiol. Immunol.* 112, 73–115
9   Finkel, M. P., Biskis, B. O. and Jinkins, P. B. (1966) *Science* 151, 698–701
10 Finkel, M. P., Reilly, C. A. Jr, Biskis, B. O. and Green, I. L. (1973) *Colston Res. Soc. Proc. Symp.* 24, 353–363
11 Van Beveren, C., van Straaten, F., Curran, T., Müller, R. and Verma, I. M. (1983) *Cell* 32, 1241–1255
12 Van Straaten, F., Müller, R., Curran, T., Van Beveren, C. and Verma, I. M. (1983) *Proc. Natl Acad. Sci. USA* 80, 3183–3187
13 MacConnell, W. P. and Verma, I. M. (1983) *Virology* 131, 367–372
14 Curran, T., Miller, A. D., Zokas, L. and Verma, I. M. (1984) *Cell* 36, 259–268
15 Curran, T. and Verma, I. M. (1984) *Virology* 135, 218–228
16 Van Beveren, C., Enami, S., Curran, T. and Verma, I. M. (1984) *Virology* 135, 229–243
17 Miller, A. D., Curran, T. and Verma, I. M. (1984) *Cell* 36, 51–60
18 Meijlink, F., Curran, T., Miller, A. D. and Verma, I. M. (1985) *Proc. Natl Acad. Sci. USA* 82, 4987–4991
19 Verma, I. M., Mitchell, R. L., Kruijer, W., Van Beveren, C., Zokas, L., Hunter, T. and Cooper, J. A. (1985) in *Cancer Cells. Vol. 3, Growth Factors and Transformation,* pp. 275–287, Cold Spring Harbor Laboratory
20 Jenuwein, T., Müller, D., Curran, T. and Müller, R. (1985) *Cell* 41, 629–637
21 Miller, A. D., Verma, I. M. and Curran, T. (1985) *J. Virol.* 55, 521–526
22 Gonda, T. J. and Metcalf, D. (1984) *Nature* 310, 249–251
23 Mitchell, R. L., Zokas, L., Schreiber, R. D. and Verma, I. M. (1985) *Cell* 40, 209–217
24 Müller, R., Curran, T., Müller, D. and Guilbert, L. (1985) *Nature* 314, 546–548
25 Greenberg, M. W. and Ziff, E. B. (1984) *Nature* 311, 433–438
26 Kruijer, W., Cooper, J. A., Hunter, T. and Verma, I. M. (1984) *Nature* 312, 711–716
27 Müller, R., Bravo, R., Burchhardt, J. and Curran, T. (1984) *Nature* 312, 716–720
28 Bravo, R., Burckhardt, J., Curran, T. and Müller, R. (1985) *EMBO J.* 4, 1193–1198
29 Kelly, K., Cochran, B. H., Stiles, C. D. and Leder, P. (1983) *Cell* 35, 603–610
30 Treisman, R. (1985) *Cell* 42, 889–902
31 Deschamps, J., Meijlink, F. and Verma, I. M. (1985) *Science* 230, 1174–1177

I. M. Verma is at Molecular Biology and Virology Laboratory, The Salk Institute, PO Box 85800, San Diego, CA 92138, USA.

Normal and activated *ras* oncogenes and their encoded products

Arthur D. Levinson

Cellular ras *genes, first identified as progenitors of the transforming genes of certain oncogenic retroviruses, have been implicated in the development of human tumors. Genes with remarkable homology to* ras *have been found throughout the plant and animal kingdom; emerging evidence suggests roles for the encoded polypeptides in the control of normal growth.*

There is compelling evidence that human cancer develops as a consequence of genetic damage. Initial suggestions were provided by epidemiologial studies indicating a relationship between tumor incidence and exposure to environmental carcinogens known for their mutagenic properties, and findings that most malignancies are characterized by the presence of cytogenic abnormalities[1]. Recently, support came in a stunning fashion with the demonstration that DNA prepared from a variety of tumors, but not normal tissues, possessed the ability to malignantly transform non-tumorigenic NIH3T3 mouse fibroblast cells when introduced by transfection techniques[2], a result establishing that discrete transforming sequences exist within the genome of at least some tumor types. Based on the ease with which transformed cells can be selected from their non-transformed counterparts, a number of novel strategies were devised whereby those genes specifically associated with the oncogenic potential of tumor cell DNA could be isolated. Strikingly, the transforming genes molecularly cloned in this fashion were often found to belong to a family of cellular genes which had first been identified on the basis of homology with the previously characterized genes (oncogenes) responsible in the *in vivo* tumorigenic activity of Harvey (Ha-*ras*) and Kirsten (Ki-*ras*) rat sarcoma viruses[2,3]. A third member of this family (N-*ras*) has never been found as a biologically active component of an acutely transforming retrovirus; it was discovered as the active transforming gene within the genome of a human neuroblastoma cell line[2,3].

Structure and activation of cellular *ras* genes

Molecular hybridization techniques provided much evidence that the molecular alterations empowering *ras* genes with tumorigenic potential consisted of changes of relatively small physical proportions. Analysis of *in vitro* recombination of wild type and mutant *ras* genes and comparative sequence analysis led to the startling demonstration that a single nucleotide substitution and concomitant amino acid change within the encoded Ha-*ras* protein represented the genetic alteration accounting for the transforming potential of DNA associated with a particular bladder carcinoma[2]. These findings stimulated efforts to define the molecular organization of the entire *ras* gene family. As a result, we know that the family shares properties beyond the common sequences that serve to define it: each of the three genes possesses four coding exons, interrupted by intervening sequences located at identical positions, which conspire to encode proteins of 188–189 amino acids[2]. Only the Ki-*ras* gene provides a modest variation on this basic theme; two versions of the fourth coding exon exist which, due to their differential utilization via alternating splicing pathways, enable the locus to encode two distinct, but closely related polypeptides[2]. The *ras* proteins are closely homologous to their viral counterparts, and differ from one another markedly only near their carboxyl termini (see Fig. 1). These and other experiments have provided compelling evidence that activated cellular *ras* genes, as defined by transfection experiments, develop by a mutational process: in all such cases to date the oncogene differs from its normal counterpart by a single critical nucleotide, always within a portion of the *ras* gene encoding p21, a 21 kDa phosphoprotein. From an analysis of a large number of such activated genes derived from tumors, it was found that changes at residues 12, 13 or 61 can activate the transforming potential of p21. By analysing randomly mutated *ras* genes, it was also demonstrated that amino acid substitution at residues 59 and 63 can activate p21 as determined by the transformation of NIH3T3 cells[4]; whether these particular changes activate p21 *in vivo* remains to be seen. Activation of p21 by alterations affecting position 12 have been studied most thoroughly. From an analysis of the transforming potential of 20 different Ha-*ras* genes, each encoding a different amino acid at this position, it was determined[5] that only a single amino acid (proline) other than that normally present (glycine) fails to activate p21 (Ref. 5). As both proline and glycine residues have an exceptional tendency to break α-helical backbones of polypeptide chains, these results raise the possibility that the activation of p21 involves the acquisition of an inappropriate function resulting from a conformation involving a continuous α-helix within this N-terminal domain.

While the vast majority of reports have indicated that *ras* genes become activated by a mutational process, this may to some extent reflect a bias of the transfection assay routinely employed to detect such events. Thus, any involvement of *ras* in tumor development due to overexpression resulting (for example) from gene amplification or epigenetic mechanisms might escape detection by conventional transfection analyses. This caveat is inspired by two considerations. First, by analogy with other proto-oncogenes where quantitative, not qualitative, changes in expression can apparently affect the course of tumor development[6]. Second, and more directly, by the demonstration that cellular p21, if sufficiently overexpressed, can promote the morphological and tumorigenic transformation of NIH3T3 cells[7]. There is some evidence that overexpression of normal *ras* genes can play a role in tumor development *in vivo*; significant amplification of the Ki-*ras* gene has been observed in cell lines derived from tumors[6], although in at least one such instance these amplified copies contain alterations known to be of an activating type.

ras proteins

Facilitated by the development of antisera from rats bearing tumors induced by transplantation of Ha-MuSV transformed cells, the product of the viral Ha-*ras* gene was identified as p21 by Ed Scolnick and colleagues[8,9] in 1979. Briefly, other key discoveries by this same research group prominently shaped the course of subsequent efforts. Viral p21 was found to possess an associated

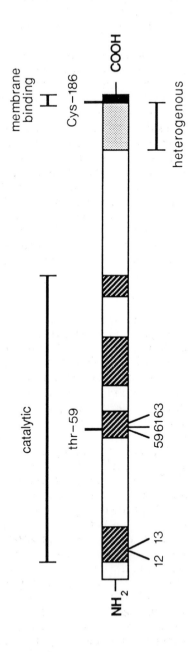

Fig. 1. *Scheme of p21. Depicted are the proposed catalytic and membrane binding domains, the heterogenous region which varies markedly between the different p21s (dotted), and the four regions within the catalytic domain (hatched) that display significant homology with other GTP binding proteins (see text). Also highlighted are the two residues subject to post-translational modification [Thr59 (some viral p21s) and Cys186] and Cys186] and the five residues (12,13,59,61,63) at which amino acid substitutions can activate the transforming potential of the polypeptide.*

guanine nucleotide binding activity and be capable of autophosphorylation using GTP as the phosphoryl donor molecule; and to reside at the inner surface of the plasma membrane as determined by immunocytochemical and physical methods[8]. The ability of p21 to bind guanine nucleotides can now be rationalized on structural grounds by virtue of its homology with a broad spectrum of otherwise unrelated GTP binding proteins from organisms as distant as *E. coli*[10,11] (see Fig. 1).

Ras proteins are subject to two potential forms of post-translational modification. After synthesis on free polysomes in the cytoplasm, p21 becomes acylated at what is believed to be Cys186, an event probably coincident with its translocation to the plasma membrane[9]. The importance of this modification can be inferred from studies using a mutated *ras* gene that encodes a protein with a different amino acid at this position: such a protein fails to attach to the membrane and is unable to transform cells[9]. The other form of post-translational processing exhibited by certain versions of viral p21 is the phosphorylation of Thr59 (Ref. 8), believed to result from the aforementioned autophosphorylating activity (Fig. 1). The failure of either normal or activated cellular forms of p21 to manifest this activity is adequately explained by the absence of this phosphoacceptor residue[12]. While one must therefore conclude that the autokinase activity is not essential for the tumorigenic potential of p21, it should also be noted that the acquisition of this phosphoacceptor site in otherwise normal p21, which unmasks this activity[12], increases the oncogenic potential of p21 (Ref. 4).

Regulation of p21

Although the function of p21 was not revealed by the identification of these properties, the similarities between p21 and a class of plasma membrane-associated polypeptides known collectively as G (or N) proteins did not go unnoticed[13]. Such G proteins are involved in signal transduction across the membrane, and are so designated to reflect their mode of regulation, which involves the binding of guanine(G) nucleotides. Their immediate function is exerted in response to the binding of GTP, an event triggered by the arrival of an appropriate signal at an associated cell surface receptor; an intrinsic GTPase is responsible for the transient nature of this activation[14]. Stimulated by the knowledge that G and *ras* proteins display common properties, combined with emerging indications of stuctural homologies[14], efforts to detect an intrinsic GTPase activity associated with p21 were initiated. Facilitated by the assembly of vectors that efficiently directed the synthesis of p21 in *E. coli*, such a GTPase activity was detected in highly purified preparations of p21 (Refs 12, 15 and 16). Suggestions that this hydrolytic activity plays a critical role in the oncogenic activation of the polypeptide came from demonstrations that an activating amino acid substitution at position 12 causes a 5- to 10-fold decrease in this GTPase activity[12,15,16]. These suggestions were supported by findings that activating mutations at positions 59 and 61 also significantly impair the p21 GTPase activity[9], and the observation that a non-activating proline substitution at position 12 actually stimulates the rate of GTP hydrolysis[17]. That an impairment of its hydrolytic activity can apparently activate p21 can be contrasted with findings that no other known property of p21, including affinity for guanine nucleotides, subcellular localization, biological half-life and capacity for autophosphorylation[9], is consistently affected by activating lesions. Taken together, these results support the notion that p21 is regulated in a manner reminiscent of G proteins, whose activity is markedly increased by agents that prevent GTP hydrolysis (Fig. 2). Whether or not the activity of p21 is likewise modulated by a dissociable subunit whose effects are exerted in a negative fashion is conjectural at present; if so, however, it follows that overexpression of p21 would result in a shift of its steady state distribution in favor of the activated species, conceivably explaining observations that cellular transformation can be promoted by normal p21 if present in sufficiently large quantities.

It remains to be determined if all structural changes that lead to a p21 with transforming ability involve an impaired GTPase function. This appears to be true for a range of substitutions involving positions 12 (Ref. 17) or 61 (Ref. 18), although non-activating substitutions at position-61 also can reduce GTPase activity[18]. Thus, while the activation of p21 may inevitably involve an impairment of GTPase function, it appears that activation is not mandated by this deficiency. It is noteworthy that while all activated p21s resulting from substitutions at positions 12 and 61 exhibit an impaired GTPase function, in neither case is there an absolute correlation between the extent of reduction in GTPase activity and the degree to which the transforming potential of the polypeptide becomes activated[17,18], attesting to the importance of properties other than that of GTP hydrolysis in this process.

Role of *ras* activations during tumor development

Although the notion that the activation of the proto-oncongenes plays a direct role in the development of cancer continues to be questioned[19], one cannot easily dismiss the overwhelming body of evidence indicating that the

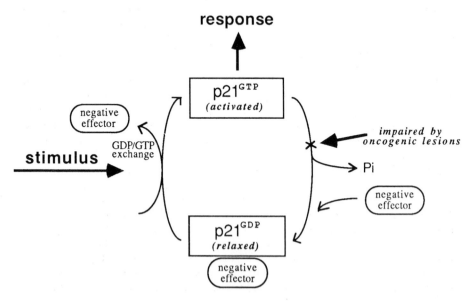

Fig. 2. *Model of p21 regulation showing the alternating relaxed and activated states of the protein, the distribution of which is in part controlled by the intrinsic rate of GTP hydrolysis. Also portrayed, by analogy with other G proteins (see text), is a putative effector that negatively regulates the activity of p21 by binding preferentially to the relaxed form.*

alterations of *ras* genes, which empower them with oncogenic potential *in vitro*, result from somatic mutations acquired during oncogenesis. In mice and rats bearing chemically induced tumors, the *ras* mutation is specific for tumor tissue; normal cells do not contain the mutation[2]. There is still some controversy as to whether *ras* mutations represent an early or late event in the development of a tumor; compelling evidence on behalf of both positions has been presented. For example, dominant transforming *ras* genes have been detected in late, but not early, passage levels of carcinogen-treated cells[2]. However, *ras* activation can also occur early in tumor development, as illustrated in the mouse skin model of chemical carcinogenesis. The DNA in transplantable mouse skin carcinomas induced by chemical carcinogens often contains an activated Ha-*ras* gene. This tumor progresses through several identifiable stages before it becomes a malignant carcinoma; the finding that a pre-malignant primary papilloma precursor also harbors the lesion[20] supports this alternative view. Similar conclusions were reached by Barbacid and co-workers, who found that a single exposure of rats to a carcinogen leads to the efficient development of mammary carcinomas within 6–12 months, the majority of which display an activated Ha-*ras* gene[21]. Since the biological half-life of the carcinogen is measured in hours, one may infer that the malignant activation of Ha-*ras* in these cases must have been an early event concomitant with the initiation of carcinogenesis.

Findings that *ras* activation can occur either early or late in tumor development can be reconciled within the context of epidemiological and experimental evidence that carcinogenesis is a multistep process probably involving the concerted action of several genes. The experimental underpinnings of this proposal stem from early work with DNA tumor viruses, in which the combined action of two or more genes was shown to be required for full elaboration of the phenotypes associated with cellular transformation[22]. These results were placed within the context of transformation by cellular oncogenes with the demonstration that the neoplastic conversion of primary rodent cells, unlike continuous cell lines, generally required the collaboration of two oncogenes[23,24]. Why might the susceptibility of different cells (e.g. primary vs continuous) to transformation by oncogenes be so dissimilar? One interpretation is that established cells are unusual in that they have previously acquired the capacity to propagate indefinitely, almost certainly the result of additional premalignant genetic alterations whose nature is presently unclear. Such alterations, it can be argued, are providing the function of certain activated oncogenes normally required for transformation of normal (i.e. primary) cells. Seen in this manner, tumor development proceeds in stages through the acquisition of discrete genetic aberrations. Although it is unclear what selective advantages might be conferred upon a particular premalignant population as a result of any individual change, the combined effects of presumably independent mutations may inevitably manifest themselves in disordered cellular growth. As such, the precise order in which a *ras* gene (or other cellular proto-oncogene) becomes activated may in some instances be of little consequence to the course of tumor development.

ras genes in lower organisms

In view of the difficulty of assigning a molecular role for p21, great excitement attended the discovery that genes with remarkable homology to *ras* are widely distributed throughout the plant and animal kingdom. These genes have been identified and characterized in such organisms as *Drosophila melanogaster, Dictyostelium, Aplysia* and *Saccharomyces cerevisiae* (Fig. 3). Fueled by an anticipation that the striking structural similarities implied a functional conservation, efforts to identify the role of these gene products in yeast by a combined genetic and biochemical approach were initiated. These revealed much about the two encoded *ras*-like proteins: the N-terminal 164 amino acids of each are 70% homologous to the mammalian protein; they bind and hydrolyse GTP, and they are essential for yeast proliferation[9]. At least some functions of *ras* proteins have been conserved over this evolutionary distance as evidenced by demonstrations that: (1) the human protein can complement yeast strains lacking RAS genes; (2) the yeast RAS2 gene product can, in a derivative form, transform mammalian cells; and (3) the GTPase activity of the yeast proteins is impaired by mutations analogous to those present in the oncogenic mammalian *ras* variants[8,9]. These findings laid the groundwork for the demonstration by Michael Wigler and his colleagues that the similarities between yeast *ras* and G proteins extend beyond structural and biochemical considerations. They found that the yeast *ras* protein can function as a GTP-dependent positive regulator of adenylate cyclase[26], leading to suggestions that mammalian p21 may function in a similiar manner. Subsequent studies indicated that the expression of human p21 in yeast similarity elevates adenylate cyclase activity[27]. Yet recent observations cast a measure of doubt on these speculations: adenylate cyclase activity in membranes derived from either normal mammalian cells, or cells transformed by v-Ha-*ras*, is unaffected by the addition of even vast quantities of purified p21 (Ref. 28). Nor does purified p21 display any potential to interact with the purified components of the G-d2s protein complex (A. Gilman, pers. commun.). While hopes that a resolution of yeast *ras* function might quickly reveal fundamental insights into the mechanism by which activated mammalian *ras* proteins transform cells have been temporarily frustrated, the identification of novel gene products that interact with yeast *ras* proteins will undoubtedly provide a wealth of reagents which may yet facilitate efforts to identify the targets of mammalian *ras* proteins.

Prospects

Despite the tremendous advances in our understanding of the structure of activated *ras* oncogenes and their involvement in tumor development, there are but the merest hints to suggest in what manner the encoded proteins act. There are suspicions that *ras* polypeptides may be involved in a pathway by which growth factors affect cellular proliferation and differentiation, not by mimicking growth factors or their receptors, but as coupling proteins that act as signal transducers in the transfer of information from cell surface receptors to intracellular targets. For the most part, this notion derives from a reluctance to accept the resemblances between p21 and other signal transducers as merely coincidental. If mammalian *ras* proteins are indeed involved in signal transduction across the plasma membrane, ascertaining the nature of the linkage between the particular cell surface receptor involved and downstream effector function will clearly be of immense importance. Since there are four known p21-*ras* proteins (one encoded by Ha-*ras*, one by N-*ras* and two by Ki-*ras*), each with distinctive C-termini, there exists the daunting possibility that while all might serve a common effector (e.g. adenylate cyclase, a cyclic nucleotide phosphodiesterase, phospholipase C), each might couple to a distinct receptor.

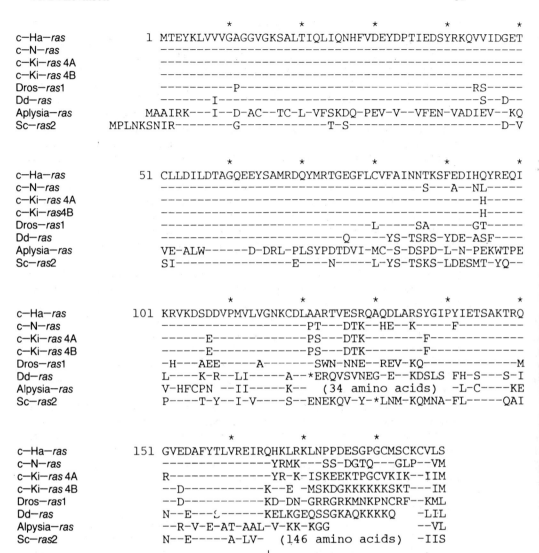

Fig. 3. *Deduced amino acid sequences of various* ras *and* ras-*like genes from human (c-Ha-*ras, *c-N-*ras *c-Ki-*ras4A, *and c-Ki-*ras4B), Drosophila melanogaster *(Dros-rasl)*, Dictyostelium discoideum (Dd-ras), Aplysia (Aplysia-ras) *and Saccharomyces cerevisiae (Sc-ras2). The original literature citations can be found in elsewhere*[3,9,25]. *Dashes represent exact correspondence with the prototype sequence (c-Ha-ras), asterisks within the sequence depict the presence of two amino acids, and blank spaces indicate the absence of corresponding residues.*

There is growing evidence that *ras* gene products function by affecting the cell cycle. Microinjected p21 will induce maturation in *Xenopus* oocytes, an event involving a release from prophase arrest[34], while endogenous p21 appears to be required for the initiation of S-phase in NIH3T3 mouse cells[29]. There is also accumulating evidence that *ras* genes can either block or promote the differentiation of various cell types *in vitro*. Perhaps most strikingly, activated p21 can mimic the effects of nerve growth factor on a rat phaeochromaocytoma cell line[30,31]; such cells cease dividing and display phenotypes considered hallmarks of differentiated sympathetic neurones. There are indications that at least some of these effects are mediated by growth factors. These are based on findings that *ras*-transformed cells can secrete highly elevated amounts of a polypeptide known as transforming growth factor α[32], and from studies in which the introduction of activated *ras* genes into estrogen-dependent human breast cancer cells renders them hormone-independent for tumor formation[33]. While the molecular basis of these effects is not known, there are suggestions that alterations in the levels of intermediates in the phosphotidylinositol turnover cycle, promoted by p21, may play a role[35].

Although our knowledge of the structure and biochemistry of the *ras* gene products is substantial, it should be apparent from even these isolated examples that we can acknowledge, but not yet comprehend, the complexity of the interplay between these proteins and the control circuits that regulate cellular metabolism and physiology. While the task of defining the molecular mechanisms by which p21 participates in tumor development represents a vital and immediate objective, a full appreciation of *ras* gene function awaits the potentially larger challenge of establishing how the encoded polypeptides participate in the control of normal cellular growth.

References

1 Sandberg, A. A. (1980) *The Chromosomes in Human Cancer and Leukemia*, Elsevier North-Holland
2 Varmus, H.E. (1984) *Annu. Rev. Genet.* 18, 553–612
3 Bishop, J. M. (1985) *Cell* 42, 23–38
4 Fasano, O. *et al.* (1984) *Proc. Natl Acad. Sci. USA* 81, 4008–4012
5 Seeburg, P. H. *et al.* (1984) *Nature* 312, 71–75
6 Alitalo, K. (1984) *Med. Biol.* 62, 304–317
7 Chang, E. H. *et al.* (1982) *Nature* 297, 479–483
8 Shih, T. Y. and Weeks, M. O. (1984) *Cancer Invest.* 2, 109–123
9 Gibbs, J. B., Sigal, I. S. and Scolnick, E. M. (1985) *Trends Biochem. Sci.* 10, 350–353
10 Halliday, K. R. (1984) *J. Cycl. Nucleotide Protein Phosphates Res.* 9, 435–438
11 McCormick, F. *et al.* (1985) *Science* 230, 78–82
12 McGrath, J. P. *et al.* (1984) *Nature* 310, 644–649
13 Shih, T. T. *et al.* (1980) *Nature* 287, 686–691
14 Gilman, A. G. (1984) *Cell* 36, 577–579
15 Sweet, R. W. *et al.* (1984) *Nature* 311, 273–275
16 Gibbs, J. B. *et al.* (1984) *Proc. Natl Acad. Sci. USA* 81, 5704–5708
17 Colby, W. W. *et al.* (1986) *Mol. Cell. Biol.* 6, 730–734
18 Der, C. J., Finkel, T. and Cooper, G. M. (1986) *Cell* 44, 167–176
19 Duesberg, P. H. (1985) *Science* 228, 669–677
20 Balmain, A. *et al.* (1984) *Nature* 307, 658–660
21 Sukamar, S. *et al.* (1983) *Nature* 306, 658–661
22 Cuzin, F. (1983) *Biochim. Biophys. Acta* 781, 193–204
23 Land, H., Parada, L. F. and Weinberg, R. A. (1983) *Nature* 304, 596–602
24 Ruley, E. (1983) *Nature* 304, 602–606
25 Madaule, P. and Axel, R. (1985) *Cell* 41, 31–40
26 Toda, T. *et al.* (1985) *Cell* 40, 27–36
27 Clark, S. G. *et al.* (1985) *Mol. Cell. Biol.* 5, 2746–2752
28 Beckner, S. K., Hattori, S. and Shih, T. Y. (1985) *Nature* 317, 71–72
29 Mulcahy, L. S., Smith, M. R. and Stacey, D. W. (1985) *Nature* 313, 241–243

30 Pragnell, I. B., Spandidos, D. A. and Wilkie, N. M. (1985) *Proc. R. Soc. London Ser B Biol. Sci.* 226, 107–119
31 Kasid, A. *et al.* (1985) *Science* 228, 725–728
32 Bar-Sagi, D. and Feramisco, J. R. (1985) *Cell* 42, 841–848
33 Noda, M. *et al.* (1985) *Nature* 318, 73–75
34 Birchmeier, C., Broek, D. and Wigler, M. (1985) *Cell* 43, 615–621
35 Fleishman, L. F., Chahuala, S. B. and Cantley, L. (1986) *Science* 231, 407–410

A. D. Levinson is at the Department of Molecular Biology, Genentech Inc., 460 Point San Bruno Boulevard, South San Francisco, CA 94080, USA.

erb-B: growth factor receptor turned oncogene

Michael J. Hayman

The erb-*B oncogene has been shown to be a deleted version of the epidermal growth factor receptor gene. These mutations are thought to cause a constitutive activation of the receptor which is then able to induce uncontrolled growth of specific cell types. Mutational analysis of the* erb-*B gene indicates that specific domains of the* erb-*B protein interact with specific cellular target proteins to cause transformation.*

The *erb*-B oncogene was first identified in an avian retrovirus that had been isolated in the early 1930s and that primarily caused the diseases erythroblastosis and fibrosarcoma. Recently, there have been several new retrovirus isolates that contain the *erb*-B gene. These isolates mainly cause erythroblastosis[1,2] but some can also cause angiosarcoma[2]. However, in the chicken the *erb*-B gene is mainly associated with erythroid leukemias. Analysis of the product of this gene rapidly revealed that it was a membrane glycoprotein, which was related by sequence analysis to the protein-tyrosine kinases[3–5]. In view of the demonstration that many growth factor receptors were also membrane-spanning tyrosine kinases, these data quite naturally led to the hypothesis that the *erb*-B gene was derived from a growth factor receptor gene, and most likely a haematopoietic growth factor receptor gene[6]. This theory had to be rapidly revised in light of the demonstration that the *erb*-B gene had extensive homology with the human epidermal growth factor receptor (EGFR) gene and was almost certainly derived from the chicken EGFR gene[7].

The demonstration that an oncogene could be derived from a growth factor receptor gene provided a key observation in our understanding of how cells can be transformed, especially since it came so shortly after the discovery that the *sis* oncogene was related to the platelet-derived growth factor gene (see p. 135). It not only influenced how we think about the mechanism by which cells can be transformed but it also opened up the possibility that other growth factors or receptors could be oncogenes in the right cellular setting. This latter possibility was quickly given validity with the demonstration that the *fms* oncogene is derived from the receptor for the haematopoietic growth factor CSF-1[8].

We know that growth factor receptors can act as oncogenes, but how they do so is unclear. In the case of erb-B we presume that the oncogene product is somehow subverting some normal feature of the EGF-receptor's mechanism of action. Unfortunately, it is not clear how the interaction of EGF with its receptor leads ultimately to cell proliferation. What is known is that upon binding of the factor to the receptor there is a stimulation of the autophosphorylation of the receptor, primarily on tyrosine 1173, which is located close to the carboxyl terminus (see Fig. 1). There is still some controversy over whether this autophosphorylation then stimulates the activity of the receptor kinase towards other substrates, since some workers are able to

EGFR   **v–erb-B**

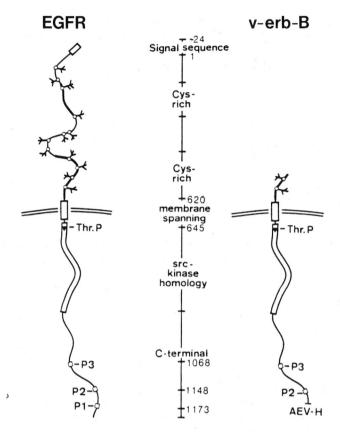

Fig. 1. *Schematic comparison of erb-B protein and the EGFR. The phosphorylated threonine residue (Thr.P) at position 654 is thought to be the target for protein kinase C. P1 represents the major site of autophosphorylation at residue 1173, P2 and P3 are the two minor sites.*

detect an increase while others are not[9,10]. After the interaction of receptor and growth factor, the receptor can be demonstrated to cluster within the plane of the membrane and subsequently be internalized. The role of these two events in the proliferative response is also unclear, but some workers feel these steps may be crucial for the activation of the kinase[11]. Therefore, it is not obvious which of these properties is important for the action of *erb*-B.

The structures of erb-B protein and EGFR, shown schematically in Fig. 1, suggest that the two gene products differ greatly. As can be seen, the erb-B protein is a dramatically truncated version of the EGFR. It has sustained a large deletion at the amino-terminal end such that only 61 amino acid residues remain compared to the 622 normally found in the external domain of the EGFR. It has also sustained a smaller carboxy-terminal deletion. These deletions have obvious mechanistic consequences, since the amino-terminal deletion almost certainly removes the EGF binding site and the carboxy-terminal deletion removes the major site of tyrosine autophosphorylation. These observations have led to the hypothesis that the deletions remove regions responsible for the regulation of the kinase activity by EGF, causing the *erb*-B gene product to be constitutively active, and that it is this property that converts the EGFR gene into an oncogene. In order to evaluate the validity of this theory we should consider the data that have been amassed on the *erb*-B gene in the avian system and also in those situations where the EGFR has been implicated in tumour formation in man.

Involvement of the EGFR in human tumours

Studies on the human EGFR had been carried out primarily on the epidermoid carcinoma cell line A431, the reason for this being that these cells expressed roughly two orders of magnitude more EGFR than most other cell lines. With the realization that the EGFR may be able to function as an oncogene, the A431 cells were examined in more detail and it was found that the reason for the high expression was that the EGFR gene was amplified approximately fifty times in these cells[12]. In addition, it was noted that a truncated version of the receptor was synthesized by the cells[13]. Interestingly, this truncation represented the external domain of the receptor and was effectively the mirror image of the *erb*-B oncogene. Examination of other squamous cell carcinomas, primarily head and neck tumours, and cell lines revealed that this amplification of the EGFR gene was quite a common occurrence but there was no good evidence for gene truncations of any kind in these other cells[14]. The EGFR gene was also found to be amplified in several brain tumours, notably tumours of glial origin[16]. Since amplification of other oncogenes is thought to be very important in the development of tumours (see p. 50 for a review on N-*myc* by Schwab[16]), it is possible that these data represent evidence for the role of the EGFR in tumour development. The mechanism of action, though obviously different from that proposed for the *erb*-B gene, could be functionally similar if, for example, over-expression also led to the constitutive activation of the kinase.

Analysis of the *erb*-B gene in avian retroviruses

The *erb*-B gene of avian erythroblastosis virus, AEV, has been studied extensively only for the last few years, but already a large body of information has been gathered from an analysis both of wild-type virus and of various virus mutants. The wild-type erb-B protein is a membrane glycoprotein which when isolated can be shown to function as a protein-tyrosine kinase with the ability both to autophosphorylate and to phosphorylate a variety of artificial exogenous substrates[17]. However, in infected cells the erb-B protein exhibits remarkably little phosphorylation on tyrosine residues, either in the presence or absence of EGF[18,19]. Notably, though, *erb*-B-transformed cells do show increased tyrosine phosphorylation on certain cellular proteins such as p36 (one of the lipocortins also phosphorylated by other tyrosine kinase oncogenes, see Brugge[20] for recent review) and p42 (Ref. 18; a substrate in EGF-, serum- or phorbol ester-stimulated fibroblasts). Thus the erb-B-protein seems to function as a constitutively activated kinase which no longer needs to undergo autophosphorylation to interact with its cellular substrates.

Mutational analysis of *erb*-B

Analysis of both conditional and non-conditional mutants of AEV has also been informative. The demonstration that mutants that are temperature sensitive for transformation are also temperature sensitive for transport of the *erb*-B gene product to the plasma membrane indicated that this was the site of action for *erb*-B. However, perhaps the most interesting mutants are the host-

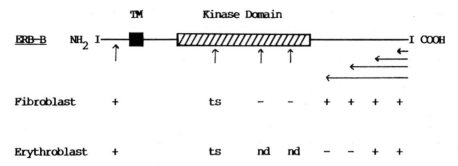

Fig. 2. *Effects of mutations in the* erb-B *gene on transformation. TM represents the position of the transmembrane region of* erb-B. *Vertical arrows indicate the position of linker insertion mutants and horizontal arrows indicate the extent of deletions from the carboxyl terminus. The effects of these mutations are indicated directly below.* −, *nontransforming;* +, *transforming; nd, not determined.*

range mutants. As mentioned earlier, AEV is capable of transforming both fibroblasts and erythroblasts, but it is possible to isolate mutants that are only able to transform one of these cell types. At present, not all of these mutants have been completely characterized although certain facts that have become apparent from the experiments carried out to date. Mutants that have lost the ability to transform erythroblasts are truncated further at the carboxyl terminus; in the case of the mutant *td359*, 108 amino acid residues have been deleted[21]. By site-directed mutagenesis it has been demonstrated recently that progressive deletion of the carboxyl terminus first weakens and then abolishes their erythroblast-transforming capacity without affecting the fibroblast-transforming capacity, as discussed by Beug *et al.*[21] Preliminary evidence indicates that these additional truncations have little effect on the tyrosine kinase autophosphorylation activity. These results suggest that a particular configuration of the carboxyl terminus is necessary to transform erythroblasts.

The other host-range mutants have recently been isolated from cases of erythroblastosis caused by the avian leukosis virus RAV-1. Injection of RAV-1, a virus lacking an oncogene, into a particular strain of chicken, L15, frequently brings about erythroid leukaemia. This is a result initially of the integration of the RAV-1 genome into the normal chicken EGFR/c-erb-B gene. This event leads to the high-level transcription of truncated forms of the c-*erb*-B mRNA which encode EGFR molecules deleted at their amino terminus[22]. During the development of the erythroid leukaemia there is a high probability that the c-*erb*-B gene sequences will be transduced into a retrovirus genome, and consequently leukaemic cells isolated from diseased birds frequently release viruses that contain parts of the c-*erb*-B gene. One of the interesting features of these viruses is that they are usually unable to transform fibroblasts in tissue culture and do not cause fibrosarcoma on injection into the muscle of young chickens[1,23]. Although only a few of these new viruses have been analysed, preliminary results indicate that the viruses can direct the synthesis of large amounts of the truncated forms of the erb-B protein. This protein is transported to the plasma membrane of the fibroblasts and has autophosphorylating activity, but is not able to transform these cells. Some of these viruses have retained the complete carboxyl terminus of the EGFR whereas others have sustained deletions that encompass the major autophosphorylation sites. These results indicate that, at present, there is no simple model which explains the role of the carboxyl terminus of the erb-B protein in transformation. They do suggest, however, that the erb-B protein transforms cells by a pleiotropic mechanism and that in different cell types the domains of the molecules are interacting with significantly different target molecules.

Recently, the other domains of the erb-B protein have also been subjected to mutational analysis. The most extensive study reported to date has addressed only fibroblast transformation[24] and these workers found that mutations within the kinase domain abolished transformation. Mutations in the amino terminus or in the extreme carboxyl terminus had no effect. Unfortunately, the effects of these mutations on the kinase activity of the protein await further study, as does the effect on erythroblast transformation. A summary of the effects of mutations on transformation is depicted in Fig. 2.

Recent studies addressing the role of glycosylation of the erb-B protein indicate that glycosylation has no direct role in transformation of either fibroblasts or erythroblasts[25,26]. Also, preliminary data indicate that although the external domain of erb-B cannot bind EGF it may play some role in transformation in that mutations at the extreme amino terminus of the protein do seem to abolish transformation (discussed in Beug et al.[21]). The effects of these mutations on biosynthesis and kinase activity, however, remain to be evaluated.

Concluding remarks

In summary, the data on transformation by *erb*-B indicate that there is an intimate interaction between the cell and this oncogene such that one molecular form of this protein can be oncogenic in certain cell types while other cells remain unresponsive. As an aside, this is a good example of the problems associated with identifying new oncogenes in human tumours, in that the indicator cell has to be very carefully chosen if one wants to be sure that all possible genes can be scored (see p. 90 for a more detailed discussion of this problem). Mechanistically, the best hypothesis for transformation by *erb*-B to date would be that the protein has to be in the plasma membrane of cells in order to function. The protein has to be altered so that the kinase activity is constitutively activated and this can be accomplished in a variety of ways but usually involves some kind of deletion. The activated protein would then interact with specific cellular target proteins, probably through the carboxy-terminal domain, and these protein–protein interactions would differ between different cell types. The kind of interaction envisaged would involve the phosphorylation of specific cellular proteins by the erb-B kinase rather than the autophosphorylation of the *erb*-B gene product itself. This rather simplistic scenario, while being consistent with the known facts, unfortunately begs the most important questions: which proteins are involved in mechanistically relevant interactions? and what are the consequences of these interactions? These are obviously the problems we have to concern ourselves with in the future if we are to understand both how the *erb*-B gene functions as an oncogene and how the EGFR causes cell proliferation. The lessons we have learned from the studies on *erb*-B and the EGFR have influenced the ways we think about cell transformation. The answers to these remaining questions promise to be equally informative.

Acknowledgements
   The author would like to thank Drs Paula Enrietto and Jennifer Knight for their help with the manuscript. The work in the author's laboratory is supported by grants CA42573 and CA28146.

References
1   Beug, H. *et al.* (1986) *J. Virol.* 57, 1127–1138
2   Tracy, S. E., Woda, B. A. and Robinson, H. L. (1985) *J. Virol.* 54, 304–310
3   Hayman, M. J. and Beug, H. (1984) *Nature* 309, 460–462
4   Privalsky, M. L. and Bishop, J. M. (1984) *Virology* 135, 356–368
5   Yamamoto, T. *et al.* (1983) *Cell* 35, 71–78
6   Beug, H. and Hayman, M. J. (1984) *Cell* 36, 963–972
7   Downward, J. *et al.* (1984) *Nature* 307, 521–527
8   Scherr, C. J. *et al.* (1985) *Cell* 41, 665–676
9   Bertics, P. J. and Gill, G. N. (1985) *J. Biol. Chem.* 260, 14642–14647
10 Downward, J., Waterfield, M. D. and Parker, P. J. (1985) *J. Biol. Chem.* 260, 14538–14546
11 Schlessinger, J. in *Oncogenes and Growth Control* (Kahn, P. and Graf, T., eds), Springer-Verlag (in press)
12 Lin, C. R. *et al.* (1984) *Science* 224, 843–848
13 Ullrich, A. *et al.* (1984) *Nature* 309, 418–425
14 Cowley, G. *et al.* (1984) in *Cancer Cells 1* (Vande Waud, G. F., Levine, A. J., Topp, W. C. and Watson, J. D., eds), pp. 5–10, Cold Spring Harbor Laboratory
15 Libermann, T. A. *et al.* (1985) *Nature* 313, 144–147
16 Schwab, M. (1985) *Trends Genet.* 1, 271–273 (and this book, pp. 50–58)
17 Kris, R. M. *et al.* (1985) *Cell* 40, 619–625
18 Gilmore, T., Declue, J. E. and Martin, G. S. (1985) *Cell* 40, 609–618
19 Decker, S. J. (1985) *J. Biol. Chem.* 260, 2003–2006
20 Brugge, J. S. (1986) *Cell* 46, 149–150
21 Beug, H., Hayman, M. J. and Vennstrom, B. in *Oncogenes and Growth Control* (Kahn, P. and Graf, T., eds), Springer-Verlag (in press)
22 Nilsen, T. W. *et al.* (1985) *Cell* 41, 719–726
23 Miles, B. D. and Robinson, H. L. (1985) *J. Virol.* 54, 295–303
24 Ng, M. and Privalsky, M. L. (1986) *J. Virol.* 58, 542–553
25 Bassiri, M. and Privalsky, M. L. (1986) *J. Virol.* 59, 525–530
26 Schmidt, J. S., Beug, H. and Hayman, M. J. (1985) *EMBO J.* 4, 105–112

M. J. Hayman is at the Department of Microbiology, State University of New York, Stony Brook, NY 11794, USA.

Mutagens, oncogenes and cancer

Mariano Barbacid

At least 15 different oncogenes have been implicated in the development of human neoplasia. Some of these oncogenes are reproducibly activated in carcinogen-induced animal tumor model systems. Emerging evidence indicates that these oncogenes can be activated during initiation of carcinogenesis as a direct consequence of the mutagenic action of the carcinogen.

Unveiling the molecular basis of cancer requires prior understanding of the pathways that control cell proliferation. Over 30 different cellular loci presumably involved in these pathways have been identified in recent years. Identification of these genes has been made possible by the existence of genes, both in acute transforming retroviruses[1] and in human and animal tumors[2-4], which are capable of inducing some of the phenotypic changes characteristic of tumor cells. These genes have been generically designated oncogenes, whereas their counterparts in normal cells are known (for lack of a more informative name) as proto-oncogenes. The list of cellular oncogenes has increased from just two in 1981 (c-*myc*, an oncogene activated by retroviral insertion in chicken bursal lymphomas and c-*mos*, a proto-oncogene turned into an oncogene by *in vitro* transcriptional activation) to over 30 in 1986 (see Refs 5 and 7 for reviews). These cellular oncogenes can become activated by insertional mutagenesis (c-*myc*, c-*erb*-B, c-*myb*, *int*-1, *int*-2, *pim*, c-*mos*), single point mutations (*ras* gene family, *neu*), chromosomal translocations (c-*myc*, c-*abl*, *bcl*-1, *bcl*-2) and gene amplification (*myc* gene family, K-*ras*, c-*abl*, c-*myb*, c-*erb*B-1, c-*erb*B-2). The properties of some of these oncogenes are reviewed in other chapters of this book.

Oncogenes in human tumors

One of the ultimate goals in understanding the intimate events that control cellular growth and differentiation is to apply such knowledge towards establishing the molecular basis of human cancer. Over the last five years, we have learned that human tumors are a fruitful source of oncogenes (see Refs 2–4 for recent reviews). By use of gene transfer assays, it has been possible to identify several oncogenes, of which the members of the *ras* gene family, H-*ras*, K-*ras* and N-*ras*, are the most prevalent. The *ras* oncogenes have been detected in ~10–15% of types of human tumors that include some of the most common forms of human neoplasia (Table 1). The *ras* genes are known to acquire their transforming properties by single point mutations in two domains of their coding sequences, most commonly in codons 12 and 61 (for a recent review see p.74, or Ref. 8). The *ras* genes code for proteins, known as p21, of 188 or 189 amino acid residues; the proteins bind GDP and GTP and have an intrinsic GTPase activity. This enzymatic activity is greatly reduced in the mutant p21 proteins coded for by the *ras* oncogenes[8]. Based on these observations and on limited sequence homology, it has been proposed that *ras* genes may code for regulatory proteins similar to G proteins. These proteins are known to exist in equilibrium between an 'active' state in which they have GTP bound and an

Table 1. Human Oncogenes[a]

Oncogene	Mechanism of activation	Type of tumor	Proportion of tumors containing activated oncogene (%)
H-ras-1	Single point mutation	Several carcinomas, melanomas	1–10
K-ras-2	Single point mutation	Several carcinomas, rhabdomyosarcoma, ALL,	1–15
	Amplification	Lung and bladder carcinomas	1
N-ras	Single point mutation	Several types of leukemias, some carcinomas, melanomas, and sarcomas	1–25
c-myc	Chromosomal translocation	Burkitt's lymphoma	100
	Amplification	SCLC, breast and colon carcinomas, PML	1–35
N-myc	Amplification	Neuroblastoma, SCLC, retinoblastoma	20–50
L-myc	Amplification	SCLC	25
c-abl	Chromosomal translocation	CML	100
bcl-1	Chromososomal translocation	B-cell lymphomas	80–100[b]
bcl-2	Chromosomal translocation	Follicular lymphoma	80–100

[a]Only includes those oncogenes frequently found in human malignancies. SCLC, small cell lung carcinoma; ALL, acute lymphocytic leukemia; PML, promyelocytic leukemia; CML, chronic myelogenous leukemia.
[b]100% refers to B-cell lymphomas with (11 : 14) chromosomal translocations.

'inactive' or 'relaxed' state in which they bind GDP. The transition from the 'inactive' to the 'active' state is accomplished by GDP/GTP exchange whereas 'deactivation' takes place by hydrolysis of the bound GTP molecule. If this model is correct, the mutations that turn *ras* genes into oncogenes would block their p21 products in their 'active' state by inhibiting intrinsic GTPase activity that should permit 'deactivation' after their putative effector role has been exerted.

Of the oncogenes found in human tumors, those belonging to the *myc* gene family are among the most frequently represented (Table 1). All Burkitt's lymphomas carry c-*myc* oncogenes activated by chromosomal translocations that alter their regulatory environment in chromosome 8 by placing them under the influence of immunoglobulin loci. In addition, the c-*myc* locus has been found to be amplified in several human tumors[2-4] including breast carcinomas, where 32% of 104 samples tested exhibited c-*myc* amplification ranging from 5- to 15-fold. Moreover, five of these breast tumors exhibited genetic rearrangements (R. Callahan, pers. commun.). The c-*myc* oncogene, as well as the related N-*myc* and L-*myc* oncogenes, are amplified in most of the highly malignant variants of small cell lung carcinomas (SCLC). N-*myc* is also amplified in over 50% of stage III and IV neuroblastomas as well as in some retinoblastomas (see p.50; Table 1). The *myc* gene family codes for nuclear proteins of an, as yet, unknown function.

Another oncogene, c-*abl*, is translocated from chromosome 9 to chromosome 22 during the generation of the Philadelphia chromosome characteristic of chronic myelogenous leukemia (CML). As a consequence of this translocation the c-*abl* locus is decapitated and fused to *bcr*, a gene of unknown function. The c-*abl* proto-oncogene codes for a protein of 145 kDa that exhibits tyrosine protein kinase activity and is associated with the plasma membrane[2-4]. Recent findings have revealed at least four alternative coding exons in the c-*abl* locus[9], thus predicting the existence of a family of c-*abl* proteins, each exhibiting a different amino-terminal sequence. There are at least two lines of evidence that suggest that this variable amino-terminal domain may play an important role in regulating the tyrosine protein kinase activity of c-*abl* proteins. The product of the v-*abl* oncogene requires amino-terminal myristilation for proper membrane anchorage and biological activity[1]. The product of the translocated *bcr*–c-*abl* oncogene is a 210 kDa protein in which the variable amino-terminal domain has been replaced by the corresponding domain of the *bcr* product (see Ref. 10 for a review). Recently, it has been speculated that the c-*abl* product might represent the cytoplasmic domain of a new class of growth factor receptors in which the external and transmembrane domain may be contributed by a different locus (e.g. the IL-2 receptor).

Activation of c-*myc* and c-*abl* oncogenes by chromosomal translocations has led some investigators to postulate that the reproducible chromosomal breakpoints, characteristic of certain human leukemias, harbor oncogenes. Croce and co-workers have isolated two loci, *bcl*-1 and *bcl*-2, that are reproducibly involved in chromosomal abnormalities of B-cell lymphomas (Table 1). The recent cloning of the T-cell receptor gene family is also making it possible to investigate whether oncogenes are activated by the translocations and inversions of chromosomes 7 and 14 involving T-cell receptor genes.

Circumstantial evidence has implicated other cellular oncogenes in the development of human neoplasia[2-4]. For instance, expression of c-*sis*, the gene coding for the B chain of the platelet-derived growth factor, is increased in human sarcoma and glioblastoma cell lines. Overexpression of this locus in NIH/3T3 cells leads to their morphological transformation. However, there is no direct evidence that the relatively low levels of c-*sis* transcripts in these human tumor cell lines contributed to their neoplastic development. Other proto-oncogenes, including c-*erb*B-1 [the gene coding for the epidermal growth factor (EGF) receptor], its close relative c-*erb*B-2, and the c-*myb* gene, have been found to be amplified and overexpressed in certain tumor cells of different lineage. So far, overexpression of the cloned c-*erb*B-1/EGF receptor gene has failed to show any detectable transforming activity in available *in vitro* assays. However, it is likely that most, if not all, genetically altered proto-oncogenes contribute to some extent to the multi-stage development of human neoplasia.

At least five new loci[2–4,7] have been identified by their ability to transform NIH/3T3 mouse cells in gene transfer assays. Among them, *trk* and *met* have been shown to be novel tyrosine protein kinases and c-*raf*-1 a transforming allele of a proto-oncogene related to the retroviral v-*raf/mil* oncogenes. Activation of these oncogenes may be of limited significance to human cancer because they occur rather infrequently. However, their isolation and subsequent characterization will provide valuable information on the different pathways involved in the regulation of cell proliferation.

Oncogenes in carcinogen-induced animal tumors

The frequent activation of *ras*, *myc* and *abl* oncogenes in human cancers, along with their well-known tumorigenic properties when transduced by retroviruses, strongly support the concept that these oncogenes are involved in the development or human neoplasia. However, formal establishment of a causal link between oncogene activation and initiation or progression of human cancer is very difficult. Human neoplasia cannot be experimentally induced or manipulated, thus making it virtually impossible to define the precise role that these oncogenes might have played in the development of those tumors in which they have been found. A fundamental criterion for studying the role of oncogenes *in vivo* is the definition of model systems in which oncogenes can be activated reproducibly within controlled experimental conditions. This criterion has now been met, by a variety of animal tumor systems, for at least four oncogenes: H-*ras*-1, K-*ras*-2, N-*ras* and *neu* (Table 2). Balmain and Pragnell first reported the presence of transforming H-*ras*-1 genes in three transplanted squamous cell carcinomas induced by treatment of mouse skin with dimethylbenz(a)anthracene (DMBA) and promoted with phorbol esters[11]. H-*ras*-1 oncogenes have also been identified in the majority of rat mammary tumors induced with a single dose of *N*-nitroso-*N*-methylurea (NMU) during sexual development[12]. Similar observations have been made in B6C3F$_1$ mouse hepatomas induced by different carcinogens[13] (Table 2). Interestingly, the H-*ras*-1 oncogene has also been identified in spontaneous liver adenomas and carcinomas of this strain[14].

Other animal tumor systems in which *ras* oncogenes have been reproducibly activated are summarized in Table 2. They include induction of mouse thymomas by X-rays or chronic NMU treatment (both K-*ras*-2 and N-*ras* become activated)[15], induction of mouse fibrosarcomas by 3-methyl-cholanthrene (3-MCA) (K-*ras*-2 is activated)[16], and induction of rat kidney mesenchymal tumors by a single dose of methyl(methoxymethyl)nitrosamine

Table 2. Oncogenes in carcinogen-induced animal tumors

Species	Carcinogen	Tumor	Oncogene	Proportion of tested tumours containing transforming gene[a] (%)	Reference
Rat	NMU	Mammary carcinomas	H-ras-1	86 (80)	6,18
	DMBA	Mammary carcinomas	H-ras-1	23 (50)	18
	DMN	Renal carcinomas	K-ras-2	40 (25)	10
	ENU	Neuroblastomas	neu	100 (3)	11
	NMU	Schwannomas	neu	70 (10)	b
	MMS	Nasal carcinomas	?	100 (8)	12
Mouse	DMBA	Skin carcinomas	H-ras-1	90 (36)	26,27
	Several	Hepatomas	H-ras-1	100 (25)	13
	X-rays	Lymphomas	K-ras-2	57 (7)	8
	NMU	Lymphomas	N-ras-1	85 (6)	8
	3-MCA	Fibrosarcomas	K-ras-2	50 (4)	9

[a]Number in parentheses indicates number of tumors tested.
[b]Our unpublished observations.

(DMN) (K-*ras*-2 is activated)[17]. Oncogenes other than members of the *ras* gene family have been identified in at least two additional animal model systems. Induction of rat tumors of the peripheral nervous system (neuroblastomas, gliomas or schwannomas) by ethyl-nitrourea (ENU)[18] or NMU (our unpublished results) leads to the reproducible activation of the *neu* oncogene. This gene directs the synthesis of a 185 kDa protein that shares extensive homology with the EGF receptor[18] and is likely to be an allele of the human c-*erb*B-2 proto-oncogene. Rat nasopharyngeal carcinomas induced by methyl-methane sulphonate (MMS) contain an unidentified transforming gene which shares no sequence homology with either *ras* or *neu* oncogenes[19].

So far, efforts aimed at correlating oncogene activation with induction of animal tumors by chemical or physical carcinogens have been limited to those oncogenes capable of transforming NIH/3T3 mouse cells in gene transfer assays. The exclusive use of this methodology probably accounts for the limited range of oncogenes detected. In fact, it is known that other oncogenes that will not score in NIH/3T3 transfection assays can also be implicated in the development of experimental animal tumors. Pristane-induced mouse plasma-cytomas consistently exhibit a c-*myc* oncogene activated by a chromosomal translocation similar to that found in human Burkitt's lymphoma (see Ref. 20 for a review). Development of new oncogene detection assays based on different biological principles should expand our knowledge of the molecular events involved in development of carcinogen-induced animal tumors.

Oncogenes as targets for carcinogens

The availability of animal model systems in which oncogenes can be reproducibly activated under controlled etiological and genetic conditions is making it possible to investigate the role of these oncogenes in the multistep process of carcinogenesis. We have examined the contribution of the etiological agent to the specific activation of a given oncogene. Substitution of NMU by DMBA as the carcinogen in the rat mammary tumor system leads to a dramatic decrease in the percentage of tumors carrying H-*ras*-1 oncogenes (Table 2). Whereas more than 85% of the NMU-induced tumors exhibit a transforming H-*ras*-1 gene, only 23% of those induced by DMBA have this oncogene. There are two basic hypotheses to explain these observations. It is possible that carcinogens can induce the same type of malignancy by independent pathways whose selection would depend on an intricate and delicate balance of factors such as carcinogen activation, delivery, cellular absorption, repair mechanisms, etc. However, it is also possible that NMU and DMBA may act upon different stages of a unique pathway affecting genes involved either upstream or downstream of H-*ras*-1. Such mutations will presumably lead to the same neoplastic phenotype. However, such putative oncogenes may not be detected by available gene transfer assays.

Perhaps the most interesting idea so far derived from studies of animal tumor systems is the possibility that oncogenes are the direct target of chemical carcinogens. It is generally accepted that most carcinogens are mutagens. A significant number of chemical carcinogens are known to form adducts with DNA bases[21]. In some cases, the modified bases are repaired by specific enzymes that remove the modifying radical (e.g. alkyl–guanosine transferases). However, in the majority of the cases these adducts are removed by excision repair mechanisms[22]. Mutations can be generated during repair procedures because of the limited fidelity of repair DNA polymerases, or if unrepaired apurinic sites serve as templates for DNA replication. In addition, some modified bases are highly mutagenic because of their miscoding properties. This is the case for O^6-methylguanine, one of the adducts derived from treatment with methylating agents such as NMU[23]. At least in bacteria, O^6-methylguanine residues are read as adenine residues by DNA polymerases, thus leading to the frequent generation of G→A transitions[24].

As mentioned previously, *ras* genes are known to acquire their transforming properties by single point mutations in their coding sequences, particularly in codons 12 and 61 (Ref. 8). Whereas *ras* genes have been shown to be activated by a variety of miscoding mutations[2–4], each of 61 H-*ras*-1 oncogenes present in NMU-induced mammary carcinomas of rats carried a G→A transition in the second nucleotide of codon 12 (Ref. 25; Table 3). As a control, the activating mutations of H-*ras*-1 oncogenes present in mammary carcinomas induced by DMBA were examined. DMBA, unlike NMU, forms large adducts with guanine and adenine residues leading to unspecified mutations. Each of these oncogenes exhibited a normal codon 12 (GGA). Their activating mutations were localized instead in the two adenine residues of codon 61 (CAA), the other 'hot-spot' for activation of *ras* oncogenes (Table 3). These findings strongly suggest that the mutagenic properties of NMU, presumably exerted through the generation of miscoding O^6-methylguanines, are directly responsible for the malignant activation of H-*ras*-1 oncogenes in this animal tumor system.

Similar results have been found in other animal tumor systems. As summarized in Table 3, induction of skin carcinomas of mice by DMBA or dibenz(c,h)acridine (DBACR) specifically involves activation of H-*ras*-1 oncogenes by an A→T transition in the second base of codon 61 (Refs 26 and 27). However, this mutation was not seen when the initiating carcinogen was replaced by *N*-methyl-*N*-nitro-*N*-nitrosoguanidine (MNNG), an alkylating carcinogen. Specific activation of H-*ras*-1 oncogenes by chemical carcinogens has also been observed in hepatomas of male B6C32F$_1$ mice[13]. In this model system, H-*ras*-1 oncogenes became activated by C→A transversions in the first base of codon 61 when *N*-hydroxy-2-acetylaminofluorene (HO-AFF) was used as the initiating carcinogen (Table 3). However, A→T mutations in the second base of the same codon were observed when the same tumors were induced by vinyl carbamate (VC) (Table 3). These findings strongly support the concept that H-*ras*-1 oncogenes are the direct targets of chemical carcinogens.

Oncogenes and the initiation of carcinogenesis

Recent evidence suggests that *ras* oncogenes may be involved in the initiation of carcinogenesis. Transforming H-*ras*-1 genes have been identified in the majority of papillomas induced by topical application of DMBA followed by treatment with tumor promoters[28]. These papillomas represent a pre-neoplastic stage because most of them will regress, only a few proceeding to fully developed carcinomas. Whereas no such pre-neoplastic stages can be defined during mammary carcinogenesis, our observations suggesting that H-*ras*-1 oncogenes are directly activated by NMU lead to similar conclusions[25]. As indicated above, a single dose of NMU is sufficient to induce these mammary tumors. Considering that NMU is a direct-acting carcinogen with very short half-life under physiological conditions, its mutagenic/carcinogenic effect must occur within hours after its application. Thus, if the G→A transitions that activate H-*ras*-1 oncogenes in these tumors are the direct effect

Table 3. Activation of H-ras-1 oncogenes by specific mutations in carcinogen-induced animal tumors

Species	Type of tumor	Carcinogen	Activating mutation[a]	Incidence of activating mutation in tumors	Reference
Rat	Mammary carcinomas	NMU	$G^{35} \rightarrow A$	61/61	25
	Mammary carcinomas	DMBA	$A^{182}/A^{183} \rightarrow N$	5/5	25
Mouse	Skin papillomas/carcinomas	DMBA	$A^{182} \rightarrow T$	33/34	26
Mouse	Skin carcinomas	DMBA	$A^{182} \rightarrow T$	3/3	27
	Skin papillomas/carcinomas	DBACR	$A^{182} \rightarrow T$	6/6	27
Mouse	Hepatocarcinomas	HO-AFF	$C^{181} \rightarrow A$	7/7	13
	Hepatocarcinomas	VC	$A^{182} \rightarrow T$	6/7	13

[a]Residue 35 corresponds to the second nucleotide of codon 12, residues 181–183 correspond to codon 61.

of the mutagenic action of NMU[25], oncogene activation must be concomitant with initiation of carcinogenesis.

The implication of *ras* oncogenes in the initiation of carcinogen-induced tumors does not exclude the possibility that *ras* oncogenes can be activated in the late stages of neoplastic development. Tumor progression is usually characterized by aneuploidy and the frequent occurrence of genetic alterations. Thus, it is likely that the single point mutations responsible for *ras* oncogene activation may also occur during tumor development. Activation of *ras* oncogenes has been observed upon prolonged cultivation of tumor cells *in vitro*[29,30] or during metastasis[31]. Unfortunately, the lack of epidemiological information on most human tumors makes it impossible at present to establish the percentage of *ras* oncogenes that might have been activated during tumor progression and those that participated in the initiation of the tumorigenic process.

Oncogene activation and cell proliferation

It is easy to understand that application of DMBA and phorbol esters to the skin of mice will lead to the development of skin carcinomas, but it is not so clear why intravenous injection of NMU will exclusively induce mammary carcinomas. There is ample documentation that NMU has access to most cell types. Thus, the active state of proliferation of the developing mammary gland at the time of the carcinogenic insult must play a fundamental role. Experimental evidence for this hypothesis was obtained by Huggins in 1961 (see Ref. 32 for a recent review). Ovariectomy of carcinogen-treated rats even a month after carcinogen treatment leads to a dramatic decrease in the incidence of mammary carcinomas. Thus, it is likely that active cell proliferation, induced either by exogenously supplied tumor promoters in the skin tumor model system or by the endogenous hormonal status of the mammary gland in the case of mammary tumors, is necessary for the phenotypic expression of *ras* oncogenes. This hypothesis also serves to explain why *ras* oncogenes failed to transform primary rat embryo fibroblasts (REF) *in vitro*, unless they had acquired continuous proliferating properties[33]. The order in which these two phenomena occur does not appear to be significant. Thus, *ras* oncogenes may participate in the initiation of carcinogenesis if activated in cells programmed to proliferate (e.g. mammary cells during female sexual development), or may play a role in tumor progression if activated in initiated cells that have already acquired continuous proliferating properties.

Future prospects

The discovery of oncogenes in human tumors has raised high expectations regarding the development of new strategies for the diagnosis and, perhaps, treatment of cancer. Considering the enormous amount of information accumulated during the last five years, there is reason for optimism. However, we must be fully aware of the tremendous difficulties that lie ahead of us. Cancer is a multistep process that probably results from accumulation of a series of genetic and/or epigenetic errors. If these lesions occur in an unlinked, independent fashion, identification of one, or even two oncogenes in a given tumor may not be sufficient to understand its molecular genesis. Establishment of new assays based on different biological criteria from those currently used today, should expand the number of available research tools by identifying new classes of oncogenes. However, in order to understand cancer in molecular terms we must combine existing information on oncogenes with the vast knowledge on the biology of neoplasia derived from studies using animal tumor systems. The results reviewed in this report are a promising step in this direction.

References

1 Bishop, J. M. (1985) *Cell* 42, 23–38
2 Varmus, H. E. (1984) *Annu. Rev. Genet.* 18, 553–612
3 Marshall, C. J. (1984) in *RNA Tumor Viruses*, Vol. 2, pp. 487–558, Cold Spring Harbor Laboratories
4 Barbacid, M. (1985) in *Oncology 1986*, pp. 3–22, Lippincott
5 Weinburg, R. A. (1985) *Science* 230, 770–776
6 Blair, D. G., Oskarsson, M., Wood, T. G., McClements, W. L., Fischinger, P. J. and Vande Woude, G. F. (1981) *Science* 212, 941–943
7 Bishop, J. M. (1985) *Trends Genet.* 1, 245–249 (and this book, pp.1–10)
8 Levinson, A. D. (1986) *Trends Genet.* 2, 81–85 (and this book, pp. 74–83)
9 Ben-Neriah, Y., Bernards, A., Paskind, M., Daley, G. Q. and Baltimore, D. (1986) *Cell* 44, 577–586
10 Adams, J. M. (1985) *Nature* 315, 542–543
11 Balmain, A. and Pragnell, I. B. (1983) *Nature* 303, 72–74
12 Sukumar, S., Notario, V., Martin-Zanca, D. and Barbacid, M. (1983) *Nature* 306, 658–661
13 Wiseman, R. W., Stowers, S. J., Miller, E. C., Anderson, M. W. and Miller, J. A. *Proc. Natl Acad. Sci. USA* (in press)
14 Reynolds, S. H., Stowers, S. J., Maronpot, R. P., Anderson, M. W. and Aaronson, S. A. (1986) *Proc. Natl Acad. Sci. USA* 83, 33–37
15 Guerrero, I., Calzada, P., Mayer, A. and Pellicer, A. (1984) *Proc. Natl Acad. Sci. USA* 81, 202–205
16 Eva, A. and Aaronson, S. A. (1983) *Science* 220, 955–956
17 Sukumar, S., Perantoni, A., Reed, C., Rice, J. M. and Wenk, M. L. *Mol. Cell. Biol.* (in press)
18 Schechter, A. L., Stern, D. F., Vaidyanathan, L., Decker, S. J., Drebin, J. A., Greene, M. I. and Weinberg, R. A. (1984) *Nature* 312, 513–516
19 Garte, S. *et al.* (1985) *Carcinogenesis* 5, 1709–1712
20 Klein, G. (1983) *Cell* 32, 311–315
21 Singer, B. and Kusmierek, J. T. (1982) *Annu. Rev. Biochem.* 52, 655–693
22 Walker, G. (1984) *Microbiol. Rev.* 48, 60–93
23 Eadie, J. S., Conrad, M., Toorchen, D. and Topal, M. D. (1984) *Nature* 308, 201–203
24 Loechler, E. L., Green, C. L. and Essigmann, J. M. (1984) *Proc. Natl Acad. Sci. USA* 81, 6271–6275
25 Zarbl, H., Sukumar, S., Arthur, A. V., Martin-Zanca, D. and Barbacid, M. (1985) *Nature* 315, 382–385
26 Quintanilla, M., Brown, K., Ramsden, M. and Balmain, A. *Nature* (in press)
27 Bizub, D., Wood, A. W. and Skalka, A. M. *Proc. Natl Acad. Sci. USA* (in press)
28 Balmain, A., Ramsden, M., Bowden, G. T. and Smith, J. (1984) *Nature* 307, 658–660
29 Brown, R., Marshall, C. J., Pennie, S. G. and Hall, A. (1984) *EMBO J.* 3, 1321–1326
30 Tainsky, M. A., Cooper, C. S., Giovanella, B. C. and Vande Woude, G. F. (1984) *Science* 225, 643–645
31 Albino, A. P., Lestrange, R., Oliff, A. J., Furth, M. E. and Old, L. J. (1984) *Nature* 308, 69–72
32 Welsch, C. W. (1985) *Cancer Res.* 45, 3415–3443
33 Land, H., Parada, L. F. and Weinberg, R. A. (1983) *Science* 222, 771–778

M. Barbacid is at the Developmental Oncology Section, Basic Research Program, Frederick Cancer Research Facility, Frederick, MD 21701, USA.

Oncogenes encoding protein kinases

Bartholomew M. Sefton

At least half of the more than 20 known proto-oncogenes encode proteins which phosphorylate polypeptide substrates. This suggests that protein phosphorylation plays a central role in the regulation of cellular multiplication, glucose metabolism and cell shape and that a surprisingly large number of protein kinases exert control over these processes in normal cells and can perturb them in malignant cells.

The eukaryotic genome harbors a remarkably large and diverse set of genes whose mutation or aberrant expression can lead to malignancy. With some logic, these are termed proto-oncogenes. The exact number of proto-oncogenes which eukaryotes inherit is unknown. More than 20 have been identified and it is clear that the end is not in sight.

The activity of most of the proteins encoded by proto-oncogenes falls into one of only four groups. The proteins encoded by the three *ras* genes are likely to modulate, together with guanosine trisphosphate, the activity of some protein in the plasma membrane, perhaps adenylate cyclase[1]. The *myb, myc* and *fos* proteins act within the nucleus[2-4] and may regulate gene expression. The *sis* protein acts as a polypeptide growth factor[5]. The fourth and largest group is the oncogenic proteins which catalyse the phosphorylation of polypeptide substrates[6,7]. These protein kinases are thought to induce malignant growth through modulation of the activity or function of cytoplasmic and plasma membrane proteins.

Fifteen oncogenes encoding protein kinases have been identified so far (Table 1). Acutely transforming retroviruses, which incorporate and transmit activated cellular proto-oncogenes at a significant frequency, have brought 12 of these to our attention. The viral *src, abl, fps (fes), yes, fgr, fms, ros, erb*B, *kit,* and *sea* genes each encode protein kinases which phosphorylate tyrosine residues exclusively[8]. The *mos* and *raf (mil* or *mht)* viral genes, in contrast, appear to encode protein kinases with a specificity for serine and threonine[9,10]. Three oncogenes encoding protein kinases with a specificity for tyrosine, *neu, trk,* and *met,* have been found by direct DNA transfection[11].

Divergence of the genes for protein kinases

The plethora of proto-oncogenes encoding protein kinases with a specificity for tyrosine does not reflect simple gene duplication. Although the catalytic domains of this class of protein are highly homologous, each protein possesses a unique domain or domains which may allow regulation of its activity or attend to the deposition of the protein in the correct site within the cell. Presumably, duplication of a gene for a primordial protein kinase gave rise to all these genes but this must have occurred very early in evolution. *Drosophila* contains clearly distinguishable *src, erb*B and *abl* genes which more closely resemble their respective vertebrate descendants than they do each other[12].

Table 1. Proto-oncogenes encoding protein kinases

Oncogene	Polypeptide product	Amino acid specificity	Reference
src	$pp^{60c\text{-}src}$	Tyrosine	
abl	$NCP150^{c\text{-}abl}$	Tyrosine	
erbB	EGF receptor	Tyrosine	
fps (fes)	$NCP98^{c\text{-}fps}$	Tyrosine	
fms	CSF-1 receptor	Tyrosine	
yes	?	Tyrosine	
fgr	?	Tyrosine	
ros	?	Tyrosine	
sea	?	Tyrosine	26
kit	?	Tyrosine	27
mos	$p37^{c\text{-}mos}$	Serine	
raf (mil)	?	Serine/Threonine	
neu	p^{185}	Tyrosine	
met	?	Tyrosine	28
trk	?	Tyrosine	29

NCP = normal cell protein; EGF = epidermal growth factor; CSF-1 = colony stimulating factor 1, also known as macrophage colony stimulating factor.

The biochemistry of transformation by the viral protein kinases

The oncogenic protein kinases induce transformation through either inappropriate or excessive protein phosphorylation. Transformation has profound effects on cells, causing alterations in growth regulation, glucose metabolism and cell shape. Our understanding of the role of protein phosphorylation in the normal regulation of these processes is, however, still fragmentary. Protein phosphorylation most obviously plays an important role in the regulation of cell division. The receptors for at least four polypeptide growth factors (epidermal growth factor, platelet-derived growth factor, insulin-like growth factor and colony stimulating factor I) are protein kinases with a specificity for tyrosine and each is activated upon the binding of the appropriate growth factor[6,7,13]. This suggests strongly that cell division can be initiated by growth factor-induced protein phosphorylation and that oncogenic tyrosine protein kinases may induce unregulated growth through the chronic phosphorylation of the normal substrates of growth factor receptors. The findings that the *erb*B and *fms* oncogenes are derived from the genes for the epidermal growth factor receptor and the colony stimulating factor I receptors, respectively[7,13], and that the *sis* oncogene is derived from the gene for platelet-derived growth factor have demonstrated the validity of this model[6,7].

Subcellular location of growth-regulatory protein kinases

The above-mentioned growth factor receptors all reside in the plasma membrane where their factor-binding sites are exposed on the cell surface and their catalytic domains reside on the cytoplasmic membrane face. One might expect, therefore, that the oncogenic protein kinases would occupy similar sites. This is true in some instances. The products of the *erb*B, *fms, src* and *neu* oncogenes are found in the plasma membrane. In two cases, association with the plasma membrane is apparently essential for transformation. Mutations that prevent deposition of the *src* protein in the plasma membrane prevent transformation[14,15]. Perhaps surprisingly, association with a membrane is not a property of all oncogenic protein kinases. The products of the *mos* and *fps* oncogenes are not bound tightly with membranes[16,17]. We may find that the transforming protein kinases can act at several sites within the cell.

Substrates of the viral tyrosine protein kinases

Once it was realized that the transforming protein of Rous sarcoma virus (RSV), pp60[src], functioned as a tyrosine-specific protein kinase *in vitro*, demonstration that the protein possessed this activity *in vivo* was surprisingly easy. The aggregate action of the endogenous tyrosine protein kinases in uninfected normal fibroblasts yields a remarkably low steady-state amount of tyrosine phosphate in protein, only 0.03% of total acid-stable, protein-bound phosphate. In marked contrast, the amount of phosphotyrosine in protein is ten-fold higher in cells transformed by RSV. Apparently, nine of every ten phosphorylated tyrosine residues in these transformed cells result from the action of pp60[src].

The fact that most proteins containing phosphotyrosine in an RSV-transformed cell are substrates of pp60[src] has facilitated greatly their identification. Eight presumptive substrates are known to date[18]. Three of these, vinculin, p81 and p36, are structural proteins. Three others, enolase, lactate dehydrogenase and phosphoglycerate mutase, are glycolytic enzymes. The remaining two, p50 and p42, are cytosolic proteins of unknown function.

Are these eight proteins the crucial substrates of the transforming tyrosine protein kinases? Probably not. Non-transforming mutants of RSV encoding variants of pp60[src] that are unable to bind to the plasma membrane still induce extensive phosphorylation of most of these eight substrates[14,15]. Additionally, at least two of the viral tyrosine protein kinases, *fms* and *ros*, induce transformation without causing the detectable phosphorylation of any of the above-mentioned eight substrates. It would appear that the crucial substrates of the tyrosine protein kinases with oncogenic potential have yet to be discovered.

The phosphorylation of phosphatidylinositol

Highly purified pp60[src] can also carry out the phosphorylation of phosphatidylinositol to phosphatidylinositol-4-phosphate *in vitro*[19]. Because this reaction is one of the steps in the conversion of phosphatidylinositol to diacylglycerol, the possibility existed that pp60[src] might stimulate directly the production of diacylglycerol. This was of note because both diacylglycerol and a number of tumour promoters induce a partial and reversible form of cell transformation[20], apparently through the activation of protein kinase C[21]. The possibility arose therefore that the important substrate of pp60[src] was phosphatidylinositol rather than cellular polypeptides. However, recent results suggest that the contribution of pp60[src] to total phosphatidylinositol phosphorylating activity in RSV-infected cells is miniscule[22] and therefore unlikely to accelerate significantly the production of diacylglycerol directly. It remains likely therefore that the crucial reaction catalysed by pp60[src] and the related viral transforming proteins is the phosphorylation of polypeptide substrates.

Mechanisms of proto-oncogene activation

The activated forms of all the proto-oncogenes encoding protein kinases function as dominant transforming genetic elements. Introduction of the activated form into cells containing two normal and functioning copies of the unaltered proto-oncogene, either by retrovirus infection or transfection of DNA, yields a cell expressing the transformed phenotype. What is the mechanism of activation? Some of the oncogenic potential of the virally encoded protein kinases is attributable to the fact that their expression is significantly higher than that of their normal counterpart. However, this is certainly not the complete explanation. In almost every case, viral oncogenes have been found either to be truncated or to have undergone mutation. This is unlikely to be mere coincidence. It suggests strongly that the products of activated proto-oncogenes have acquired dominant transforming activity through structural alteration. This could involve changes which either increase the intrinsic enzymatic activity of the protein or relieve an inhibition of enzymatic activity by deletion of regulatory domains. Examples of both are likely to be found.

There is growing evidence that resident proto-oncogenes encoding protein kinases play a role in neoplasias which are induced by agents other than retroviruses. Most striking, perhaps, is the finding that the *abl* gene undergoes rearrangement, as the result of chromosome translocation, in a significant majority of human chronic myelogenous leukemias. This rearrangement results in replacement of the normal aminoterminus of the *abl* protein with a domain encoded by another gene, termed *bcr* (Ref. 23). Activation of the *neu* oncogene, perhaps by mutation, occurs reproducibly in ethylnitrosourea-induced neuroblastomas of BDIX rats[11]. Finally, the transcription of the *mos* gene has been found to have been activated by insertion of a movable genetic element in one murine plasmacytoma[24].

New oncogenic protein kinases

The *raf* and *mos* oncogenes, both of which may encode proteins possessing serine and threonine protein kinase activity, are relatively new members of the family of oncogenes thought to encode protein kinases. This is not because they are newly discovered. Indeed, the fact that *mos* encodes a protein having sequence homology with the cAMP-dependent protein kinase has been known for several years[25]. Rather, uncertainty as to the nature of the enzymatic activity of these proteins is due mainly to the fact that neither shows tyrosine protein kinase activity. Until recently, it was widely believed that all growth regulatory protein kinases would prove to have such a specificity. Realization that tumor promoters may act by activating protein kinase C, a serine and threonine-specific protein kinase, has made more acceptable the idea that other types of protein kinase have oncogenic potential. Indeed the possibility that the gene for protein kinase C may be a proto-oncogene must be kept in mind.

Unequivocal identification of the substrates of viral serine or threonine protein kinases in transformed cells will be an even more formidable task than the identification of the substrates of the tyrosine protein kinases has been. All normal cells contain high endogenous concentrations of serine and threonine protein kinases and the contribution of an introduced viral enzyme to the total activity in transformed cells will be insignificant. Some of the substrates of viral serine and threonine protein kinases will almost certainly prove to differ from those of the viral tyrosine protein kinases. This should make the study of these two oncogenes all the more interesting.

References

1   Toda, T. *et al.* (1985) In yeast, *ras* proteins are controlling elements of adenylate cyclase. *Cell* 40, 27–36
2   Klempnauer, K.-H. *et al.* (1984) Subcellular localization of proteins encoded by oncogenes of avian myeloblastosis virus and avian leukemia virus E26 and by the chicken c-*myb* gene. *Cell* 37, 537–547

3   Abrams, H. D., Rohrschneider, L. R. and Eisenman, R. N. (1982) Nuclear location of the putative transforming protein of avian myelocytomatosis virus. *Cell* 29, 427–439

4   Curran, T., Miller, A. D., Zokas, L. and Verma, I. M. (1984) Viral and cellular *fos* proteins: a comparative analysis. *Cell* 36, 259–268

5   Doolittle, R. F. *et al.* (1983) Simian sarcoma virus onc gene, v-*sis*, is derived from the gene (or genes) encoding a platelet-derived growth factor. *Science* 221, 275–277

6   Sefton, B. M. and Hunter, T. (1984) Tyrosine protein kinases. *Adv. Cyclic Nucleotide & Protein Phosphorylation Res.* 18, 195–226

7   Hunter, T. and Cooper, J. A. (1985) Protein-tyrosine kinases. *Annu. Rev. Biochem.* 54, 897–930

8   Sefton, B. M. The viral tyrosine protein kinases. (1986) *Curr. Top. Microbiol. Immunol.* 123, 39–72

9   Moelling, K. *et al.* (1984) Serine- and threonine-specific protein kinase activities of purified *gag-mil* and *gag-raf* proteins. *Nature* 312, 558–561

10 Maxwell, S. A. and Arlinghaus, R. B. (1985) Serine kinase activity associated with Moloney murine sarcoma virus-124-encoded p37^{mos}. *Virology* 143, 321–333

11 Schechter, A. L. *et al.* (1984) The *neu* oncogene: an *erb-B*-related gene encoding a 185 000-M_r tumour antigen. *Nature* 312, 513–516

12 Hoffmann, F. M. *et al.* (1983) Nucleotide sequences of the *Drosophila src* and *abl* homologs: conservation and variability in the *src* family oncogenes. *Cell* 35, 393–340

13 Scherr, C. J. *et al.* (1985) The c-*fms* proto-oncogene product is related to the receptor for the mononuclear phagocyte growth factor, CSF-1. *Cell* 41, 665–676

14 Cross, F. R. *et al.* (1984) A short sequence in the pp60^{src} N-terminus is required for pp60^{src} myristylation and membrane association, and for cell transformation. *Mol. Cell. Biol.* 4, 1834–1842

15 Kamps, M. P., Buss, J. E. and Sefton, B. M. (1986) Rous sarcoma virus transforming protein lacking myristic acid phosphorylates known polypeptide substrates without inducing transformation. *Cell* 45, 105–112

16 Papkoff, J., Nigg, E. A. and Hunter, T. (1983) The transforming protein of Moloney murine sarcoma virus is a soluble cytoplasmic protein. *Cell* 33, 161–172

17 Feldman, R. A., Wang, E. and Hanafusa, H. (1983) Cytoplasmic localization of the transforming protein of Fujinami sarcoma virus: salt-sensitive association with subcellular components. *J. Virol.* 45, 782–791

18 Cooper, J. A. and Hunter, T. (1984) Regulation of cell growth and transformation by tyrosine-specific protein kinases: the search for important cellular substrate proteins. *Curr. Top. Microbiol. Immunol.* 107, 125–162

19 Sugimoto, Y. *et al.* (1984) Evidence that the Rous sarcoma virus transforming gene product phosphorylates phosphatidylinositol and diacylglycerol. *Proc. Natl Acad. Sci. USA* 81, 2117–2121

20 Driedger, P. E. and Blumberg, P. M. (1977) The effect of phorbol diesters on chicken embryo fibroblasts. *Cancer Res.* 37, 3257–3265

21 Nishizuka, Y. (1983) Phospholipid degradation and signal translation for protein phosphorylation. *Trends Biochem. Sci.* 8, 13–16

22 Sugimoto, Y., and Erikson, R. L. (1985) Phosphatidylinositol kinase activities in normal and Rous sarcoma virus-transformed cells. *Mol. Cell. Biol.* 5, 3194–3198

23 Shtivelman, E. *et al.* (1985) Fused transcript of *abl* and *bcr* genes in chronic myelogenous leukaemia. *Nature* 315, 550–554

24 Kuff, E. L. *et al.* (1983) Homology between an endogenous viral LTR and sequences inserted in an activated cellular oncogene. *Nature* 302, 547–548

25 Barker, W. C. and Dayhoff, M. O. (1982) Viral *src* gene products are related to the catalytic chain of mammalian cAMP-dependent protein kinase. *Proc. Natl Acad. Sci. USA* 79, 2836–2839

26 Hayman, M. J., Kitchener, G., Vogt, P. K. and Beug, H. (1985) The putative transforming protein of S13 avian erythroblastosis virus is a transmembrane glycoprotein with an associated protein kinase activity. *Proc. Natl Acad. Sci. USA* 82, 8237–8241

27 Besmer, P. *et al.* (1986) A new acute transforming feline retrovirus and relationship of its oncogene v-*kit* with the protein kinase gene family. *Nature* 320, 415–421

28 Dean, M. *et al.* (1986) The human *met* oncogene is related to the tyrosine kinase oncogenes. *Nature* 318, 385–388

29 Martin-Zanca, D., Huges, S. H. and Barbacid, M. (1986) A human oncogene formed by the fusion of truncated tropomyosin and protein tyrosine kinase sequences. *Nature* 319, 743–748

B. M. Sefton is at the Molecular Biology and Virology Laboratory, The Salk Institute, PO Box 85800, San Diego, CA 92138, USA.

Immortal genes

Susumu Ohno

Base sequences of certain genes in the mammalian and avian genomes are constructed in a way that endows them with a measure of immortality. Provided that the number of bases in the oligomeric unit is not a multiple of three, coding sequences that are repeats of base oligomers become impervious to the two most dysfunctioning mutational base changes that cause premature chain terminations and reading frameshifts. Oncogene coding sequences as a group appear to have descended from the above type, thus, still possessing a measure of immortality.

In a previous article (*Trends in Genetics* 1, 160–164, 1985) I showed that with unhindered spontaneous mutation rates of the order of 10^{-9} per base pair per year, genes that become dispensable do not readily disappear from the mammalian and avian genomes; their estimated half-life is 50 million years. Here, I show that the base sequences of certain genes are constructed in a way that endows them with a measure of immortality.

Many oncogenic retroviruses and their cellular counterparts in the host genome are now known. Nevertheless, v-*src* of avian Rous sarcoma virus must be considered as the prototype oncogene, for it was in Rous sarcoma virus that its transforming function was first assigned to a single viral gene that specified pp[60v-src] polypeptide with tyrosine-specific kinase activity. Therefore, I shall confine most of my discussion to v-*src* and c-*src*. My already expressed view on vertebrate cellular oncogenes[1] is that those which encode autocrine (endogenous) growth factors of various kinds are evolutionary relics of the past. Needless to say, unicellular eukaryotes have no choice but to depend upon autocrine growth factors, and even growth and differentiation of many multicellular eukaryotes such as insects appear to be cell autonomous, thus suggesting continued dependence upon autocrine factors. With development of the cardiovascular system, vertebrates have forfeited the cell autonomous mode of growth and differentiation. Accordingly, the functions of autocrine growth factors were replaced by endocrine and paracrine growth factors and their specific plasma membrane receptors. While many of the genes for these new endocrine and paracrine growth factors and genes for their receptors were derived either in part or in whole from cellular oncogenes, the oncogenes themselves became evolutionary relics. For example, the tyrosine-specific kinase function of c-*src* and a few other cellular oncogenes is now carried out by an internally protruding portion of the plasma membrane receptor for EGF (epidermal growth factor) as well as that for insulin. If cellular oncogenes are still actively used, their contributions should be limited to the very early stage of embryonic development, before the developmental mobilization of endocrine and paracrine growth factors. Even without the evolutionary consideration noted above, one would still expect many cellular oncogenes to be readily dispensable due to their sheer functional redundancy. Indeed, it has already been shown in *Saccharomyces cerevisiae*, where autocrine growth factors are still of vital importance, that only one of the two c-*ras* related gene loci in the genome is required, the other being readily dispensable[2].

I shall now focus on v-*src* and c-*src*, for they are the rightful prototype of all other oncogenes. The c-*src* coding sequence of the chicken is not really homologous *sensu stricto* with v-*src* coding sequence of Rous sarcoma virus; the last 13 codons of v-*src* are entirely different from codons 515 to 532 of c-*src*. Consequently, while the pp$^{60c\text{-}src}$ polypeptide chain has 532 amino acids pp$^{60v\text{-}src}$ has only 526 (see Fig. 1). Takeya and Hanafusa identified the non-coding segment corresponding to codons 515 to 526 of v-*src* in the chicken genome roughly 920 bp downstream of the c-*src* coding sequence[3]. It is likely that, because of their carboxy terminal sequence differences, pp$^{60c\text{-}src}$ and pp$^{60v\text{-}src}$ do not function in quite the same way (Fig. 1). Indeed, it has been shown that the incorporation of a single copy of v-*src* into the genome will transform the rat fibroblast cell line. Transfection of the same cell line with chicken c-*src* had no appreciable effect, even though these transfected cells were producing pp$^{60c\text{-}src}$ in quantities at least three times that required for transformation by pp$^{60v\text{-}src}$ (Ref. 4). Thus, we can only conjecture about the normal function, if any, of c-*src* in avian and mammalian species.

The first question to ask about v-*src* and other viral oncogenes concerns the selective advantage gained by retroviruses possessing these transforming genes. Aside from plants all eukaryotes can be considered as direct or indirect parasites of plants. One trait favored by natural selection for all forms of parasitic organism is an appropriate degree of functional incompetence. Herbivores as direct 'parasites', for example, should not crop grasses too close to the roots, and their digestive system should be sufficiently ineffective to leave enough nutrients in their dung to fertilize the very grasses they feed upon. Carnivores that feed upon herbivores as indirect parasites should have hunting skills which are barely sufficient to catch the very young, injured, diseased or feeble but not sufficient to catch herbivores in their prime. Since the vertical transmission through germ cells of their hosts rather than the horizontal transmission via infections appears to be the favored mode of propagation of retroviruses, the worst of their predicaments would be to kill their hosts in their reproductive prime. What, then, can they gain by having v-*onc* genes? It appears that natural selection has largely been ignoring v-*src* of Rous sarcoma virus.

Missense and samesense base substitutions that separate the chicken c-*src* from v-*src* of SR-A strain as well as PR-C strain of Rous sarcoma virus are indicated in Fig. 1. Codons after the 514th should not be compared, for the reason already given. In the 514 remaining codons, chicken c-*src* and SR-A v-*src* differ from each other by 9 missense base substitutions and 8 samesense substitutions. Differences between chicken c-*src* and PR-C v-*src* are considerably greater; 21 missense base substitutions and 8 samesense substitutions[3]. If all randomly sustained single-base substitutions are allowed to accumulate in coding sequences, in the absence of natural selection, the ratio between missense and samesense mutations of 2.77 : 1.00 is expected; 21 missense to 8 samesense is 2.625 : 1.00. Thus, it appears that v-*src* of Rous sarcoma virus has largely been ignored by natural selection as it offers no particular selective advantage to the possesser.

More revealing were differences between SR-A v-*src* and PR-C v-*src*. These two v-*src* differed from each other by as many as 26 missense substitutions and 12 samesense substitutions. Thus, differences between c-*src* and two v-*src* were no greater than differences between two v-*srcs* of different strains of Rous sarcoma virus. Aside from the 3' terminal 12 codons, which are derived from a noncoding segment far downstream of c-*src*, there appear to be few characteristics that set apart all the v-*src* of various Rous sarcoma strains from c-*src*. This suggests that, since the birth of Rous sarcoma virus, v-*src* gene has not exactly

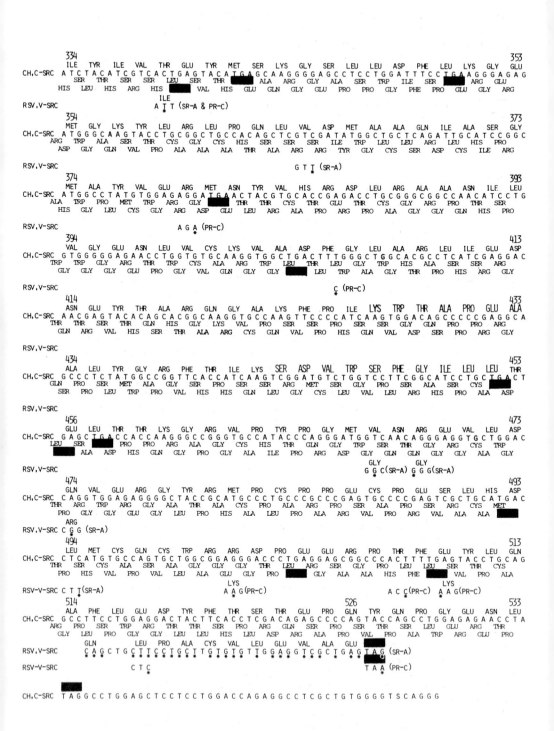

been leading an independent existence. Rather it appears that v-*src* has been lost from the viral genome from time to time and that the virus regained a new v-*src* as a fresh recruit directly from the chicken c-*src*.

Put more succinctly, experimenters in cancer research have been recognizing only those which either maintained original v-*src* or regained a freshly recruited v-*src* as Rous sarcoma virus, ignoring 'v-*src*-less' variants which should be better adapted parasites. In fact, a new transformation-competent Rous sarcoma virus can be recovered from a tumor developed in a chick infected with a transformation-defective mutant of Rous sarcoma virus[3]. Thus, within a single host generation a fraction of the transformation defective Rous sarcoma virus abandoned its mutationally dysfunctional v-*src*, and replaced it with a new v-*src* freshly derived from host c-*src*.

If c-*src* in the chicken genome is of a dubious functional significance and v-*src* does not confer a significant selective advantage to its viral possesser why do c-*src* and v-*src* persist? A crucial point is that certain coding sequences are constructed such that they are relatively impervious to normally dysfunctioning mutational base changes; in a sense they have a measure of immortality. In fact, without a degree of immortality in the first set of coding sequences in the primeval world[1] the emergence of the first cell would have been quite impossible. The assembly of that first cell would have required the presence in the prebiotic world of a minimal, but unknown, variety of coding sequences. The accumulation in the prebiotic world of these coding sequences would have required the qualitative stability of those formed earlier, in spite of subsequent base changes. As far as coding sequences are concerned, two kinds of mutational base change are most dysfunctioning. The first is a base substitution that changes an amino acid-specifying codon to a chain terminator. Unless this occurs very near to the 3′ end of the coding sequence, a shorter mutant polypeptide will be ineffective. The second is a deletion or an insertion of a number of bases that is not a multiple of three. This causes a frameshift, i.e. an alteration of amino acid sequence downstream, and usually ends up in premature chain termination as well. Provided the number of bases in the oligomeric unit is not a multiple of three, the coding sequences that are repeats of base oligomers become impervious to these most dysfunctioning base changes, thus gaining functional immortality. This is illustrated in Fig. 2a on repeats of the tridecameric unit sequence, C A G C A G C C T G C G A which was thought to be the ultimately primordial building block sequence of c-*src*, and therefore v-*src*[1]. Decameric, nonameric and octameric portions of the above tridecameric unit recur in the coding sequence of c-*src* as well as v-*src* (Figs 1 and 3).

Fig. 1. The 3′ terminal 37.5% of the coding sequence of c-src *of the chicken identified by Takeya and Hanafusa[3] is shown in ten rows.* pp$^{60c\text{-}src}$ *amino acid sequences encoded by the utilized reading frame of* c-src *are shown above the rows of bases, whereas amino acid residues encodable by two unused reading frames are shown in two rows below bases in small capital letters. Each chain terminator of every reading frame is identified by a black box. Mutational base substitutions that separate* v-src *of two (SR-A and PR-C) strains of Rous sarcoma virus from* c-src *are shown below each row and their origins are identified as either SR-A or PR-C. Only missense base substitutions are accompanied by corresponding amino acid residues. The 3′ 12 codons of both* v-src *below codon 514 are not derived from the corresponding codons of* c-src; *this segment is derived from a non-coding segment roughly 920 bp downstream of* c-src *coding sequence in the chicken genome[3].*

(a)   Wild type

```
Arg   Gln   Gln   Pro   Ala   Thr   Ala   Ala   Cys   Asp
 G A/C A G C A G C C T G C G A/C A G C A G C C T G C G A/C A
   Asp   Ser   Ser   Leu   Arg   Gln   Gln   Pro   Ala   Thr
     Thr   Ala   Ala   Cys   Asp   Ser   Ser   Leu   Arg   Gln
```

```
Ser   Ser   Leu   Arg   Gln
 G C A G C C T G C G A/C A
   Ala   Ala   Cys   Asp
     Gln   Pro   Ala   Thr
```

(b)   1st silencing mutation

```
Arg   Gln   Gln   Pro   Ala   Thr   Ala   Ala   ▓▓▓▓
 G A/C A G C A G C C T G C G A/C A G C A G C C T G A G A/C A
                                                     ▪
```

```
G C A G C C T G C G A/C A
```
                                        2nd resurrecting deletion

```
Arg   Gln   Gln   Pro⌐
 G A/C A G C A G C C T G⤬G A/C A G C A G C C T G A G A/C A
                    └─Gly   Gln   Gln   Pro   Glu   Thr
```

```
G C A G C C T G C G A/C A
   Ala   Ala   Cys   Asp
```

Fig. 2. Repeats of the tridecameric unit sequence C A G C A G C C T G C G A give tridecapeptidic periodicity to a polypeptide chain (a). This sequence is inherently impervious to frameshifting deletions and insertions (b).

Inasmuch as 13 is not a multiple of three, three consecutive copies of the tridecameric sequence, totaling 39 bases, give the tridecapeptidic periodicity to a polypeptide chain encoded by this repeated coding sequence (see Fig. 2a). This is to be contrasted with repeats of a longer pentadecameric unit ($N = 3 \times 5$) which can give only a pentapeptic periodicity to its polypeptide. The very fact that within a given reading frame, the unit is already translated in all three different reading frames implies that if one reading frame of this type of coding sequences is open, the other two are automatically open as well; the coding sequence of this type encodes three polypeptide chains of the identical periodicity in its all three reading frames. Thus, this kind of coding sequences is impervious both to a premature chain termination which affects only one of the three reading frames and to frameshifting insertions and deletions[1]. For example, let us assume that Cys codon T G C of the first reading frame shown immediately above the tridecameric repeats has sustained a single base substitution to become a chain terminator T G A as shown in Fig 2b. This would shorten the polypeptide chain encoded by the first reading frame probably silencing it functionally. But the other two reading frames also open would continue to encode polypeptide chains of the identical tridecapeptidic periodicity. Hence the immortality of such a coding sequence. Even if the first reading frame was the only one utilized, each of the other two reading frames lacking an in-phase chain initiator A T G, the silencing would only be temporary. This is because for either a single base insertion or deletion occurring upstream of a mutationally created T G A, such as a deletion of middle C from Ala codon G C G of the first reading frame (see Fig. 2b) would allow a shift to the third reading frame still open. By such a frameshift, the tripeptidic periodicity of a resurrected polypeptide chain would show a disturbance confined only to one period, (see Fig. 2b). Hence the inherent imperviousness to frameshifting deletions and insertions embodied in such a coding sequence.

In most modern coding sequences, both unused reading frames are full of chain terminators occurring at the expected intervals of every 20 or 21 codons. This suggests that either they have descended from oligomeric repeats of the unit sequence with multiples of three of bases or they have diverged too far and almost completely lost their original periodicity. By contrast, most oncogene coding sequences are characterized by possession of one or both long, unused open reading frames which is correlated with easily recognizable remnants of internal repetitiousness within their coding sequences[1]. In the case of c-src, the first of the two unused reading frames is open for the first 240 codons[3]. Even with regard to the 3' 38% of the c-src coding sequence shown in Fig. 1, the first of the two unused reading frames identified immediately below each row of base sequence contains only five chain terminators; an average of one every 46 codons. Accordingly, there were two open stretches in this unused reading frame: one of 71 codons (rows 3 to 6 of Fig. 1) and the other of 77 codons (the last four rows of Fig. 1). Even with regard to the second of the two unused reading frames, the average interval between chain terminators was 47 codons. Because of their ultimate origin from repeats of ($N = 3n \pm 1$ or 2) base oligomers, oncogene coding sequences appear to retain long, open stretches in their unused reading frames, which gives them a measure of immortality.

In fact, the inherent imperviousness of v-src coding sequence of Rous sarcoma virus to base substitutions, frameshifting deletions and insertions has amply been demonstrated by the first ever sequenced v-src published in 1980[5]. This v-src coding sequence differed from the chicken genomic c-src coding sequence[3], not only by 11 samesence and 17 missense base substitutions but also by five single base deletions and one double base deletion as well as by 17 single base insertions and two double base insertions. Accordingly, this v-src coding sequence switched to one or the other normally unused reading frames of c-src 14 times. Yet all the functionally critical active site sequences for its tyrosine specific phosphorylase activity were conserved. Such then is an extent of immortality conferred by the possession of long open reading frames in its unused phases. It should be recalled that normally a mere single base deletion or insertion suffices to silence a common coding sequence of vertebrates.

I shall end with the observed instance of v-src gene resurrecting itself from the dead by using a segment of the long, unused open reading frame noted above. In

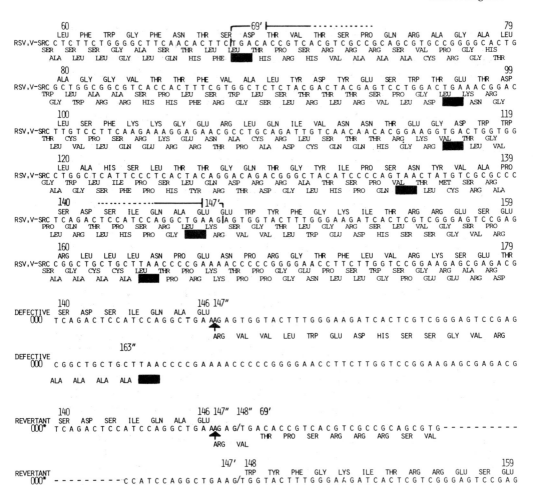

Fig. 3 *The top six rows represent a portion of a particular* v-src *coding sequence studied by Mardon and Varmus[5] encoding residues 60 to 187 of* pp[60v-src], *shown above each row of bases. Amino acid residues encodable by two unused reading frames are shown in two rows below bases using smaller capital letters. The first of the two unused reading frames shown immediately below bases is open along the entire stretch. Rows 7 and 8 identified as 000 reveal an insertion of A (identified by an arrow) between Glu 146 codon GAA and Glu 147 codon GAG as the cause of mutational silencing of* v-src. *This insertion caused the reading frame to shift to the second of the two unused reading frames, which happened to have a chain terminator TAA, 17 codons downstream; thus, a functionless short polypeptide chain that ended in Ala 163 was produced. The last two rows identified as 000* reveal a duplicative insertion of the 239 base segment identified in rows 1 to 4 of this figure into the position indicated by a slash in the second row from the bottom that resurrected* v-src. *Within the inserted segment, the reading frame shifted from the second of the unused to the first of the unused from Thr 69 downward, and a resulting double frameshift restored the original utilized reading frame to Trp 148 and thereafter. By this duplicative insertion, a new 607 residue* pp[60v-src] *regained its tyrosine-specific kinase activity, therefore, its transforming property.*

the rat cell line transformed by the genomic incorporation of a single copy of Rous sarcoma v-*src*, Mardon and Varmus[6] isolated a mutant that had lost the transformed phenotype and identified its cause as the mutational insertion of A between two Glu codons GAA and GAG of positions 146 and 147 (see two rows identified as 000 of Fig. 3). Thus, a shift in the reading frame to the second of the two unused reading frames occurred and this second unused reading frame happened to contain the chain terminator TAA, 17 codons downstream of the insertion. Accordingly, a mutated v-*src* began to encode a functionless 163 residue polypeptide chain. So far, the story is very familiar. Within this mutated transformation-defective cell line, a secondary mutant which had regained the transformed phenotype appeared[6]. Thus, once silenced, v-*src* resurrected itself by a second mutational event which was a duplicative insertion of a 239 base segment (representing roughly codons 68 to 146 of the utilized reading frame) into the position three bases downstream of the previously inserted A, as shown in the last two rows identified as 000* of Fig. 3. Since this inserted segment was now translated in the first of the two unused reading frames, the resulting double frameshifts restored the original reading frame to Trp 148 and downward. Accordingly, this doubly mutated v-*src* now encoded a 607 residue polypeptide chain that regained the tyrosine-specific kinase activity. This type of resurrection of v-*src* would have been impossible unless its (and therefore c-*src*'s) ultimate ancestor was a repeating ($N = 3n \pm 1$ or 2) base oligomer. First, there would not have been a 97 codon unused open reading frame which was a part of the longer 240 codon alternative open reading frame. Secondly, the insertion of a new amino acid sequence (97 residues or so long) into the enzyme molecule would surely have interfered with the enzyme's activity. Fortunately, this first of the two unused reading frames originally specified the same periodical polypeptide chain as the utilized reading frame of v-*src*; thus, a new inserted 97 residue amino acid sequence was similar to that of the amino-terminal sequence of v-*src*[1]. For example, residues 11 to 18 of pp$^{60v\text{-}src}$ are Pro–Ser–Gln–Arg–Arg–Ser–Leu which is quite homologous with the heptapeptidic sequence Pro–Ser–Arg–Arg–Ser–Val from the inserted segment translated in the first of the two unused reading frames (the top and second from the last rows of Fig. 3). As to the internal repetitiousness, the head and the tail of the inserted segment translated from the first of the two unused reading frames are capped by the identical tetrapeptidic sequence, Thr–Pro–Ser–Arg (rows 1 and 4 of Fig. 3).

References

1 Ohno, S. (1984) Repeats of base oligomers as the primordial coding sequences of the primeval earth and their vestiges in modern genes. *J. Mol. Evol.* 20, 313–321

2 Tatchell, K., Chalett, D. T., DeFoe-Jones, D. and Scolnick, E. M. (1984) Requirement of either of a pair of *ras*-related genes of *Saccharomyces cerevisiae* for spore virility. *Nature* 309, 523–527

3 Takeya, T. and Hanafusa, H. (1983) Structure and sequence of the cellular gene homologous to the RSV *src* gene and the mechanism for generating the transforming virus. *Cell* 32, 881–890

4 Parker, R. C., Varmus, H. E. and Bishop, J. M. (1984) Expression of v-*src* and chicken c-*src* in rat cells demonstrates qualitative differences between pp$^{60v\text{-}src}$ and pp$^{60c\text{-}src}$. *Cell* 37, 131–139

5 Czenilofsky, A. P. *et al.* (1980) Nucleotide sequence of an avian sarcoma virus

oncogene (*SRC*) and proposed amino acid sequence for gene product. *Nature* 287, 198–203

6   Mardon, G. and Varmus, H. E. (1983) Frameshift and intragenic suppression mutations in a Rous Sarcoma provirus suggest *SRC* encodes two proteins. *Cell* 32, 871–879

S. Ohno is at the Beckman Research Institute of the City of Hope, 1450 East Duarte Road, Duarte, CA 91010, USA.

Oncogenes, processed genes and safety of genetic manipulation

Ditta Bartels, Hiroto Naora and Atuhiro Sibatani

Recent findings in eukaryote molecular biology[1] prompt us to revise our ideas on heredity, and developmental and evolutionary biology. Such a revision should encompass mutations caused by insertion, lateral gene transfers, reverse transcription, and the gene family concept (including pseudogenes and processed genes), as well as movable genetic elements.

Retroviruses and oncogenes

The emerging picture of biology should also include another set of newly acquired views, namely those concerning oncogenes[2-8] and retroviruses[9,10]. Retroviruses have an intronless RNA genome, which replicates by way of reverse transcription into double-stranded DNA. This proviral DNA usually integrates into the host's genetic material and becomes transcribed. Furthermore, the retroviruses may incorporate certain genes from their hosts, in particular oncogenes. For this and other reasons the retroviruses are often tumorigenic agents. Long terminal repeats (LTR) which are part of the retroviral provirus, are instrumental in the various steps of the virus replication cycle. Whereas circular DNA intermediates also participate in the replication events, the virus's ultimate form is a linear integrated sequence containing almost complete LTRs at both ends. In this respect, the genomic retroviral DNA differs from the circular as well as from the integrated form of polyoma virus DNA, which lacks such terminal repeated sequences.

The oncogenes comprise a set of related distinct genes which are normal and apparently essential components of the mammalian and avian genome, and are usually expressed at very low levels. However, oncogenes can become part of retroviral genomes, and thereafter they are transcribed at greatly enhanced levels and propagated through the viral replication cycle. These events are set in motion when retroviral DNA happens to insert itself into the eukaryote host genome in the vicinity of an oncogene. Retroviruses which contain oncogenes are acutely tumorigenic when injected into animals.

In general the cellular oncogenes (c-*onc*) contain introns, but when they become reintegrated into the host genome following their passage through the retrovirus replication cycle, they will have undergone gene splicing due to post-transcriptional modification and hence they appear as 'processed' genes without introns. It seems that oncogenes can be expressed either in the c-*onc* state with introns, or in the proviral v-*onc* state without introns.

Additionally, cellular oncogenes may also be activated through diverse carcinogenic events and fully expressed in a malignant tumour without the intervention of a retrovirus. Both retroviral v-*onc* DNA as well as c-*onc* DNA obtained from cancer cells can transform cultured NIH 3T3 cells. But the oncogenes of normal cells, though sometimes differing from the c-*onc* genes of cancer cells in only one nucleotide[11,12], have little transforming potential. Obviously the presence or absence of introns in an oncogene is not crucial to the process of cell transformation. Whereas activation of the c-*onc* gene by a retrovirus may occur through the molecular control element of the LTR, other mechanisms of activation must also exist. This conclusion can be drawn since the viral control element is missing in non-virus-generated tumours, and since the orientation and the position of the integrated viral or non-viral control element seem not to be specific[2,13].

Such novel aspects of the eukaryote genome and of oncogenes are reported almost daily in the literature and discussed at meetings. At the same time there is, however, a curious lack of comment about the implications of these findings for the issue of safety in genetic manipulation.

Methylation of genomes

There can be little doubt that these exciting new findings are a direct outcome of molecular biologists employing recombinant DNA techniques. Nevertheless, the emerging information also has a bearing on the assessment of safety in recombinant DNA research. In this context we should consider the activation mechanism of the Moloney murine leukaemia (MML) retrovirus which is stably integrated into the genome of the mouse substrain *Mov-3* (Ref. 14). The integrated provirus has been shown to be inactive in an infection assay, but it acquires infectivity when the relevant genomic fragment is cloned in *E. coli*. Moreover, the change from a non-infectious to an infectious state is associated with the demethylation of specific cytosine residues in the DNA. Thus, the originally inactive, methylated proviral DNA produces non-methylated, infectious DNA as a result of bacterial cloning.

Polyoma DNA revisited

These experiments with MML retrovirus are somewhat reminiscent of those cloning experiments in which polyoma virus DNA was used to test the safety of recombinant DNA work. It will be recalled that anxiety about the hazards of gene splicing related primarily to the possibility that infection and/or tumorigenesis might be brought about by *E. coli* harbouring a harmful viral genome. This could result either from the intended cloning of pathogenic DNA or, unwittingly, through shot-gun experiments in which random fragments of DNA harbouring latent but potentially oncogenic sequences are used. This concern was expelled with a sigh of relief, when polyoma virus DNA cloned in *E. coli* gave largely negative results in its various pathogenicity tests.

The polyoma virus was chosen because its pathogenicity is restricted to rodents, and because of the ease with which viral protein can be immunologically detected[15]. Polyoma DNA, integrated into plasmid or bacteriophage vectors and then cloned in *E. coli*, was tested for viral infectivity (tested *in vivo* by mouse feeding or injection, and *in vitro* by fibroblast transfection), and also for tumorigenicity (tested by injection into new-born hamsters)[15–18].

Following their cloning in bacteria, only the vectors containing head-to-tail polyoma dimers displayed some infectivity, whereas the vectors containing a polyoma monomer were quite active in inducing tumours. All the vectors became inactive when they were encapsulated in bacteria.

The negative results obtained from the viral-infectivity experiments were to be expected. Polyoma DNA is a circular duplex and its digestion by restriction enzymes is certain to inactivate some viral genes. Thus, bacterially cloned polyoma DNA is likely to be defective in one of the virus genes; hence, virus production will not readily ensue. However, when a polyoma DNA dimer is inserted into the cloning vector, a recombination event can occur, resulting in the production of an intact viral genome. Infectivity which necessitates virus production and hence an intact viral genome, is thus expected in the case of a dimer, but not in the case of a monomer.

By contrast, tumour induction can take place in the absence of the replicative integrity of the viral genome[17,19]. Thus, vectors harbouring a defective monomer of polyoma DNA were as active in tumorigenesis as the native supercoiled DNA itself. Surprisingly, cleavage by various restriction enzymes actually increased tumorigenicity. This was particularly pronounced in the case of the enzyme XbaI which is known to destroy one of the T-antigen genes involved in viral replication. Here, cleaved viral DNA was 100% tumorigenic (28/28 with 0.5 μg DNA).

Interpretation of experiments

The polyoma safety-testing experiments were interpreted as follows: in no case does the cloning of viral DNA increase infectivity to over and above that of the original viral DNA, and in most cases cloning actually reduces or abolishes infectivity. Thus, the belief arose that cloned DNA, whether it is incorporated in self-replicating entities or is present in isolated form, is no more dangerous than the original pathogen itself and is usually much safer than the latter, when one compares equivalent quantities in terms of the multiplicity of the biologically active material. It then follows that any biological experiment involving a pathogen's DNA can be more safely conducted with a cloned genome of the pathogen than with the original organism. But it should be noted that one can expand the potentially infectious material more easily by cloning it in E. coli than by propagating the pathogen itself in a more complex system.

One can argue that the relative safety of the cloned polyoma DNA is at least partially due to the fact that for cloning purposes the circular viral genome must first be converted into linear form by artificial means, thus usually destroying the integrity of some viral gene. Furthermore, the recombination by which the intact viral genome is recovered from the vector harbouring a monomer viral DNA (either before or after its entrance into the host cell) is quite a rare event (cf. Ref. 20)

The relevance of retroviruses in relation to the safety of recombinant-DNA research lies in the fact that being linear, the retroviral genome need not be cleaved for cloning purposes, and therefore cloning does not destroy the native genomic order. Moreover, the viral genome need not be tandemly duplicated, nor excised from the vector or host chromosome for transcription to occur, and yet transcription alone is sufficient for the retrovirus to go into the next replication cycle. Hence, the complication which is inherent in gene splicing of circular-DNA viruses such as polyoma does not pertain to retroviruses. Furthermore, the latent provirus of a retrovirus is intronless; this removes one barrier to the expression of eukaryote genes in prokaryote cells, a point which is repeatedly mentioned in recent discussions on the safety of gene technology. Accordingly retroviral DNA which carries an oncogene or any other processed gene without distorted base sequences may be expressed in prokaryote hosts so that the gene-coded protein is produced. The same argument may apply to cloned cDNA of cancerous cells in which some oncogenes are actively transcribed.

If we compare the situation between polyoma and retroviruses, we observe the following. Polyoma virus DNA was chosen to test the safety of recombinant-DNA research because of convenience, rather than for its a priori theoretical suitability. But if we consider the linear nature of the retroviral genome, its characteristically different mode of replication, its high affinity for the host genome, and the putative insertions of human oncogenes into retroviruses, then the inclusion of retroviruses in safety-testing, especially with respect to viral infection, becomes imperative. It is clear that there is a need to reassess the conclusions reached in 1979 with respect to the biological safety of gene splicing. Future tests should include oncogenic retrovirus genomes or even some small RNA virus genomes converted to their DNA form by artificial reverse transcription.

In view of these considerations let us turn back to the experiments with MML retrovirus[14]. Prior to its cleavage from the plasmid vector, the cloned proviral DNA already had 20% infectivity when compared with active viral DNA. This was at least 17 times higher than the control data. Fragmentation of the cloned DNA by treatment with restriction enzyme *Eco*RI increased infectivity even further. Thus, from the point of view of infectivity and probably also of tumorigenicity, cloned DNA is not always an innocuous substance, especially after it has been treated with appropriate restriction enzymes. In this context, it is important to note that DNA and its cleavage by restriction enzymes are routinely handled outside of the physical containment area of the laboratory. We also note that, unexpectedly, DNA is quite stable in the soil[21], although it is easily destroyed in acid.

In 1979, Martin[22] actually admitted that his group's results with polyoma virus DNA could not be applied to retroviruses. However, at the time he was unable to test the infectivity of cloned retrovirus DNA in animals, as he felt constrained by the US regulations pertaining to the usage of potential vectors in mammalian cells. Since then the inhibiting regulatory requirements have been relaxed considerably, and no practical objections now obstruct risk-assessment experiments involving retroviruses.

Is gene expression density-dependent?

As mentioned above, the oncogenes of normal cells may be activated without the intervention of retroviruses. A theory is now being developed, according to which the spatial distribution of genes influences their expression, so that the individual gene requires a certain territory around itself or a minimum gene density in the DNA sequence for its full expression[23]. Similar opinions have been expressed[24]. A pseudogene of *Xenopus* 5S rRNA, which is normally untranscribed, can be transcribed when isolated from the neighbouring active 5S rRNA gene[25]. Similarly, recent findings indicate that a chromosomal translocation may activate one of the human oncogenes, apparently without the involvement of the transcriptional control machinery[13]. In fact, the DNA of normal vertebrate cells can acquire transforming activity following digestion with restriction enzymes, especially after secondary transfection[14]. In essence this process may be regarded as the molecular cloning of oncogenes in animal cells. Furthermore, it has been pointed out[6] that the transformation of cells by retroviruses may activate a separate oncogene which is not linked to the infecting retrovirus genome. Thus, we have to keep in mind the possibility that oncogenes from normal cells may become actively tumorigenic once they are cloned in either bacterial or in animal cells.

At present the possibility cannot be completely dismissed that the cloning of retroviral DNA could lead to the production of virus particles in bacterial cells, due to the intronless nature of the viral genome. This uncertainty, however, can be removed rather easily by appropriate tests and need not remain a complicating factor in the safety issue. Considering the diverse nature of oncogenes, it is impossible to ascertain how far one can generalize about their infectious and tumorigenic properties. It seems that we are faced with the old uncertainty of 1974 concerning the possible biohazard of experiments involving eukaryote genomes. However, now we are in a better position than at the start of the debate in so far as we can specify the type of possible biohazard that may ensue.

Conclusions and recommendation

The scientific community became sceptical of the reality of biohazards in recombinant DNA work, when it was revealed that eukaryote genes are generally interspersed by introns and hence cannot be expressed in prokaryotes. However, the frequency of processed genes without introns in higher animals[1,26] clearly indicates that we are now back at the point of departure. During the intervening period of 4 years most of the stringency conditions which were initially incorporated in various local and national guidelines have been scrapped. Until more is known about the expression of cloned processed genes in bacteria, uncertainty about the biohazard of cloning animal DNA will remain. It might also be expected that, in animal and human genomes, many oncogene families have not only pseudogenes with introns, but also processed genes of normal sequence without introns, which may become active after cloning in prokaryotes. Incidentally, a human retrovirus causing adult T-cell leukaemia, endemic to south-western Japan, has now been demonstrated in peripheral blood lymphocytes of some healthy persons[27]. Similar human retroviruses are now known from other parts of the world[28].

Finally, the scientific community seems to have become rather wary of again involving itself in the debate on the hazards of gene manipulation[29]. The question arises as to whether we raised a false alarm too often, or whether we are simply carried away by the profound biological insights which are currently being generated by gene manipulation. One may compare the shrill voice of past years levelled against charges of possible hazard with the deafening silence which prevails at present. This is neither logical nor consistent behaviour for scientists who urged that rationality be adhered to on all sides.

If specialists in molecular biology find it difficult to grasp the essence of recent findings, which by their nature are so complex and fast-moving, how difficult does criticism become for transdisciplinary scientists, for science critics and for the lay public? It is surely time to call again for a system of review of the hazards involved in various aspects of our work. The arguments need to be based on pertinent experiments conceived in the light of current knowledge. For some time to come the scope of such experiments should be steadily expanded to cover a wider range of pathogens. This is a commonplace biological precaution, and considering the rapid pace of development in molecular biology, such a review should take place on a regular basis.

Conclusion

Since 1983 a number of findings regarding oncogene DNA have come to light which make it considerably more urgent to conduct risk assessment studies in this area. As yet no such studies have been carried out, and the suggestions developed here could provide a suitable starting point.

References
1   Dover, G. A. and Flavell, R. G., eds (1982) *Genome Evolution*, Academic Press, New York
2   Bishop, J. M. (1982) *Sci. Am.* 246(3), 69–78

3   Weinberg, R. A. (1982) *Trends Biochem. Sci.* 7, 135–136
4   Rigby, P. W. J. (1982) *Nature (London)* 297, 451–453
5   Parada, L. F., Tabin, C. J., Shih, C. and Weinberg, R. A. (1982) *Nature (London)* 297, 474–478
6   Cooper, C. M. (1982) *Science* 218, 801–806
7   Santos, E., Tronick, S. R., Aaronson, S. A., Pulciani, S. and Barbacid, M. (1982) *Nature (London)* 298, 343–347
8   Shimotohno, K. and Temin, H. M. (1982) *Nature (London)* 299, 265–268
9   Varmus, H. E. (1982) *Science* 216, 818–820
10 Weiss, R. A. (1982) *Virus Persistence, Proc. Symp. Soc. Gen. Microbiol.* (Mahy, B. W. J., Minson, A. C. and Darby, G. K., eds), Vol. 33, pp. 267–288, Cambridge University Press, Cambridge
11 Tabin, C. J., Bradley, S. M., Bargmann, C. I., Weinberg, R. A., Papageorge, A. G., Scolnick, E. M., Dhar, R., Lowy, D. R. and Chang, E. H. (1982) *Nature (London)* 300, 143–149
12 Reddy, E. P., Reynolds, R. K., Stantos, E. and Barbacid, M. (1982) *Nature (London)* 300, 149–152
13 Marx, J. L. (1982) *Science* 218, 983–985
14 Harbers, K., Schneike, A., Stuhlmann, H., Jähner, D. and Jaenisch, R. (1981) *Proc. Natl Acad. Sci. USA* 78, 7609–7613
15 Israel, M. A., Chan, H. W., Rowe, W. P. and Martin, M. A. (1979) *Science* 203, 883–887
16 Chan, H. W., Israel, M. A., Garon, C. F., Rowe, W. P. and Martin, M. A. (1979) *Science* 203, 887–892
17 Martin, M. A., Chan, H. W., Israel, M. A. and Rowe, W. P. (1979) *Recombinant DNA and Genetic Experimentation* (Morgan, J. and Whelan, W. J., eds), pp. 195–203, Pergamon Press, Oxford
18 Fried, M., Ball, W., Weissmann, C., Klein, B., Murray, K., Greenaway, P. and Tooze, J. (1979) *Recombinant DNA and Genetic Experimentation* (Morgan, J. and Whelan, W. J., eds), pp. 205–208, Pergamon Press, Oxford
19 Israel, M. A., Simmons, D. T., Hourihan, S. L., Rowe, W. P., and Martin, M. A. (1979) *Proc. Natl Acad. Sci. USA* 76, 3713–3716
20 Binétruy, B., Meneguzzi, G., Breathnach, R. and Cuzin, F. (1982) *EMBO J.* 1, 621–628
21 Stotzky, G. (1981) Cited by Novick, R. P. (1982) *Plasmid* 7, 105–106
22 Martin, M. A. (1979) *Recombinant DNA and Genetic Experimentation* (Morgan, J. and Whelan, W. J., eds), p. 209, Pergamon Press, Oxford
23 Naora, H. and Deacon, N. H. (1982) *Differentiation* 21, 1–6
24 Brown, A. L. (1982) *Nature (London)* 298, 793–794
25 Miller, J. R. and Melton, D. A. (1981) *Cell* 24, 829–835
26 Marx, J. L. (1982) *Science* 216, 969–970
27 Gotoh, Y., Sugamura, K. and Hinuma, Y. (1982) *Proc. Natl Acad. Sci. USA* 79, 4780–4782
28 Popovic, M., Reitz, M. S., Jr, Sarngadharan, M. G., Robert-Guroff, M., Kalyanaraman, V. S., Nakao, Y., Miyoshi, I., Minowada, J., Yoshida, M., Ito, Y. and Gallo, R. C. (1982) *Nature (London)* 300, 63–66
29 Watson, J. D. and Tooze, J. (1981) *The DNA Story*, Freeman, San Francisco

Ditta Bartels is at the School of History and Philosophy of Science, University of New South Wales, 2033, Australia. Hiroto Naora is at the Molecular Biology Unit, Research School of Biological Sciences, The Australian National University, PO Box 475, Canberra, ACT 2601, Australia. Atuhiro Sibatani is at the Kansai Medical University, 18–89 Uyamahigashi Osaka 573, Japan.

Addendum – *D. Bartels, H. Naora and A. Sibatani*

The conclusion we came to in our above paper was that before 1983 adequate risk assessment studies had not been carried out to determine whether or not laboratory manipulations with oncogenes were safe. On the basis of the scientific evidence available, it seemed to us imperative that such risk assessment work should be conducted. This basic situation has not changed in the meantime. But the oncogene research findings obtained in the intervening period point more specifically at the types of risk assessment studies which should be undertaken.

Safety testing of oncogene DNA

It is now well known that oncogene DNA transforms not only the precancerous NIH3T3 cells, but also normal cells[30]. This raises the question of whether the accidental injection of oncogene DNA into laboratory workers, say activated *ras* together with activated *myc*, could also result in a cancerous outcome. It should be recalled that the injection of v-*src* into chickens gives rise to small tumour nodules[31].

In the interest of laboratory safety an experimental program should therefore be set up in which various combinations of activated oncogenes are injected into animals, using not only immunologically competent, but also immunologically deficient organisms such as nude mice. In these experiments the initial objective should be to achieve the production of tumours in the injected animals. On the basis of the findings obtained, it will then be possible to assess the likely risks to laboratory workers engaged in the manipulation of oncogenes, and to design appropriate protective measures so that this work is not impeded.

Safety testing of enhancers

It is now also known that enhancer elements are very important in cancer causation, and yet the safety implications of this have not been considered. For example, the microinjection of certain *myc*-enhancer constructs into mouse embryos invariably brings about the development of lymphoid malignancies[32]. Since injection into live animals is more relevant to risk assessment than micro-injection into embryos, constructs bearing enhancers should be submitted to risk assessment studies involving their injection into live animals. As before, the objective of the work should be to determine the conditions *for* cancer induction, so that appropriate protective measures can then be applied.

It should be noted that in these suggested risk assessment experiments what is at stake is the potential hazard posed to laboratory workers by oncogene DNA and/or by enhancer DNA *per se*, and not by recombinant organisms containing such genetic material.

Safety testing of bacteria producing oncogene proteins

But this is not to say that recombinant organisms containing oncogene DNA can invariably be assumed to be safe. The production of oncogene proteins can now be achieved at very high rates of efficiency in *E. coli*[33]. On the basis of certain assumptions decided upon at the 1980 NIH Workshop of Risk Asssess-ment at Pasadena[34], it can be calculated that in the case of an accident, if oncogene expression vectors are transferred from laboratory bacteria to all the *E. coli* of the gut, but not to any of the other 99% of gut bacteria, then about 25 mg of oncogene protein would be produced in the gut per day.

We do not know whether these oncogene proteins could survive in the gut and penetrate the mucosal barrier. We also do not know whether these proteins could produce a carcinogenic event in the mucosal cells or be transported by the bloodstream to a target site in the bladder or the bone marrow and result in cancer there. But these questions are amenable to experimental investigation, and the effort should be made to determine whether laboratory work with high efficiency producers of oncogene proteins is safe. It is also relevant that the vectors employed in this work are not pBR322 which had been tested for transmissibility to gut *E. coli* and found to be safe[35]. The vectors employed currently have not been tested in this way.

References

30 Land, H., Parada, L. F. and Weinberg, R. A. (1983) *Nature* 304, 596–606
31 Fung, Y. K. T., Crittenden, L. B., Fadly, A. M. and Kung, H. J. (1983) *Proc Natl Acad. Sci. USA* 80, 596–606
32 Adams, J. M., Harris, A. W., Pinkert, C. A., Corcoran, L. M., Alexander, W. S., Cory, S., Palmiter, R. D. and Brinster, R. L. (1985) *Nature* 318, 533–538
33 Lautenberg, J. A., Ulsh, L., Shih, T. Y. and Papas, T. S. (1983) *Science* 221, 858–860
34 Workshop on Recombinant DNA Risk Assessment, Pasadena, California (1980) *Recomb. DNA Tech. Bull.* 3, 111–128
35 Levy, S. B., Marshall, B. and Onderdonk, A. (1980) *Science* 209, 391–394

Growth factors

Growth factors and oncogenes

Antony Burgess

The regulation of the production of normal cells of the skin, blood and intestine has attracted considerable interest since the very earliest days of tissue culture[1,2]. The proliferation of normal cells has long been known to depend on specific proteins – called growth factors. However, the experimental systems were so complex and poorly understood, that only the persistence of a few biochemists kept the rather complex field of growth factor chemistry moving forward[3]. Now, after the discovery of the retroviral oncogenes[4] and their cellular equivalents[5], it is our knowledge of growth factors[6-12], their receptors[9] and their mode of action[11,12], which is paving the way for understanding the functional nature of the molecular lesions which give rise to cancer cells[13-16]. Each cellular system has its unique features but here I discuss some of the similarities in the molecular regulation of proliferation and differentiation in both normal and transformed cells from several different tissues.

What are growth factors?

Although all of the essential components of culture media could be described as growth factors, there are sets of proteins which appear to be responsible for the proliferation and differentiation of the cells in specific tissues. Perhaps the most extensively studied are epidermal growth factor (EGF)[11], nerve growth factor (NGF)[17] and T-cell growth factor[9,10,18]. The amino acid sequences of EGF and NGF have been known for a decade[19,20], but it was not until 1983 that detailed structural information for other growth factors such as platelet-derived growth factor[14,21] (PDGF), the regulators of blood cell growth, e.g. T-cell growth factor (also called interleukin-2, IL-2[9,10,22]), and the colony stimulating factors[23,24] became available.

The different tissue-specific growth factors appear to have little in common structurally (although even the early reports searched for amino acid sequence homologies between molecules such as NGF and insulin). However, 'growth' factors can be grouped together functionally because they all stimulate DNA synthesis in cultures of the appropriate target cells. For some tissues, the growth factors are not only required for stimulating the proliferation of the immature cells, but also for the survival of these cells[9,25-27]. Once under the influence of the growth factor, those target cells which require growth factor for survival, appear to be capable of tissue-specific differentiation programmes. As well as stimulating the progenitor cells, the mature cells of some lineages are activated by the appropriate growth factors[27-29]. It is now envisaged that these proteins are not only required for the viability of the progenitor cells, but may act to increase the functional effectiveness of mature cells such as macrophages[27,29] and neutrophils[28].

At present, our knowledge of the regulation of stem cell differentiation, self-renewal and commitment[8,30] limits our ability to understand the function of the growth factors. However, it is apparent that for the haemopoietic and epithelial tissues there is a set of self-renewing stem cells which do not appear to be influenced by any of the growth factors purified to date. Once the multipotential stem cells have undergone the initial divisions leading to commitment along a specific lineage, the cells become dependent on the presence of the appropriate growth factor for their survival *in vitro*[9,18,26]. It is almost as though the growth factors rescue the committed progenitor cells from immediate cell death – thus, the modulation of the growth factor concentration allows for the exquisite control of cell production in a specific tissue. *In vitro*, the presence of the appropriate growth factor, e.g. granulocyte-macrophage (GM) colony stimulating factor (CSF) appears sufficient for both the proliferation and associated differentiation of the progenitor cells but it is almost certain that production of cells in each lineage is controlled by at least two growth factors. As the progenitor cells differentiate they are still able to respond to or bind the appropriate growth factor. Indeed, the more mature nucleated blood cells have more receptors for GM-CSF, G-CSF and M-CSF. It is to be expected that the amplified signal resulting from the higher concentration of growth factor receptor complex will lead to molecular responses different from those following progenitor cell stimulation by growth factors.

It is interesting to note that other than the growth factors, the transforming viruses are the only other agents capable of rescuing the committed progenitor cells from cell death. Indeed, it is possible to overcome the absolute dependence of some cell lines on their appropriate growth factor (e.g. the epidermal cell line MK-1 dependence on EGF) by infecting the cells with an acutely transforming retrovirus[31]. In some way, the oncogenic viruses must either produce (or induce) a protein (oncogene product) normally activated via the growth factor receptor complex and which can mimic the action of the growth factor[13,14,32,33].

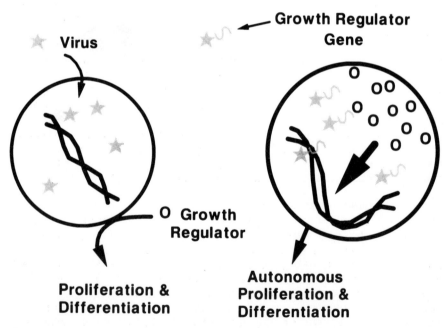

Fig. 1. *What would happen if a retrovirus acquired a growth factor gene? If growth factor viruses infected immortalized, growth factor-dependent cells of the appropriate lineage, an autocrine neoplasia would be initiated.*

What are the likely functions of oncogene products?

It may be too early to ask this question, as our knowledge of the control of normal mammalian cell division is still rather primitive. However, by applying a bias to the answer (namely, that the function of the oncogene products will be related to the mechanism of action of the growth factors) several laboratories have already uncovered some most exciting biology and biochemistry[10-15,33]. The melding of our knowledge of the retroviruses[4], oncogenes[13-15] and growth factor function[9,17,18] has revolutionized our understanding of cellular growth control in both normal and neoplastic cells.

Any structural or enzymic protein which might perturb or simulate some aspects of the action of a growth factor might be expected to have oncogenic potential. Thus an oncogene product could be:
- the growth factor to which the cell normally responds (autocrine model)[34];
- an altered form (or an increased number) of the receptor(s)[15,34], such that the target cell always appears to be in the stimulated state;
- a change in the molecular nature or concentration of an intracellular substrate for the growth factor receptor[33,35,36], so that the molecular state of the cytoplasm appears to be signalling for the initiation of DNA synthesis even in the absence of growth factor (candidates for the substrates of the receptor kinases appear to be cytoskeletal components, or enzymes which modify cytoskeletal proteins, closely associated with the inner surface of the cell membrane[37-39]);
- a nuclear protein involved in activation of eukaryotic chromatin (either by direct DNA binding or by altering the nuclear matrix[40]).

Already there is evidence supporting the notion that schemes such as these are involved in the neoplastic transformation of specific cell types. Indeed the molecular causes of both primary tumour transformations (due to spontaneous mutation or genetic rearrangement) appear to be similar to the known mechanisms of viral transformation.

Can retroviral oncogene products be thought of as perturbed analogues of the different molecules involved when a growth factor 'induces' the proliferation of a normal cell? Unfortunately, our molecular knowledge of the mechanism of action of the tissue-specific growth factors and the functions of the retroviral oncogenes is still scanty[13-15,33] so this hypothesis is difficult to explore in detail, but there is sufficient preliminary evidence to explore the ramifications of this oncogene product–growth factor relationship. Undoubtedly many neoplasias will involve more than one molecular lesion. It may be difficult to determine the primary neoplastic lesion, but it is important to study the effect(s) of these lesions on the normal biochemical pathways activated by the growth factors[34,35].

Growth factors and autocrine tumours

It is over 20 years since the first autocrine models of tumourigenesis were proposed, but 1983 brought some stunning molecular support for this hypothesis[13,14]. Early in the year, after almost a decade of protein chemistry which has resulted in the purification of PDGF[41,42], some initial amino acid sequence analysis was reported[21]. Due to some remarkably sensitive, accurate and skilful analyses, this amino acid sequence of PDGF had been eked out from a mixture of four peptides[21]. Almost at the same time the nucleotide sequence corresponding to the coding region of the transforming gene v-*sis* from the Simian sarcoma gene was published[43], but the two sets of data remained unconnected for almost four months. During this time, more extensive amino acid sequence data for PDGF was derived independently[14]. Two laboratories searching the most up to date libraries of amino acid sequences realized, simultaneously, that the PDGF and v-*sis* proteins were closely related[13,14]. The considerable interest in these observations has already led to the identification of the PDGF which is secreted by cells transformed with the v-*sis* oncogene[44]. Obviously, experiments have been designed to try and inhibit the autocrine action of PDGF (e.g. antibodies against PDGF) on Simian sarcoma virus (SSV) transformed fibroblasts, but no successful reports of growth inhibition have appeared as yet.

Interestingly, the intracellular protein phosphorylation patterns of fibroblasts stimulated by PDGF or transformed by SSV show distinct differences (Hunter, T., unpublished observations). It will be important to prove exactly the mechanism by which the v-*sis* gene product leads to transformation (e.g. does it interact with the PDGF receptor) or whether there are other virally associated changes which also contribute to the state of transformation.

Although the tumour-derived (also called transforming) growth factors (TGF-1, also called TGF-2) can be produced by virally transformed cells these molecules are not virally encoded and indeed one of the first TGFs to be purified was isolated from a spontaneous human melanoma cell line[45]. It has been proposed that viral transformation activates a growth factor gene leading to autocrine stimulation and consequently neoplasia. After a considerable effort, one form of TGF-1 was purified[45] and the complete amino acid sequence has now been determined[46,47]. TGF-1 is structurally and functionally related to epidermal growth factor (EGF)[46]. Although this homology is weak at both the N-terminus and C-terminus, the amino acid sequence of the TGF-1 decapeptide loop III is closely related to EGF:

i.e.   C* H S G* Y* V* G* V R* C*

where an asterisk indicates a homology with the amino acid in the equivalent position for a known EGF sequence. TGF-1 and mEGF bind with the same affinity (K_d approximately 2.7×10^{-9}M) to a single class of receptors (i.e. the EGF receptor) on A431 epidermioid carcinoma cells[46]. TGF-1 has now been fully synthesized by a solid phase technique and the synthetic TGF-1, prepared from the amino acid sequence data has the same biological activity as the purified molecule[48].

Thus, epithelial cells with proliferative potential, which secrete TGF-1 (or EGF), might be expected to become transformed. Unfortunately, much of this system is clouded by our poor knowledge of the biological action of epithelial growth factors. In particular, the role of EGF in directly stimulating the proliferation of normal epithelial cells (rather than inducing maturational events) is still far from clarified. It is more than likely that several other epithelial growth factors yet to be properly characterized[49] are capable of stimulating the proliferation of foetal and/or adult stem cells. Perhaps the EGF dependent-TGFs (also called TGF-2 or TGF-β) represent this class of molecules. Again, antibodies against the different TGFs will help provide useful information about the existence and function of these other epithelial growth factors. It is particularly important in this context to determine the tissue specificity of the epithelial and fibroblastoid growth factors. For example, there are some indications that TGF-2 may act conjointly with EGF to stimulate fibroblast proliferation, but that epithelial cells are inhibited by this molecule.

Similarly, although PDGF is known to be involved in regulating the proliferation of 'fibroblastoid' cells, the effects of PDGF are not equivalent to transformation. However, if PDGF is supplemented with TGF-2 and a platelet-derived EGF-like protein[50], viral (or oncogenic) transformation can be mimicked. Perhaps, sarcomas arise as a result of the cumulative effects of at least two mutations, one of which short-circuits the action of TGF-β and/or the 'EGF-like' growth factors and the other which leads to the necessary (but not sufficient) autocrine production of PDGF.

Several other growth factor modulated transformation systems have been described[51]. Perhaps the most convincing of these is the transformation of early erythroid cells using the Friend-murine leukaemia virus (F-MuLV)[51]. The cell line (IW32) appears to be derived from mature cells of the erythroid lineage which are still capable of proliferation (CFU-E). The F-MuLV transformed cells resemble erythroblasts but produce erythropoietin (the normal growth factor known to control both proliferation and differentiation in this compartment of the erythroid system). The authors are careful to note that whilst the cells produce erythropoietin and presumably have specific receptors for this growth factor, there is no direct proof that the secreted erythropoietin is responsible for the proliferation of IW32. At present amino acid sequence information has only been 'reported' for a part of human erythropoietin. But antibodies are available which apparently bind to murine erythropoietin and it would be interesting to know if excess antibody (or microinjected antibody) could prevent IW32 proliferation.

The autocrine 'stimulation' of progenitor cell proliferation (or rescue from the irreversible progression to cell death due to differentiation) still poses at least one dilemma. If the only lesion associated with these neoplastic cells is the inappropriate production of their own growth regulator, why is it that the normal differentiation programme (which would lead to cell death) appears to be blocked? There must be other molecular changes associated with the growth regulatory pathways in IW32 cells. Otherwise the erythropoietin should induce terminal differentiation of these leukaemic erythroblasts. Other growth factors are known to be involved in the proliferation of early erythroid cells[8], so perhaps the other lesion(s) is concerned with the function of these molecules. The autocrine production of a growth factor may represent a secondary event which confers a further proliferative advantage to a preneoplastic cell resulting in the final stage of neoplasia.

Of course, there could be other molecular lesions which prevent the cells responding normally[52,53]. However, it is known that high concentrations of growth factors (e.g. GM-CSF) retard maturation and promote proliferation[25]. Perhaps constitutive production leads to concentration of the growth factor at the cell surface at levels sufficiently high to induce proliferation at the expense of almost any maturation. There are several other possibilities, but one of the most intriguing is that the tumour cells may be producing a growth factor capable of both intracellular and extracellular functions and, furthermore, that it is the high intracellular concentration of growth factor which perturbs the balance between proliferation and differentiation resulting in neoplastic cells.

Growth factor receptors: receptor tumours

Many growth factors bind to specific cell surface receptors on their target cells but is this the end of their direct involvement in stimulating cell division? It has been proposed that the primary function of growth factors is to activate these receptors, which then initiate the intracellular reactions necessary to stimulate cell division. Several of the growth factor receptors are now known to be capable of catalysing the phosphorylation of tyrosine residues[11,54] on both membrane and cytoplasmic proteins. The tyrosine kinase activity of the growth factor receptors is known to be dependent on the binding of the appropriate growth factor[11,54]. It was quickly realized that this enzymic activity was identical to the enzymic activity of the transforming product of the first retrovirus to be described[2], the Rous sarcoma virus, pp60[src] (Ref. 55). Further, there was a strong correlation between the ability of the pp60[src] to act as a tyrosine kinase and its ability to transform cells. The tyrosine kinase activity of the growth factor receptors appears to be an integral part of their function in stimulating cellular proliferation, but there are many substrates (both membrane and cytoplasmic) and it has been difficult to find a molecular scheme to explain which tyrosine phosphorylations are responsible for cell division[35].

The homologous functions of pp60[src] and the EGF receptor suggested another mechanism by which neoplastic transformation could occur – that excess or altered growth factor receptors could result in the alteration in the proportion of phosphorylated derivatives of the intracellular proteins controlling cell division. Is pp60[src] directly related to the EGF receptor? The initial experiments using antibodies against pp60[src], failed to immunoprecipitate the EGF receptor; however these antibodies must have formed complexes with the EGF receptor as they were substrates for the receptor kinase. Recently, Schlessinger *et al.* have succeeded in precipitating the EGF receptor using antibodies raised against two distinct regions of pp60[src] (the tyrosine phosphorylation site and a C-terminal region peptide). These antibodies not only precipitated the EGF receptor from crude membrane preparations but also radio-iodinated pure EGF receptor.

The human EGF receptor has now been purified to homogeneity and the amino acid sequences for several of the tryptic peptides have already been determined[15]. The amino acid sequences for each of six peptides isolated from the EGF receptor were homologous to part of the hypothetical sequence of the chicken v-erbB protein. For the peptides sequenced, 89% of the amino acid residues were in homologous positions for v-erbB and the EGF receptor. This observation has now been extended, as the entire cDNA clone for the EGF receptor has been sequenced[56]. It appears that the progenitor avian erythroblastosis virus (AEV) has acquired the intracellular domain and part of the trans-membrane domain of the EGF receptor[56]. It has been suggested that it is the inappropriate expression of this intracellular domain (i.e. the tyrosine kinase domain) of a truncated (epidermal) growth factor receptor which is responsible for the transforming properties of AEV (Ref. 15)*.

Thus, an alteration in the concentration of growth factor receptors appears to be associated with a number of tumours. The proliferative response of growth factor dependent cells depends not only on the concentration of the growth factor, but also on the display, surface density and turnover of the growth factor receptors. This has been studied most elegantly in the influence of TCGF (IL-2) on T-lymphocytes[9,10,18,57]. However, the amplification of the EGF receptor gene in a number of tumour cell lines also indicates that perturbed receptor production is directly involved in epithelial tumours. Interestingly, more than 30% of human gliomas are known to be associated with the amplification of the EGF receptor gene[77].

Although many attempts have been made to detect autocrine production of TCGF by T-lymphomas none has been successful. Perhaps an investigation of the receptor status and the interactions between the TCGF receptor and its intracellular substrates will prove more fruitful. Particularly interesting results may be available from the study of virally derived T lymphomas or carcinomas[31].

---

*The tyrosine kinase activity of the erbB molecule has only recently been detected (Schlessinger, J., unpublished observations; Baldwin, G. S., Savin, K. and Kemp, B., unpublished observations).

Intracellular mediators of growth factor 'stimulation'

How do growth factors function? How does the inappropriate expression of 'oncogene' products lead to uncontrolled cellular proliferation? The answers to these questions are not yet available and the section that follows simply represents a sketch of several hypothetical scenarios which serve as models to illustrate the striking progress in our understanding of the function of the growth factors and oncogene products.

Growth factor modulated expression of oncogene products

There are now several reports linking the expression of proto-oncogene (c-*onc*) products with the mechanism of action of growth factors[58]. Activation of both T-lymphocyte proliferation and fibroblast proliferation is associated with increased production of c-myc[59]. Indeed, at least some of the genetic rearrangements in murine T-lymphomas are associated with direct activation of the c-*myc* gene by inserted retroviral sequences[60]. However, increased expression of c-*myc* is not sufficient to transform fibroblasts. Thus fibroblasts which have been engineered to express levels of c-*myc* threefold higher than are observed in transformed cells do not necessarily display a transformed phenotype[7]. The expression of oncogene products appears to be related to both the proliferation and maturation state of a cell. For example, the myelomonocytic leukemia WEHI-3B(D $^+$) expresses high levels of c-*myc* and c-*myb* (Ref. 61) but when induced to differentiate using both G-CSF (Ref. 6) and actinomycin D the expression of both c-*myb* and c-*myc* decreased[61]. This change in expression of c-*myb* and c-*myc* appeared to be associated with late maturation (differentiation) events rather than the initiation of differentiation[61]. Similarly, the induction of c-*fos* expression in this system appeared to be associated with the production of mature macrophages[61] rather than the initial signals for leukaemic cell differentiation. Interestingly, induction of 'c-fos-like' molecules has been observed during the stimulation of fibroblasts by PDGF[16].

Perturbation of the concentration or distribution of proteins normally associated with the growth factor initiated-mitogenic cascade might be expected to uncouple the regulation of cell growth. Similarly, a mutation of one of these molecules which changes its enzymic specificity could be expected to uncouple these growth regulatory pathways. Indeed the first human oncogene to be identified (c-*ras*)[5] appeared to be in an activated state as a result of a specific mutation. However, extensive comparison of the mutated and normal c-*ras* products (p21) indicated that the subcellular localization, post-translational modification and dGTP binding of both the normal and 'onc' p21 proteins was identical[62]. But, a recent report has detected a difference in the ability of these two p21 proteins to catalyse the hydrolysis of GTP and has suggested that the function of p21 may be closely linked to the G-proteins associated with the adenylate cyclase system.

Oncogene products and the cytoskeleton

At least some of the oncogene products appear to be closely related to or are capable of modifying cytoskeletal proteins such as vinculin[38] and tubulin[39]. An analysis of some of the recent reports on the relationship of the oncogene products to cytoskeletal proteins[37,63,64] has interesting implications for the mechanism of action of the growth factors. It is now known that: at least one of the fusion products from the transforming gene of Gardner-Rasheed feline sarcoma virus[63] contains actin sequences; the *ras* gene product (p21) maps on the yeast genome between the actin and tubulin genes[63] (there also appears to be another nucleotide sequence in yeast which is related to v-*ras*[H] but the location and significance of this gene is not yet clear[64]); the polyoma middle T antigen contains an amino acid sequence (L.E$_6$.Y...)[34] which is associated with the ability of this molecule to transform cells. The tyrosine residue in this sequence is the site of phosphorylation of the middle T antigen. Interestingly, one of the epithelial growth factors, gastrin, is also homologous to this region of the middle T antigen of polyoma virus[34]. (Perhaps, the first indication of an intracellular role for a peptide growth factor.)

A computer search of two protein sequence data banks indicated that sequences of the gastrin-polyoma middle T type ...E$_5$.X.Y.... (where X can be any amino acid) or ...Z$_5$.X.Y... (where Z can be Glu or Gln) are not common (less than four sequences in 30 000 heptapeptides searched) and it is interesting to list some of the other proteins in the data banks with acidic or amide sequences preceding a tyrosine residue:

human growth hormone[65]	QEFEEAY
human c-myc[41]	DEEENFY
v-myc[41]	EEEEENFY
p21[66]	QEEY
tubulin[67]	EEEGEEEY
erythrocyte band 3 protein[68]	EENLEQEEY

There were also two other molecules with amino acid sequences similar to c-myc in the vicinity of Tyr (Ref. 41), in which the acidic or amide sequences were predominantly on the carboxyl side of the tyrosine residue:

Ela[69]	YQEADD
Actin[70]	DYEQELE

This structural association between some 'growth factors' (gastrin, growth hormone), oncogene products (polyoma middle T antigen, c-myc, v-myc, p21) and the cytoskeletal proteins (actin, tubulin[37] and the band 3 protein) and at least one of the cytokeratins (Steinert, P., unpublished observations) suggests several models for the action of growth factors and one of the possible mechanisms by which oncogene products may interfere with cellular proliferation.

If cellular proliferation depends on the topography of the cytoskeleton and/or nuclear matrix and in particular the association of these proteins with the plasma membrane or nuclear membrane – then growth factors may act simply to perturb the formation of that cytoskeleton or nuclear matrix e.g. by inducing the phosphorylation of specific cytoskeletal (intermediate filament or nuclear matrix) proteins (thus interfering with the formation of the cytoskeleton, nuclear matrix or the anchorage of these structures to the plasma or nuclear membranes). There have been several reports concerning the phosphorylation of intermediate filaments[71] and interference with this phosphorylation is associated with a transformed phenotype. Presumably only a small proportion of the cytoskeletal and intermediate filament proteins would need to be phosphorylated (i.e. those molecules near the plasma or nuclear membranes) to perturb the topography of the cytoskeleton or nuclear matrix. Thus the phosphorylation of critical tyrosine residues on the c-ras, 'middle T-like' or nuclear proteins such as c-myc could be associated with a breakdown of the quaternary structure of the cytoskeleton or nuclear matrix. This would account for the dramatic redistribution of proteins such as tubulin, c-myc and c-myb during differentiation[72]. Similarly mutations in the vicinity of the tyrosine phosphorylation site (e.g. v-myc and c-myc) could alter either the polymerization of nuclear matrix structural proteins or the stable interaction of such structural proteins with the cytoplasmic or nuclear membrane.

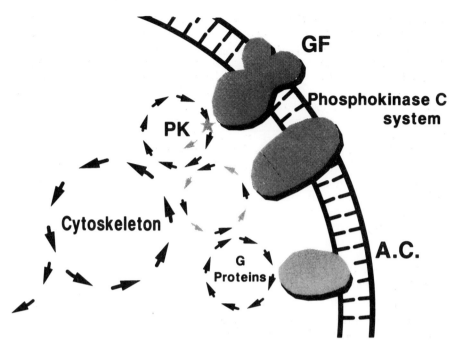

Fig. 2. The cell surface growth factor receptors are linked to cytoplasmic protein kinases (PK) and thus to the adenylate cyclase system. Cytoskeletal proteins at the cell membrane are candidate substrates for the activated PKs and may be involved in signal transmission.

The growth factor mediated phosphorylation of tyrosine residues, suggested to be important for the maintenance of the cytoskeletal (or nuclear matrix) – membrane interactions – is turned over rapidly. Thus, a continuous, and adequate, source of membrane associated ATP would be required to maintain a cytoplasmic and nuclear topography leading to cell division. Normal progenitor cells may be dependent on their specific growth factor simply because the growth factor–receptor complex is intimately associated with the production of ATP. This naïve view of growth factor action is supported by experiments which show that growth factor dependent cell lines[10] (i.e. cells which die if the growth factor is removed) essentially stop the synthesis of ATP if the growth factor is removed[73]. One report indicates that in these systems the growth factor can be partially replaced by an exogenous ATP regenerating system. Normal haemopoietic progenitor cells, which are also growth factor dependent, also cease to phosphorylate proteins when the growth factor is removed (Stanley, I. J., unpublished observations). Protein phosphorylation reactions are intimately associated with the ability of cells to proliferate[37]. It is interesting to note that by using either of two inorganic oxides of vanadium to inhibit intracellular tyrosine phosphatases, it is possible to stimulate DNA synthesis[74]. Since vanadate has also been reported to perturb the distribution and function of the intermediate filaments[75] it is most tempting to think that the disruption of the cytoskeleton by oncogene products is closely related to the changes in protein phosphorylation associated with growth factor stimulation of DNA synthesis.

The mechanisms by which the oncogene products interfere with the cytoskeleton may be expected to vary. For example, there may be excess of peptide sequences homologous to regulator sites which compete in the phosphorylation reactions controlling the polymerization of the cytoskeleton at the plasma membrane (e.g. polyoma middle T)[33,36] or excess of the nuclear matrix proteins. There may be inappropriate activation of the growth factor dependent kinase (e.g. an erbB-like kinase) which causes inappropriate or excessive phosphorylation[15] of cytoskeletal proteins, or alters the structure of a normal substrate of a kinase, thus changing the ratio of phosphorylated and unmodified forms of the protein (e.g. v-myc and c-myc) and consequently the ability of the proteins to polymerize.

These observations also suggest that growth factors might be able to act by mechanisms other than via membrane receptor activation. Molecules such as gastrin[33] and growth hormone could be expected to have intracellular potency by specifically competing for interactions between some of the cytoskeletal proteins. It would be interesting to know if transfected genes (capable of expressing products such as gastrin or growth hormone) can perturb cellular proliferation by increasing the cytoplasmic (or nuclear) concentrations of the protein. The use of peptide analogues designed to compete with the substrates of the growth factor activated tyrosine kinases should provide an interesting route for the development of new reagents to control cell growth.

Much of the structural information about growth factors and many of the oncogene products has been published within the past two years. Several interesting observations suggest that there is a close relationship between retroviral oncogene function and growth factor production[76] and function. This year is already seeing many more fascinating additions to our knowledge of their function, but the coming together of these two fields has been one of those rare events in science which will be regarded as a turning point in cell biology. The discovery of new oncogenes, the availability of purified growth factor receptors and growth factor cDNA clones, is certain to maintain the current level of excitement in cancer biology for many years to come.

References
1   Ellerman, V. and Band, O. (1980) *Zentralbl. Bakteriol. Parasitenkde Infektionskr.* **46**, 1595
2   Rous, P. (1911) *J. Exp. Med.* **13**, 397
3   Cohen, S. (1960) *Proc. Natl Acad. Sci. USA* **46**, 302
4   Bishop, J. M. (1983) *Cell* **32**, 1018–1020
5   Der, C. J., Krontiris, T. G. and Cooper, G. M. (1982) *Proc. Natl Acad. Sci. USA* **79**, 3637–3640
6   Nicola, N. A., Metcalf, D., Matsumoto, M. and Johnson, J. R. (1983) *J. Biol. Chem.* **258**, 9017–9023
7   Baserga, R., ed. (1981) *Tissue Growth Factors,* Springer-Verlag, Berlin
8   Burgess, A. W. and Nicola, N. A. (1983) *Growth Factors and Stem Cells,* Academic Press, Sydney
9   Robb, R. J. (1984) *Immunol. Today* **5**, 203–209
10 Morgan, D. A., Ruscetti, F. W. and Gallo, R. C. (1976) *Science* **193**, 1007–1008
11 Cohen, S. (1982) in *Accomplishments in Cancer Research* (Fortner, J. G. and Rhoads, J. E., eds), p. 76, Lippincott, Philadelphia
12 Stiles, C. D. (1983) *Cell* **33**, 653–655
13 Doolittle, R. F., Hunkapiller, M. W., Hood, L. E., Devare, S. G., Robbins, K. C., Aaronson, S. A. and Antoniades, H. A. (1983) *Science* **221**, 275–277
14 Waterfield, M. D., Scrace, G. T., Whittle, N., Stroobant, P., Johnsson, A., Wasteson, A., Westermark, B., Heldin, C. H., Huang, J. S. and Deuel, T. F. (1983) *Nature (London)* **304**, 35–39

15 Downward, J., Yarden, Y., Mayes, E., Scrace, G., Totty, N., Stockwell, P., Ullrich, A., Schlessinger, J. and Waterfield, M. D. (1984) *Nature (London)* 307, 521–527
16 Armelin, H. A., Armelin, M. C. S., Kelly, K., Stewart, T., Leder, P., Cochran, B. H. and Stiles, C. D. (1984) *Nature (London)* 310, 655–660
17 Bradshaw, R. A. (1978) *Annu. Rev. Biochem.* 47, 191
18 Gillis, S. and Smith, K. A. (1977) *Nature (London)* 268, 154–156
19 Savage, C. R. Jr., Inagami, T. and Cohen, S. (1973) *J. Biol. Chem.* 247, 7612–7621
20 Angeletti, R. H. and Bradshaw, R. A. (1973) *Proc. Natl Acad. Sci. USA* 68, 2417–2420
21 Antonaides, H. N. and Hunkapillar, M. W. (1983) *Science* 220, 963–965
22 Taniguchi, T., Matsui, H., Fujita, T., Takaoka, C., Kashima, N., Yoshimoto, R. and Hamuro, J. (1983) *Nature (London)* 302, 305–310
23 Fugn, M. C., Hapel, A. J., Ymer, S., Cohen, D. R., Johnson, R. M., Campbell, H. D. and Young, I. G. (1984) *Nature (London)* 307, 233–237
24 Gough, N. M., Gough, J., Metcalf, D., Kelso, A., Grail, D., Nicola, N. A., Burgess, A. W. and Dunn, A. R. (1984) *Nature (London)* 309, 763–767
25 Metcalf, D. (1977) in *Hemopoietic Colonies,* Springer-Verlag, Berlin
26 Sachs, L. (1978) *Nature (London)* 274, 535–539
27 Tushinsky, R. J., Oliver, I. T., Guilbert, L. J., Tynan, P. W., Warner, J. R. and Stanley, E. R. (1982) *Cell* 28, 71–81
28 Burgess, A. W. and Metcalf, D. (1977) *J. Cell. Physiol.* 90, 471–484
29 Hamilton, J. A., Stanley, E. R., Burgess, A. W. and Shadduck, R. K. (1980) *J. Cell. Physiol.* 103, 435–445
30 Lajtha, L. G. (1983) in *Stem Cells* 1 (Potten, C. S., ed.), Churchill Livingstone, Edinburgh
31 Weissman, B. E. and Aaronson, S. A. (1983) *Cell* 32, 599–606
32 Todaro, G. J., Fryling, C. and De Larco, J. E. (1980) *Proc. Natl Acad. Sci, USA* 77, 5258–5262
33 Baldwin, G. S. (1982) *FEBS Lett.* 137, 1–5
34 Erikson, E., Shealy, P. J. and Erikson, R. C. (1981) *J. Biol. Chem.* 256, 11381–11384
35 Hunter, T. and Cooper, J. A. (1981) *Cell* 24, 741–752
36 Ito, Y., Hamagishi, Y., Segawa, K., Dalianis, T., Appella, E. and Willingham, M. (1983) *J. Virol.* 48, 709–720
37 Birchmeier, W. (1981) *Trends Biochem. Sci.* 6, 234–237
38 Wang, K., Ash, J. F. and Singer, S. J. (1975) *Proc. Natl Acad. Sci. USA* 72, 4483–4486
39 Willingham, M., Yamada, S. S., Bechtel, P. J., Rutherford, A. V. and Pastan, I. H. (1981) *J. Histochem. Cytochem.* 29, 1289–1301
40 Colby, W. W., Chen, E. Y., Smith, D. H. and Levinson, A. D. (1983) *Nature (London)* 301, 722–725
41 Antoniades, H. N. (1981) *Proc. Natl Acad. Sci. USA* 78, 7314–7317
42 Heldin, C. H., Westarmark, B. and Wateson, A. (1981) *Science* 193, 907
43 Devare, S. G., Reddy, E. P., Robbins, K. C., Andersen, P. R., Tronick, S. R. and Aaronson, S. A. (1982) *Proc. Natl Acad. Sci, USA* 79, 3179–3182
44 Chiu, I. M., Reddy, E. P., Givol, D., Robbins, K. C., Tronick, S. R. and Aaronson, S. A. (1984) *Cell* 37, 123–129
45 Marquardt, H. and Todaro, G. J. (1982) *J. Biol. Chem.* 257, 5220–5225
46 Marquardt, H., Hunkapiller, M. W., Hood, L. E. and Todaro, G. J. (1984) *Science* 223, 1079–1082
47 Derynk, R., Roberts, A. B., Winkler, M. E., Chen, E. Y. and Goeddel, D. V. (1984) *Cell* 38, 287–297
48 Tam, J. P., Marquardt, H., Roseberger, D. F., Wong, T. W. and Todaro, G. J. (1984) *Nature (London)* 309, 376–378
49 Nexø, E., Hollenberg, M. D., Figueroa, A. and Pratt, R. M. (1980) *Proc. Natl Acad. Sci. USA* 77, 2782–2785

50 Assoian, R. K., Grotendorst, G. R., Miller, D. M. and Sporn, M. B. (1984) *Nature (London)* 309, 804–806
51 Tambourin, P., Casadevall, N., Choppin, J., Lacombe, C., Heard, J. M., Fichelson, S., Wendling, F. and Varet, B. (1983) *Proc. Natl Acad. Sci. USA* 80, 6269–6273
52 Land, H., Parada, L. F. and Weinberg, R. A. (1983) *Nature (London)* 304, 596–602
53 Ruley, H. E. (1983) *Nature (London)* 304, 602–606
54 Heldin, C. H., Ek, B. and Ronnstrand, L. (1983) *J. Biol. Chem.* 258, 10054–10061
55 Hunter, T. and Sefton, B. M. (1980) *Proc. Natl Acad. Sci. USA* 77, 1311–1315
56 Ullrich, A., Coussens, L., Hayflick, J. S., Dull, T. J., Gray, A., Tam, A. W., Lee, J., Yarden, Y., Libermann, T. A., Schlessinger, J. *et al.* (1984) *Nature (London)* 309, 418–425
57 Cantrell, D. A. and Smith, K. A. (1984) *Science* 224, 1312–1316
58 Naharro, G., Robbins, K. C. and Reddy, E. P. (1984) *Science* 223, 63–66
59 Kelly, K., Cochran, B. H., Stiles, C. D. and Leder, P. (1983) *Cell* 35, 601–605
60 Corcoran, L. M., Adams, J. M., Dunn, A. R. and Cory, S. (1984) *Cell* 37, 113–122
61 Gonda, T. J. and Metcalf, D. (1984) *Nature (London)* 310, 249–251
62 Finkel, T., Der, C. J. and Cooper, G. M. (1984) *Cell* 37, 151–158
63 Gallwitz, D., Donath, C. and Sander, C. (1984) *Nature (London)* 306, 704–707
64 De Feo-Jones, D., Scolnick, E. M., Koller, R. and Dhar, R. (1983) *Nature (London)* 306, 707–709
65 Niall, H. D., Hogan, M. L., Sauer, R., Rosenblum, I. Y. and Greenwood, F. C. (1971) *Proc. Natl Acad. Sci. USA* 68, 866–869
66 Dhar, R., Ellis, R. W., Shih, T. Y., Oroszlan, S., Shapiro, B., Maizel, J., Lowy, D. and Scolnick, E. (1982) *Science* 217, 934–936
67 Postingl, H., Krauns, E., Little, M. and Kempf, T. (1981) *Proc. Natl Acad. Sci. USA* 78, 2757–2761
68 Kaul, R. K., Murthy, S. N., Reddy, A. G., Steck, T. L. and Kohler, H. (1983) *J. Biol. Chem.* 258, 7981–7990
69 Perricaudet, M., le Moullec, J. M. and Tiollais, P. (1980) *Nature (London)* 288, 174–176
70 Zakut, R., Shani, M., Givol, D., Neuman, S., Yaffe, D. and Nudel, U. (1982) *Nature (London)* 298, 857–859
71 Steinert, P. M., Wantz, M. L. and Idler, W. W. (1982) *Biochemistry* 21, 177–183
72 Klempnauer, K. H., Symonds, G., Evan, G. I. and Bishop, J. M. (1984) *Cell* 37, 537–547
73 Whetton, A. D. and Dexter, T. M. (1983) *Nature (London)* 303, 629–631
74 Smith, J. B. (1983) *Proc. Natl Acad. Sci. USA* 80, 6162–6166
75 Wang, E. and Choppin, P. W. (1981) *Proc. Natl Acad. Sci. USA* 78, 2363–2367
76 Koury, M. J. and Pragnell, I. B. (1982) *Nature (London)* 299, 638–640
77 Lax, I., Kris, R., Sasson, I., Ullrich, A., Hayman, M. J., Beug, H. and Schlessinger, J. (1985) *EMBO J.* 4, 3179–3182

A. Burgess is at the Ludwig Institute for Cancer Research, Melbourne Tumour Biology Unit, Post Office Royal Melbourne Hospital, Victoria 3050, Australia.

Oncogenes and growth control

Tony Hunter

*Retroviral oncogenes are known to have been acquired from normal cells. Two of these oncogenes were derived from genes for proteins which function in cellular growth control pathways. The v-*sis *oncogene encodes a protein closely related to platelet-derived growth factor, while the v-*erb-B *oncogene encodes a truncated form of the epidermal growth factor receptor.*

The proliferation of cells, at least in culture, is regulated largely by extracellular agents, among the most important of which are the polypeptide growth factors. These factors interact with specific cell-surface receptors which in turn deliver intracellular signals ultimately leading to DNA synthesis and cell division. Uncontrolled proliferation is a hallmark of tumor cells. The recent characterization of oncogenes implicated in tumorigenesis has stimulated an intensive investigation into the molecular mechanisms underlying the loss of growth control. Almost all oncogenes are altered versions of normal cellular genes and their products are presumed to work at least in part by mimicking the products of the cellular genes from which they arose.

A priori there are three sites in a growth control pathway at which oncogenic proteins can intercede to deliver a growth stimulus. Firstly, the protein might itself mimic a growth factor. The interaction of such a protein with a suitable receptor could stimulate cell growth in an autocrine fashion. Secondly, the oncogenic protein might imitate an occupied growth factor receptor and thus provide a mitogenic signal in the absence of exogenous growth factors. Thirdly, the oncogenic protein might act on an intracellular growth control pathway, uncoupling it from the need for an exogenous stimulus.

It turns out that there are oncogenic proteins of all three types. The identification of oncogenes whose products clearly fit into the first two categories came from comparison of the predicted amino acid sequences of the oncogenic proteins with those of purified growth factors or growth factor receptors. Until recently the only growth factors whose primary sequences had been determined were epidermal growth factor (EGF) and the two insulin-like growth factors (IGF), IGF-1 and IGF-2. Their sequences did not match those of any of the known oncogene products. When the partial sequence of human platelet-derived growth factor (PDGF) was obtained, however, it immediately became apparent that there was a strong homology between the predicted product of the v-*sis* oncogene of simian sarcoma virus (SSV) and PDGF[1-3].

The v-*sis* oncogene and PDGF

PDGF is a disulphide-bonded dimer of about 30 kDa. Preparations of human PDGF contain two distinct but related chains. It is not known whether they form a heterodimer or whether there is a mixture of two homodimers, but the latter seems most likely because purified porcine PDGF has only a single type of chain corresponding to the B chain of human PDGF[4]. It is the PDGF B chain which is very closely related to the COOH-terminal part of the predicted v-*sis* protein. The NH$_2$-terminal sequence of the B chain is recognizable immediately following a Lys–Arg dipeptide in the v-*sis* protein[1,2] (see Fig. 1). Although little is known about the synthesis of PDGF and its sequestration into the α-granules of platelets, the B chain seems to be made from a larger precursor in which the Lys–Arg sequence serves as a processing site. Three of the 100 residues sequenced in the human B chain differ from those of the equivalent region of the v-*sis* protein[5]. These appear to be species differences and, as we will see, probably unnecessary for the transforming activity of the v-*sis* gene. In all likelihood therefore the c-*sis* gene is the cellular gene which encodes the B chain of PDGF[5-7]. The complete structure of the c-*sis* gene at its 5' end has not yet been determined, so that the exact size of the c-*sis* protein, the presumptive precursor of the B chain, is still unknown.

The cellular sequences acquired by SSV have been inserted into the gene for the retroviral envelope protein (*env*) near the 3' end of the genome[3]. In the parental virus this gene is expressed as a surface glycoprotein from a spliced subgenomic mRNA. The 5' end of the *env* gene appears to be intact in SSV and there is evidence that the v-*sis* protein is expressed from a subgenomic mRNA which presumably uses the *env* mRNA splice acceptor site. Since the *env* and v-*sis* genes are in the same reading frame, the primary v-*sis* translation product will contain the *env* protein signal sequence (Fig. 1). It is therefore likely to be synthesized on membrane-bound polysomes and transported into the lumen of the endoplasmic reticulum. Since the v-*sis* protein lacks an obvious membrane anchor sequence it has the potential to be secreted, particularly in cells lacking the α-granule storage system.

What is known about the protein products of the v-*sis* gene? Using antibodies directed against synthetic peptides corresponding to v-*sis* sequences it has been shown that SSV-transformed cells make a glycosylated v-*sis* protein of 28 kDa, which is likely to be the primary translation product lacking the signal sequence[3,8]. This protein is rapidly dimerized to a 56 kDa form which is then processed proteolytically in a series of steps giving rise to a 24 kDa dimer[8,9]. All these products are also recognized by anti-PDGF serum. A small fraction of the v-*sis* protein is found in the culture supernatant of SSV-transformed cells[10].

Given the homology between PDGF and the v-*sis* gene products, the obvious

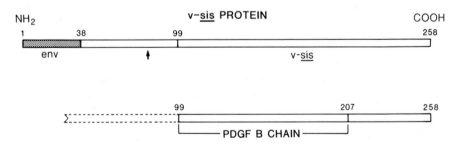

Fig. 1. The predicted structure of the v-sis gene translation product is shown. This is based on the sequence of SSV[3] and the likely initiation site for the v-sis protein[13]. The primary translation product would have 38 amino acids derived from the viral env gene and 220 amino acids encoded by v-sis sequences. Presumably the env protein signal sequence would be cleaved from this protein, but its true NH₂ terminus has not been determined. The single potential glycosylation site is indicated. The structure of the B chain of human PDGF[1,2,5] is aligned with the v-sis protein. Its NH₂ terminus corresponds to residue 99, and this is created by cleavage of a longer precursor of unknown size. Most of the human B chain terminates at position 207 (Ref. 5), again as a result of cleavage of a precursor which would extend to residue 258.

question is whether any of the v-*sis* proteins have growth factor activity and mimic PDGF. Lysates from SSV-transformed cells possess mitogenic activity for normal fibroblasts which can be partially neutralized by anti-PDGF antibodies[9]. Furthermore the culture medium of most SSV-transformed cells contains a PDGF-like mitogenic factor[10,11]. The ability of the v-*sis* protein synthesized in bacteria to compete with PDGF for binding to PDGF receptors is an additional indication of a functional similarity[12].

All these data are consistent with the hypothesis that the mature v-*sis* gene product enters the cellular secretion pathway and interacts with the PDGF receptor to cause the unrestricted growth of SSV-transformed cells in an autocrine fashion. The proof that this is the mechanism of growth stimulation is harder to attain, although there are strong indications that this is indeed the case. Anti-PDGF antibodies partially inhibit the growth of some but not all SSV-transformed cell lines[11]. The cells whose growth is unaffected are those which secrete the least 'PDGF-like' growth factor. In these cases it is possible that the v-*sis* protein interacts with the PDGF-binding domain of newly synthesized PDGF receptors in an intracellular compartment (e.g. the Golgi or a transport vesicle) and that the liganded receptors are immediately internalized when they reach the cell surface. The fact that mutants with deletions in the putative *env* gene-derived signal peptide sequence of the v-*sis* gene are non-transforming shows that the v-*sis* protein must enter the cellular secretion pathway to transform[13]. The presence of PDGF receptors appears to be required for transformation by the v-*sis* protein, since SSV-induced tumors are restricted to cell types which have PDGF receptors (e.g. glial cells, myoblasts and fibroblasts). SSV-transformed cells also display fewer functional PDGF surface receptors than their parental cells, as expected if some receptors are occupied with the v-*sis* protein[11].

There are two other important issues. Since the activation of many proto-oncogenes depends on structural mutations, one might ask whether the v-*sis* protein transforms because it has an altered structure with respect to authentic PDGF. Assuming that porcine PDGF is typical, we can discount the possibility that the v-*sis* protein transforms because it is a homodimer rather than a heterodimer. The necessity for coding mutations can also be ruled out. Mouse fibroblasts can be transformed either by a suitably expressed human c-*sis* cDNA clone[14] or by human c-*sis* genomic sequences themselves[15].

If the v-*sis* protein is identical to PDGF, why does the former but not the latter induce the transformed phenotype? One possibility is that autogenous 'PDGF' is more effective than exogenous PDGF. Alternatively, chronic production of PDGF throughout the cell cycle could in some way provide a different signal to that induced by acute external administration. There are potential natural precedents for this idea. While in general the cells which make growth factors are distinct from those that bear the cognate receptors, placental cytotrophoblast cells have PDGF receptors and also secrete a PDGF-like factor. These cells grow extremely rapidly and in many senses have properties of transformed cells. Their phenotype might in part be a result of an autocrine mechanism involving PDGF. A similar situation may exist with rapidly growing embryonic smooth muscle cells.

Another interesting question is whether the growth of any natural tumor is the result of an autocrine mechanism, particularly one involving the activation of the c-*sis* gene. Many tumor cells secrete growth factors. In certain combinations these factors confer a reversible transformed phenotype on normal established cells and they are known as transforming growth factors (TGF). Among the

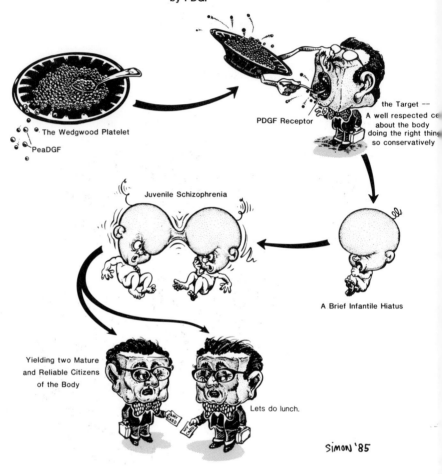

"HOW TO STIMULATE A DESIRABLE TARGET AND STILL MAINTAIN A SENSE OF DECORUM"
by PDGF

The Wedgwood Platelet

PeaDGF

PDGF Receptor

the Target --
A well respected ce
about the body
doing the right thing
so conservatively

Juvenile Schizophrenia

A Brief Infantile Hiatus

Yielding two Mature
and Reliable Citizens
of the Body

Lets do lunch.

Simon '85

(1) Synthesis of v-*sis* protein on membrane bound ribosomes.
(2) Transport of v-*sis* protein to cell surface via Golgi apparatus.
(3) Release of v-*sis* protein from cell.
(4) Interaction of secreted v-*sis* protein with surface PDGF receptor followed by internalization through coated pits.
(5) Delivery of mitogenic signal.

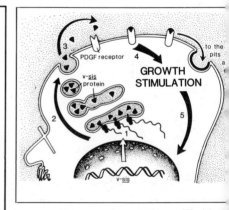

"HOW I DO THAT VOODOO I DO SO WELL" by SSV

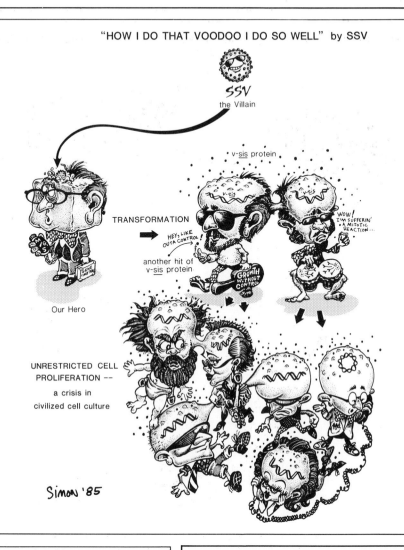

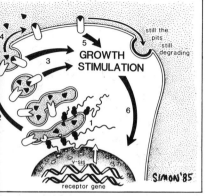

(1) Simultaneous synthesis of v-*sis* protein and PDGF receptor on membrane-bound ribosomes.

(2) Interaction of v-*sis* protein and PDGF receptor intracellularly during transport to surface.

(3) Delivery of mitogenic signal by internal v-*sis* protein/PDGF receptor complexes.

(4) Release of v-*sis* protein from cell.

(5) Interaction of v-*sis* protein with surface PDGF receptor followed by internalization through coated pits.

(6) Delivery of mitogenic signal.

TGFs are the EGF-related, TGFα, and the unrelated TGFβ. Because TGFα and TGFβ together induce growth in agar of suitable indicator cells, it has been proposed that these TGFs may be instrumental in inducing the transformed phenotype of cells which secrete them. A number of cells, including virally transformed cells and some human osteosarcoma lines, secrete PDGF-like growth factors some of which may be c-*sis* gene products. PDGF or PDGF-like growth factors can accentuate the effect of TGFα and TGFβ in stimulating growth of normal cells in agar, but by themselves are not very potent. So it is currently unclear whether PDGF-like factors are responsible for the growth phenotype of any tumor cell type. (For a review of TGF, see p. 157.)

Are other oncogene products growth factors?
    Are there additional oncogene products which might act as growth factors? No other oncogenic protein is known to be secreted, and from their predicted structures this would in most cases be precluded by the absence of a signal sequence. So far therefore the v-*sis* protein seems to be unique. Nevertheless it is entirely possible that the genes for other growth factors might act as oncogenes if they were expressed in an appropriate fashion. The availability of several cloned growth factors (e.g. EGF, TGFα, IGF-1, IGF-2) makes it feasible to test this. There are hints of yet further links between growth factors and oncogenes. For instance the middle-sized tumor antigen of polyoma virus shows an intriguing amino acid sequence homology to the peptide hormone gastrin[16], but the significance of this homology is unclear.

The v-*erb*-B oncogene and the EGF receptor
    The second connection between oncogenes and growth control emerged from a study of the structure of the EGF receptor. Comparison of the sequences of several tryptic peptides derived from the EGF receptor, purified from the human tumor cell line A431, showed an almost perfect match with the predicted product of the v-*erb*-B oncogene of avian erythroblastosis virus (AEV)[17,18]. This homology has been confirmed by the isolation and sequencing of cDNA clones for the EGF receptor from the A431 line. Thus it seems extremely likely that the v-*erb*-B gene was derived from the chicken EGF receptor gene[19–21].
    The EGF receptor is the best characterized growth factor receptor. It is a 175 kDa glycoprotein which has been purified to homogeneity. The receptor has an intrinsic protein-tyrosine kinase activity which is stimulated several-fold upon binding EGF[22]. Increased protein-tyrosine kinase activity can be detected in EGF-treated cells in the form of new phosphotyrosine-containing proteins. Although there is as yet no formal proof it seems reasonable to suppose that such phosphorylations play a role in the mitogenic signal. Proteolysis studies show that about 115 kDa of the receptor is on the outside of the cell, forming a heavily glycosylated EGF-binding domain. About half the 1186 amino acid receptor lies inside the cell[19] (see Fig. 2). A 250 amino acid stretch of this internal domain has a striking homology with the catalytic domain of the *src* gene family of protein-tyrosine kinases, in keeping with the known enzymic activity of the receptor. The internal and external domains of the EGF receptor are separated by a 26 amino acid region which lacks charged residues and which is presumed to be anchored in the membrane.
    Residues 551–1154 of the human EGF receptor show over 90% identity with the predicted sequence of the chicken v-*erb*-B gene product[18,19], a remarkable degree of similarity considering the evolutionary distance between humans and

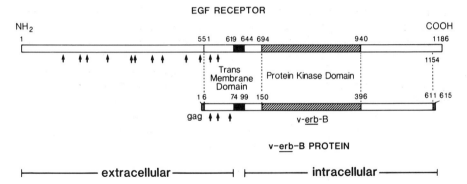

Fig. 2. *The predicted structure of the human EGF receptor is shown with the amino acid numbering starting at the residue determined to be the NH₂ terminus of the mature protein[19]. The primary translation product has a 24 amino acid signal sequence which is removed proteolytically. The v-erb-B protein is aligned with EGF receptor and is depicted as the product of a spliced mRNA based on the sequence of AEV-H (Ref. 18). It is comprised of six amino acids of the viral gag gene joined to 609 amino acids encoded v-erb-B gene sequences. Presumably this protein contains a signal sequence which is cleaved, but its true NH₂ terminus has not been determined. In both cases the potential glycosylation sites in the external domains are shown.*

chickens. The v-*erb*-B protein thus appears to be a truncated form of the EGF receptor, which lacks most of the external EGF-binding domain, but which retains the proposed membrane anchor domain (Fig. 2). The v-*erb*-B gene product is a glycoprotein present in infected cells in various forms. *In vitro*, the primary translation product of the v-*erb*-B mRNA is about 61 kDa, but in infected cells this protein is glycosylated post-translationally yielding an immature glycoprotein of 64–68 kDa[23,24]. This protein is membrane-associated and appears to accumulate in the Golgi apparatus *en route* to the surface of the cell. In the Golgi, the carbohydrate side-chains are further modified and a fraction of the v-*erb*-B protein is found on the cell surface as a 75–80 kDa protein. Cells infected with conditional mutants of AEV do not display v-*erb*-B protein on the cell surface at the restrictive temperature[25]. From this it has been inferred that the surface form plays an important role in the transformed phenotype.

The crucial question is whether the surface form of the v-*erb*-B protein mimics an occupied EGF receptor in stimulating the growth of erythroblasts. A priori one might imagine that the truncated v-*erb*-B membrane protein, in the absence of the regulatory domain, would behave like a constitutively activated EGF receptor. There are several problems with this idea in its simplest form. Unlike the EGF receptor it has been difficult to demonstrate that the v-*erb*-B proteins have protein-tyrosine kinase activity *in vitro*, although recent reports show that such an activity can be detected under some conditions[26,27]. In cells transformed by other viruses which encode members of the *src* gene family of protein-tyrosine kinases the elevated intracellular protein-tyrosine kinase activity is evinced as an increase in total cellular phosphotyrosine. A number of proteins containing phosphotyrosine have been identified in such cells, some of which may prove to play a role in the transformed phenotype. In contrast, in AEV-transformed cells there is only a slight increase in cellular phosphotyrosine levels. This might be sufficient to explain transformation if it involved a restricted but crucial set of substrates. Although fibroblasts transformed by AEV do contain some of the same phosphotyrosine-containing proteins which are found newly phosphorylated in EGF-treated normal fibroblasts, this question cannot be settled until protein-tyrosine kinase substrates critical for mitogenesis have been identified. Secondly, erythroblasts are not known to possess EGF receptors, so that even if the v-*erb*-B protein mimics an activated EGF receptor this would not be a normal growth signal for these cells. Some other growth factor receptors, however, have ligand-activated protein-tyrosine kinase activities, including the PDGF and insulin receptors. Perhaps an erythroid growth factor receptor, such as that for erythropoietin, is a protein-tyrosine kinase with specificities similar to the v-*erb*-B protein.

Several types of human tumor show abnormalities in EGF receptor expression. Many squamous cell carcinomas and gliomas have very high concentrations of EGF receptor protein. In some cases this is apparently a result of amplification of the entire EGF receptor gene. Whether the altered expression of EGF receptors played a part in tumorigenesis in these cases is unclear.

Are other oncogenes derived from growth factor receptor genes?

Rather few growth factor receptors have been characterized at the molecular level, so one cannot determine how many might be related to oncogenic proteins. Presuming, however, that the receptors will mostly be transmembrane glycoproteins there are only two other known oncogenic proteins which are reasonable candidates. The first is the v-*fms* protein, which is the transforming protein of the McDonough strain of feline sarcoma virus (SM-FeSV). The intact protein is a hybrid containing sequences derived from the viral *gag* gene at its NH$_2$ terminus. As with the v-*erb*-B gene, several v-*fms* gene products are derived by modification and processing of a single primary translation product[28]. They are all membrane-associated glycoproteins. A major 120 kDa v-*fms* product is affiliated with intracellular membranes, while a minor 140 kDa form is found on the cell surface[28,29]. The predicted structure of the v-*fms* gene product is very similar to that of the EGF receptor, with a large extracellular domain, a single membrane anchor sequence and a cytoplasmic domain containing a region homologous to the catalytic domain of the *src* gene family of protein-tyrosine kinases. Although the v-*fms* proteins display protein-tyrosine kinase activity *in vitro*, no new tyrosine phosphorylation events are detected in SM-FeSV-transformed cells. There is evidence from site-directed mutations, however, that both membrane association and expression on the cell surface are required for transformation. In addition the surface form of the v-*fms* protein accumulates in coated pits in a manner reminiscent of growth factor receptors[29]. Very recently the c-*fms* protein has been identified as a receptor for the myeloid cell growth factor, colony stimulating factor 1 (CSF-1). The CSF-1 receptor has protein-tyrosine kinase activity which is stimulated by binding CSF-1. Thus, the surface form of the v-*fms* protein could mimic the occupied CSF-1 receptor[30].

The second oncogenic protein with claims to be a growth factor receptor is the product of the recently characterized *neu* gene, the oncogene detected in a series of rat neuro/glioblastomas. The *neu* gene encodes a 185 kDa surface glycoprotein which has an associated protein-tyrosine kinase activity. Although no sequence data are yet available on the *neu* gene, a weak relationship between it and the v-*erb*-B gene can be detected by hybridization[31]. A product very similar to that of the *neu* gene is found on normal fibroblasts and this can be distinguished from the EGF receptor. It seems likely that the *neu* protein is an altered form of a growth factor receptor, but proof awaits the demonstration of a ligand binding site. One candidate is the PDGF receptor which has both a very similar size and an associated protein-tyrosine kinase activity.

Other connections between oncogenes and growth control

The third type of oncogene product is one that intercedes in a cellular growth control pathway at a postreceptor stage. While it is not the aim of this review to deal with such oncogenic proteins, there are several candidates. For instance the *src* family of oncogenes, including the *yes*, *fgr*, *fps/fes*, *ros* and *abl* oncogenes, all encode proteins with protein-tyrosine kinase activity. These enzymes might phosphorylate proteins which are normally targets for the growth factor-activated receptor protein-tyrosine kinases and thus provide a continuous intracellular mitogenic stimulus. Evidence is also emerging that *ras* proteins may transduce signals from cell surface receptors by regulating adenylate cyclase and hence cAMP levels. Finally there is a series of oncogenes including the *myc*, *myb* and *fos* genes, whose products are nuclear. Both the c-*myc* and c-*fos* genes are very rapidly induced upon PDGF treatment of resting fibroblasts. This, coupled with the nuclear location of these proteins, suggests that the c-*myc* and c-*fos* proteins might play a role in regulating the expression of other genes needed for the mitogenic response. From the diverse and numerous connections between growth control and oncogenes which have already come to light we can anticipate that other revealing links will emerge.

Acknowledgements

I am grateful to my colleagues in the Molecular Biology and Virology Laboratory for their constructive criticisms.

References

1   Waterfield, M. D., Scrace, G. T., Whittle, N., Stroobant, P, Johnsson, A., Wasteson, A., Westermark, B., Heldin, C-H., Huang, J. S. and Deuel, T. F. (1983) *Nature* 304, 35–39
2   Doolittle, R. F., Hunkapiller, M. W., Hood, L. E., Devare, S. G., Robbins, K. C., Aaronson, S. A. and Antoniades, H. N. (1983) *Science* 221, 275–277
3   Devare, S. G., Reddy, E. P., Robbins, K. C., Andersen, P. R., Tronick, S. R. and Aaronson, S. A. (1983) *Proc. Natl Acad. Sci. USA* 80, 731–735
4   Stroobant, P. and Waterfield, M. D. (1984) *EMBO J.* 3, 2963–2967
5   Johnsson, A., Heldin, C-H., Wasteson, A., Westermark, B., Deuel, T. F., Huang, J. S., Seeburg, P. H., Gray, A., Ullrich, A., Scrace, G., Stroobant, P. and Waterfield, M. D. (1984) *EMBO J.* 3, 921–928
6   Chiu, I–M., Reddy, E. P., Givol, D., Robbins, K. C., Tronick, S. R. and Aaronson, S. A. (1984) *Cell* 37, 123–129
7   Josephs, S. F., Guo, C., Ratner, L. and Wong-Staal, F. (1984) *Science* 223, 487–490
8   Robbins, K. C., Antoniades, H. N., Devare, S. G., Hunkapiller, M. W. and Aaronson, S. A. (1983) *Nature* 305, 605–608
9   Deuel, T. F., Huang, J. S., Huang, S. S., Stroobant, P. and Waterfield, M. D. (1983) *Science* 221, 1348–1350
10   Owen, A. J., Pantazis, P. and Antoniades, H. N. (1984) *Science* 225, 54–56
11   Huang, J. S., Huang, S. S. and Deuel, T. F. (1984) *Cell* 39, 79–87
12   Wang, J. Y. J. and Williams, L. T. (1984) *J. Biol. Chem.* 259, 10645–10648
13   Hannink, M. and Donoghue, D. J. (1984) *Science* 226, 1197–1199
14   Josephs, S. F., Ratner, L., Clarke, M. F., Westin, E. H., Reitz, M. S. and Wong-Staal, F. (1984) *Science* 225, 636–639
15   Gazit, A., Igarishi, H., Chiu, I.-M., Srinivasan, A., Yaniv, A., Tronick, S. R.,

      Robbins, K. C. and Aaronson, S. A. (1984) *Cell* 39, 89–97
16   Baldwin, G. S. (1982) *FEBS Lett.* 137, 1–5
17   Downward, J., Yarden, Y., Mayes, E., Scrace, G., Totty, N., Stockwell, P., Ullrich, A., Schlessinger, J. and Waterfield, M. D. (1984) *Nature* 307, 521–527
18   Yamamoto, T., Nishida, T., Miyajima, N., Kawai, S., Ooi, T. and Toyoshima, K. (1983) *Cell* 35, 71–78
19   Ullrich, A., Coussens, L., Hayflick, J. S., Dull, T. J., Gray, A., Tam, A. W., Lee, J., Yarden, Y., Libermann, T. A., Schlessinger, J., Downward, J., Mayes, E. L. V., Whittle, N., Waterfield, M. D. and Seeberg, P. H. (1984) *Nature* 309, 418–425
20   Xu, Y.-H., Ishii, S., Clark, A. J. L., Sullivan, M., Wilson, R. K., Ma, D. P., Roe, B. A., Merlino, G. T. and Pastan, I. (1984) *Nature* 309, 806–810
21   Lin, C. R., Chen, W. S., Kruijer, W., Stolarsky, L. S., Weber, W., Evans, R. M., Verma, I. M. and Rosenfeld, M. G. (1984) *Science* 224, 843–848
22   Buhrow, S. A., Cohen, S. and Staros, J. V. (1982) *J. Biol. Chem.* 257, 4019–4022
23   Hayman, M., Ramsay, G., Savin, K., Kitchener, G., Graf, T. and Beug, H. (1983) *Cell* 32, 579–588
24   Privalsky, M., Sealy, L., Bishop, J. M., McGrath, J. and Levinson, A. (1983) *Cell* 32, 1257–1267
25   Hayman, M. and Beug, H. (1984) *Nature* 309, 460–462
26   Gilmore, T., DeClue, J. E. and Martin, G. F. (1985) *Cell* 40, 609–619
27   Kris, R. M., Lax, I., Gullick, W., Waterfield, M. D., Ullrich, A., Fridkin, M. and Schlessinger, J. (1985) *Cell* 40, 619–625
28   Anderson, S. J., Gonda, M. A., Rettenmeier, C. W. and Sherr, C. J. (1984) *J. Virol.* 44, 696–702
29   Manger, R., Najita, L., Nichols, E. J., Hakomori, S-I. and Rohrschneider, L. (1984) *Cell* 39, 327–337
30   Rettenmeir, C. W., Sacca, R., Roussel, M. F., Look, A. T. and Stanley, E. R. (1985) *Cell* 41, 665–676
31   Schecter, A. L., Stern, D. F., Vaidyanathan, L., Decker, S. J., Drebin, J. A., Greene, M. I. and Weinberg, R. A. (1984) *Nature* 312, 513–516

T. Hunter is at the Salk Institute, PO Box 85800, San Diego, CA 92138, USA.

Peptide growth factors

Graham Carpenter and Stanley Cohen

Interaction of growth factors with target cells involves the rapid internalization of ligand–receptor complexes. The receptor possesses intrinsic tyrosyl protein kinase activity which may, in part, mediate the biological activities of the peptide factors. Sequence data indicates that growth factors and/or their receptors are related to oncogene products some of which also possess tyrosyl kinase activity.

In the past eight years much effort has been directed toward understanding, in biochemical terms, the mechanisms by which extracellular peptides produce biological responses in target cells. In particular, studies on the influence of growth factors on the regulation of cell proliferation have been rewarding and have even led to re-evaluations of the mechanism of action of some of the more 'classical' hormones. Not only have novel intracellular pathways for hormone–receptor complexes been traced, but evidence has also accumulated that some hormone receptors are bifunctional transmembrane molecules with a catalytic function (protein tyrosine kinase activity) that is enhanced when the hormone is bound. In view of the authors' perspective, studies with epidermal growth factor (EGF) will be highlighted and significant progress with other factors will be noted.

Hormone metabolism

The possibility that peptide hormones might enter the intracellular compartments was not seriously considered by most investigators prior to the mid-1970s. Notwithstanding a few reports and speculations to the contrary, the prevailing opinion was that peptide hormones (unlike their chemically distant but biologically similar cousins, the steroids) bound to receptors at the cell surface in a reversible fashion and did not actively or passively permeate the cell membrane. Quantitative chemical evidence that ^{125}I-EGF was actively internalized and degraded by cultured human fibroblasts was provided in 1976[1] and subsequently confirmed with morphological techniques[2,3]. It is now generally accepted that the binding of a great many peptide hormones to surface receptors is followed by rapid vesicular internalization and lysosomal degradation of the peptides. The fate of the internalized receptors is less clear, although much of the internalized EGF receptor in cultured fibroblasts is now known to be degraded[4].

Despite this endocytic pathway being a well-recognized route in many hormonal systems, it is currently understood primarily in morphological terms. However, biochemical techniques and increasingly sophisticated morphological procedures are being applied to the analysis of these pathways. The acidic environment of nearly all endosomal compartments has been documented, but its biochemical regulation and physiological meaning have not been defined. Since many ligand–receptor complexes are dissociated at low pH, this may be an important step in those systems that involve separate processing of ligand and receptor. The sorting of intracellular traffic, such as the separation of LDL and EGF receptors, which have different fates (recycling and degradation, respectively) but are co-internalized within the same endocytic vesicle[5], suggests sophisticated biochemical mechanisms.

It is generally agreed that hormone-laden endocytic vesicles, formed at the membrane primarily in coated pit areas, ultimately fuse with lysosomal bodies, wherein degradation of the ligand, and in some cases the receptor, occurs. Prelysosomal modifications of ligand and receptor probably occur, but have not been defined. Likewise, the exact route from coated pit to lysosome, which may occur very rapidly, is obscure, but may involve intermediate stops in other organelles, such as the Golgi. Debate continues as to whether or not free, intracellular, ligand-bearing endosomes contain clathrin[6,7]. The weight of evidence, however, suggests the transient existence of intracellular, clathrin-coated vesicles.

A critical question in this area is whether the intracellular processing of hormones and their receptors is related to, or necessary for, the generation of biological responses to the hormone. In the case of growth factors, considerable effort has been expended to investigate the role of endocytosis in the stimulation of DNA synthesis. Our opinion is that no clear experimental evidence exists to answer this important question.

Activation of protein phosphorylation

A major advance in growth factor studies was the demonstration, in 1979, of a direct effect of EGF on a chemical reaction in a cell-free system[8]. When EGF was added to a membrane preparation in the presence of ATP, the rapid activation of protein phosphorylation occurred. This system enabled biochemical tools to be applied to the mechanism of EGF action. In a short time, the EGF receptor was highly purified by affinity chromatography and demonstrated to retain EGF-sensitive protein kinase activity[9]. The isolated receptor is a glycoprotein with a molecular mass of 170 000 (Ref. 10). Several studies have since demonstrated, by immunological[10] and ATP affinity labeling[11] techniques, that the EGF-sensitive protein kinase activity is intrinsic to the 170 000 receptor molecule. Evidence for the existence of similar protein kinase effector systems is now associated with an increasing number of peptide hormones that influence cell growth: platelet-derived growth factor (PDGF), insulin, insulin-like growth factor, and somatomedin-C.

Data from these systems suggest that the generation of a 'second messenger' by the peptide hormones occurs through a receptor–effector system that is contained in one protein molecule and involves direct activation of a protein kinase domain by the hormone. The classic studies of Sutherland and his colleagues have defined a related mechanism in which elevated protein kinase activity is produced indirectly by peptide hormones, through the intermediate activation of cyclic nucleotide systems. In these systems, which generally involve acute biological responses to the hormones, the effector activity (adenyl cyclase) is physically separable from the receptor. Hormone-induced coupling of the two proteins in the membrane is thought to activate the system.

An exciting development in the characterization of the EGF-sensitive protein kinase was the finding that substrates were phosphorylated exclusively at tyrosyl residues[12], an activity previously thought to be associated only with the protein products of oncogenes. The general occurrence of tyrosine kinases in both hormonal and viral systems capable of regulating cell proliferation has created a possible biochemical point of merger (or intersection?) for two seemingly dissimilar disciplines. The crucial questions now being asked of both systems are: what are the direct intracellular substrates of these kinases, and which substrates are physiologically important to the process of growth control. The approaches being tried include: (1) the identification of proteins whose phosphorylation pattern *in vivo* is altered by hormones or transforming viruses[13], (2) the addition of purified proteins of known function to *in vitro* phosphorylation assays, and (3) the *in vitro* identification of proteins that have an affinity for the hormone–receptor complex formed *in vivo*[14]. Each approach has its own difficulties and merits, but so far the former have been dominant. Further investigation may link the hormonal activation of protein kinase activity with the endocytosis of hormone–receptor (kinase) complexes. Are hormonal phosphorylations generated solely at the plasma membrane or is the kinase translocated to other sites within the cell?

In addition to phosphotyrosine, the EGF receptor labeled *in vivo* also contains significant quantities of phosphoserine and phosphothreonine. Since only phosphotyrosine has been detected in autophosphorylation reactions with the purified receptor, it would seem that other kinases may phosphorylate the receptor at serine and threonine residues. It has been suggested that protein kinase C may participate in these phosphorylations. However, no regulatory role for any phosphorylation site on the EGF receptor has been assigned.

Growth factor genes

Molecular biological techniques have recently been applied to growth factor systems. In the last year, nucleic acid sequences for EGF, nerve growth factor (NGF), and insulin-like growth factor (IGF-I) have been cloned and sequenced. The cloned cDNA for mouse β-NGF suggests the presence of a prepro-hormone of 25 000 to 34 000 molecular mass[15,16]. The sequence predicts a long extension at the amino-terminus of the polypeptide and a very short (two amino acids) extension at the carboxyl-terminus. Assignment of the exact size of the amino-terminal segment is difficult as the cDNA sequence suggests three possible open reading frames. Analysis of the isolated gene for human β-NGF indicates a high degree of homology to the mouse cDNA and the presence of one intron, located within the sequence for the amino-terminal extension[16].

Dibasic amino acid cleavage sites are located at each end of the NGF sequence and at two other sites. Whether the fragments generated by processing the prepro-NGF represent other biologically active peptides is not known, but the generation of multiple peptide hormones from a common polypeptide precursor has become a not uncommon event. The processed peptides need not have similar physiological functions. IGF-I, also known as somatomedin-C, is also synthesized in the form of a precursor protein, as deduced by the sequence of cloned cDNA, having a 25 amino acid peptide N-terminal to the IGF sequence and a carboxyl-terminal peptide of 35 amino acids[17].

The cloned mouse EGF cDNA has been sequenced[18,19] and suggests the presence of a very large EGF precursor with a molecular mass of approximately 130 000. The amino-terminal segment (976 amino acids) of the EGF precursor contains sequences that might produce seven EGF-like peptides. The carboxyl-terminal segment of the precursor is 188 amino acids long. Thus, there would seem to be an enormous potential in this precursor of 1217 amino acids to generate a family of peptides related in some way to EGF, which contains 53 amino acids. A chemically synthesized gene for human EGF has been constructed, cloned and expressed in both *E. coli* and yeast[20,21]. Also, the human gene for the EGF receptor has been mapped to the p13→q22 region of chromosome 7 (Ref. 22).

Growth factor families

Although the occurrence of bioactive 'factors' seems widespread in biological systems and in the scientific literature, the chemical identification of these factors has proceeded slowly, with a substantial attrition rate. The advances in purification and sequencing techniques for microgram quantities of protein, however, have started to produce chemical data about some of these peptides. These data, in combination with data deduced from nucleic acid sequences and the results of competitive binding assays, suggest the presence of growth factor families.

The 'insulin family' includes insulin, the insulin-like growth factors, relaxin, and nerve growth factor. An 'EGF family' has begun to develop with sequence analysis of transforming growth factors (TGF). The transforming growth factors can be isolated from normal as well as malignant cells or tissues and are capable of inducing anchorage-independent growth of otherwise non-transformed, anchorage-dependent cells[23]. This biological effect, in most instances, is due to the action of two distinct proteins, designated α-TGF and β-TGF (Ref. 24). The α peptide competes with ^{125}I-EGF in radioreceptor assays and mimics the biological activities of EGF in cell culture, but is not neutralized by antibodies to EGF. The production of biological responses to these TGFs requires binding of the α-TGF to the EGF receptor, and binding of the β-TGF to an as yet unidentified receptor. The first 45 N-terminal residues of α-TGF show an overall limited, but significant, degree of homology with EGF (Ref. 25). However, the positions of the potential disulfide bonds and the sequences near these cysteine residues are quite similar in both peptides. The sequence of α-TGF is more similar to the EGF sequence than to the sequences for the other potential peptides in the large, 130 000 mol. mass EGF precursor. The significance of TGFs *in vivo* should become subject to investigation as larger quantities of purified peptides become available. It should be pointed out that the natural biological function(s) of EGF in the intact animals is not understood and little progress in this important area has been made in the last ten years. The use of cloned EGF cDNA probes should, however, facilitate the mapping of the EGF gene and the identification of cells which produce EGF mRNA.

The 'PDGF family', also, has increased as a result of protein and nucleic acid sequence analysis. The N-terminal partial protein sequence of human PDGF has revealed a very high degree of homology to the protein product, as determined by its nucleic acid sequence, of the *sis* gene of the simian sarcoma virus[26,27]. Since the *sis* gene is known to be the transforming gene of this virus, these sequence similarities suggest a relationship between oncogenes and growth factor genes and, perhaps, functional similarities among their protein products.

Recently, it has been reported that there exists a high degree of homology between the sequences of certain peptides derived from the EGF receptor and the deduced sequence of the erb B oncogene product[30]. This finding suggests that other oncogene products also may be related to growth factor receptors and conceivably exert their biological effects by alterations of normal receptor functions.

Nuclear events

Investigations of peptide hormone actions on specific events in the nucleus have started to yield useful data. A number of groups have begun to identify DNA sequences that are rapidly and selectively expressed following the exposure of cultured cells to growth factors. A ten-fold increase in RNA sequences related to VL30 elements has been detected in cells treated with EGF[28]. Although the function of these VL30 elements is not known, they are a class of repetitive sequences related to retrovirus sequences and transposable elements. The rapid induction of RNA sequences for the c-*myc* proto-oncogene by PDGF has also been demonstrated[29]. It seems probable to us that the activation of the transcription of overlapping families of RNA transcripts may be a general phenomenon for both peptide and steroid hormones that regulate cell growth.

An intriguing concept relative to the hormonal control of nuclear activity arises from the observation that purified EGF receptor and purified *src* kinase have an ATP-dependent interaction with DNA[31]. In the presence of ATP, these proteins are able to nick supercoiled DNA, converting it to a relaxed form. The possibility exists that this enzymatic activity is both a nicking and closing activity reminiscent of DNA topoisomerases. It remains to be demonstrated, however, whether this activity is intrinsic to these proteins or is produced by other associated proteins present as trace contaminants. Should the DNA nicking activity be shown to be inherent in these proteins, then the ligand-dependent process of internalization of hormone–receptor complexes may represent a mechanism to facilitate the translocation of this plasma membrane protein to the nucleus, where it could interact directly with the genome. Such a mechanism implies that the receptor itself is the 'second messenger' molecule for hormone-induced mitogenesis.

References

1 Carpenter, G. and Cohen, S. (1976) *J. Cell Biol.* 71, 159–171
2 Haigler, H. T., McKanna, J. A. and Cohen, S. (1979) *J. Cell Biol.* 81, 382–395
3 Schlessinger, J., Shechter, Y., Willingham, M. C. and Pastan, I. (1978) *Proc. Natl Acad. Sci. USA* 75, 2659–2663
4 Stoscheck, C. M. and Carpenter, G. (1984) *J. Cell Biol.* 98, 1048–1053
5 Carpentier, J. L., Gorden, P., Anderson, G. W., Goldstein, J. L., Brown, M. S., Cohen, S. and Orci, L. (1982) *J. Cell Biol.* 95, 73–77
6 Pastan, I. and Willingham, M. C. (1983) *Trends Biochem. Sci.* 8, 250–254
7 Helenius, A., Mellman, I., Wall, D. and Hubbard, A. (1983) *Trends Biochem. Sci.* 8, 245–250
8 Carpenter, G., King, L. Jr and Cohen, S. (1979) *J. Biol. Chem.* 254, 4884–4891
9 Cohen, S., Carpenter, G. and King, L. Jr (1980) *J. Biol. Chem.* 255, 4834–4842
10 Cohen, S., Ushiro, H., Stoscheck, C. and Chinkers, M. (1982) *J. Biol. Chem.* 257, 1523–1531
11 Buhrow, S. A., Cohen, S. and Staros, J. V. (1982) *J. Biol. Chem.* 257, 4019–4022
12 Ushiro, H. and Cohen, S. (1980) *J. Biol. Chem.* 255, 8363–8365
13 Cooper, J. A. and Hunter, T. *Curr. Top. Microbiol. Immunol.* (in press)
14 Fava, R. A. and Cohen, S. (1984) *J. Biol. Chem.* 259, 2636–2645
15 Scott, J., Selby, M., Urdea, M., Quiroga, M., Bell, G. I. and Rutter, W. J. (1983) *Nature* 302, 538–540
16 Ullrich, A., Gray, A., Berman, C. and Dull, T. J. (1983) *Nature* 303, 821–825
17 Jansen, M., van Schaik, F. M. A., Ricker, A. T., Bullock, B., Woods, D. E., Gabbay, K. H., Nussbaum, A. L., Sussenbach, J. S. and Van den Brande, J. L. (1983) *Nature* 306, 609–611
18 Gray, A., Dull, T. J. and Ullrich, A. (1983) *Nature* 303, 722–725
19 Scott, J., Ureda, M., Quiroga, M., Sanchez-Pescador, R., Fong, N., Selby, M., Rutter, W. J. and Bell, G. I. (1983) *Science* 221, 236–240
20 Smith, J., Cook, E., Fotheringham, I., Pheby, S., Derbyshire, R., Eaton, M. A. W., Doel, M., Lilley, D. M. J., Pardon, J. F., Patel, T., Lewis, H. and Bell, L. D. (1982) *Nucleic Acids Res.* 10, 4467–4482
21 Urdea, M. S., Merryweather, J. P., Mullenbach, G. T., Coit, D., Heberlein, U., Valenzuela, P. and Barr, P. J. (1983) *Proc. Natl Acad. Sci. USA* 80, 7461–7465
22 Kondo, I. and Shimizu, N. (1983) *Cytogenet. Cell Genet.* 35, 9–14
23 DeLarco, J. E. and Todaro, G. T. (1978) *Proc. Natl Acad. Sci. USA* 75, 4001–4005
24 Roberts, A. B., Anzano, M. A., Lamb, L. C., Smith, J. M., Frolik, C. A., Marquardt, H., Todaro, G. J. and Sporn, M. B. (1982) *Nature* 295, 417–419

25 Marquardt, H., Hunkapiller, M. W., Hood, L. E., Twardzik, D. R., DeLarco, J. E., Stephenson, J. R. and Todaro, G. (1983) *Proc. Natl Acad. Sci. USA* 80, 4684–4688

26 Waterfield, M. D., Scrace, G. T., Whittle, N., Stroobant, P., Johnsson, A., Wasteson, A., Westermark, B., Heldin, C. H., Huang, J. S. and Durel, T. F. (1983) *Nature* 304, 35–39

27 Doolittle, R. F. Hunkapiller, M. W., Hood, L. E., Devare, S. G., Robbins, K., Aaronson, S. A. and Antoniades, H. N. (1983) *Science* 221, 275–277

28 Foster, D. N., Schmidt, L. J., Hodgson, C. P., Moses, H. L. and Getz, M. J. (1982) *Proc. Natl Acad. Sci. USA* 79, 7317–7321

29 Kelley, K., Cochran, B. H., Stiles, C. D. and Leder, P. (1983) *Cell* 35, 603–610

30 Downward, J., Yarden, Y., Mayes, E., Scrace, G., Totty, N., Stockwell, P., Ullrich, A., Schlessinger, J. and Waterfield, M. D. (1984) *Nature (London)* 307, 521–527

31 Mroczkowski, B., Mosig, G. and Cohen, S. (1984) *Nature* 309, 270–273

Graham Carpenter and Stanley Cohen are at the Department of Biochemistry, Vanderbilt University School of Medicine, Nashville, TN 37232, USA.

Fibroblast growth factors: broad spectrum mitogens with potent angiogenic activity

Kenneth A. Thomas and Guillermo Gimenez-Gallego

Fibroblast growth factors (FGFs) are protein mitogens, found in brain and pituitary, that induce division of a wide variety of cells in culture. Interest has focused on FGFs, in part, because of their mitogenic activity for vascular endothelial cells in culture and their ability to induce blood vessel growth in vivo.

The discovery of substances that control the growth of animal cells and the mechanism by which they work is currently one of the major focuses of research in the biochemical sciences. With the recently discovered correlations between growth factors and oncogenes[1], this work is motivated in large part by the belief that lesions in these growth control systems are the underlying causes of cancers. Two recently purified mitogens, acidic and basic FGF, are the focus of attention of numerous research groups.

The scientific origin of FGFs is almost 50 years old. Around 1940, crude brain homogenates were reported to be a plentiful source of substances that stimulated primary fibroblasts to divide in culture[2,3]. The activity was uniquely high in the central nervous system compared to a variety of other organs that were examined. In 1973, Armelin[4] found that pituitary extracts also had potent mitogenic activity for Balb/c 3T3 'fibroblasts', a cell line of uncertain differentiated state. In the 1970s, Gospodarowicz and colleagues[5] partially purified FGF activities from both pituitary and brain, based on mitogenic activity for the Balb/c 3T3 cell line. They showed that these presumably pure preparations induced division of a wide variety of cells of mesodermal origin including vascular endothelial cells, a phenotype that had previously been difficult to propagate in culture.

Originally, only a single type of brain-derived FGF, proposed to arise from limited proteolysis of myelin basic protein *in vivo,* was thought to exist. The mitogen was claimed to be inactivated at its assumed basic isoelectric point, since no biological activity could be recovered with the myelin basic protein fragments after isoelectric focusing. By 1980, however, an active FGF with an acidic isoelectric point, clearly not a fragment of myelin basic protein, was identified in these partially purified preparations of FGF from brain[6]. Shortly thereafter, the basic mitogen from pituitary also was shown to be distinct from the inactive contaminating protein that comprised the bulk of the partially purified pituitary preparations[7]. In the past few years both acidic and basic FGF have been identified in brain and pituitary preparations. Once it was clear that these protein preparations were impure, efforts were renewed to obtain homogeneous FGF from both sources.

Purification of FGFs
Acidic FGF

The method of partial purification of FGF from brain employed salt fractionation, cation exchange and gel filtration chromatography of brain homogenates.

We now know that the original identification of FGF from bovine brain by isoelectric focusing of these partially purified preparations[6] generated acidic FGF (aFGF) that was greater than 90% pure, since nearly all the contaminants are found in the basic pH region. Quantitative removal of ampholytes and residual minor protein impurities was achieved on custom-made C_4 HPLC columns[8]. These columns have subsequently been produced commercially and successfully used for the high efficiency purification of many proteins.

The brain-derived aFGF was estimated to be greater than 99% pure based on high sensitivity, silver-stained, SDS-polyacrylamide electrophoretic gels. The purified protein has an isoelectric point range of 5–7 and electrophoreses in SDS gels as a close doublet with polypeptide masses, calculated from the complete amino acid sequences[9], of 15.9 and 15.2 kDa. After resolution on shallow gradient elution from C_4 HPLC columns, both forms were found to have very similar amino acid compositions. We concluded, and later confirmed by amino acid sequencing[10], that they were microheterogeneous forms of the same protein.

Either aFGF, or closely related molecules, have recently been independently purified and reported by at least three other laboratories. Lobb and Fett[11] have purified aFGF from brain and denoted it heparin-binding growth factor α, from its binding to heparin-Sepharose. Both aFGF and eye-derived growth factor II compete with hypothalamus-derived endothelial cell growth factor in radioreceptor and monoclonal antibody based immunoassays[12]. Other acidic endothelial cell mitogens from the central nervous system, notably retinal-derived growth factor[13], might ultimately be added to this converging list of aFGF or aFGF-like proteins*. Growth factors that are very similar, if not identical, to either aFGF or bFGF are listed in Table 1.

*For simplicity and clarity, results reported for heparin-binding growth factor α (HBGFα) and endothelial cell growth factor (ECGF) are reported using the aFGF nomenclature in this review.

Table 1. Growth factors probably related to FGFs

Acidic FGF

Endothelial cell growth factor (ECGF)
Eye-derived growth factor II (EDGF II)
Heparin-binding growth factor α (HGFα, HBGFα)
Brain-derived growth factor (BDGF)
Retinal-derived growth factor (RDGF)
Astroglial growth factor 1 (AGF 1)

Basic FGF

Eye-derived growth factor I (EDGF I)
Heparin-binding growth factor β (HGFβ, HBGFβ)
Chondrosarcoma-derived growth factor
Cartilage-derived growth factor (CDGF)
Hepatoma-derived growth factor
Astroglial growth factor 2 (AGF 2)

Substantial progress also has been made toward the purification of aFGF from pituitary. Armelin and colleagues have obtained very active preparations of a 12–15 kDa acidic pituitary mitogen[14].

Basic FGF

Bovine pituitary bFGF of ~15 kDa was obtained by Lemmon and Bradshaw[15] in greater than 90% purity. The bFGF was purified using initial steps similar to those for the partially purified FGF from pituitary and brain (salt fractionation, ion exchange and gel filtration) followed by electrophoresis and elution from acidic polyacrylamide gels. The amino acid composition of this purified material proved that it could not be derived from myelin basic protein. Bohlen *et al.*[16] also purified to homogeneity a highly active pituitary bFGF (15.8 kDa, pI 9.6) using the same initial steps followed by chromatography on a Mono S cation exchange column. The relationship between the material of Lemmon and Bradshaw and that of Bohlen and colleagues remains to be determined. Given the identical source, similar mass, pI, activity and amino acid compositions, they are likely to be closely related, if not identical, proteins.

Heparin affinity purification of FGFs

Recently aFGF and bFGF have both been shown to bind avidly to heparin affinity columns[11,17,18]. This has simplified the purification protocols and led to an improved recovery of FGFs; however, the purified aFGF contains slightly more contaminating proteins than does aFGF obtained by the classical purification techniques combined with reversed-phase HPLC.

The rationale for trying heparin affinity chromatography arose from the mitogenic activity of the FGFs for vascular endothelial cells in culture. Based on the observation that mast cells were usually present in the vicinity of growing vascular capillaries *in vivo*, Folkman and colleagues tested known products of these cells in angiogenic assays. The mast cell product, heparin, was found to enhance the activity of crude tumor angiogenesis factor in promoting vascular endothelial cell chemokinesis *in vitro* and capillary growth *in vivo* but, by itself, it was inactive[19]. Heparin was subsequently shown to augment the ability of partially purified aFGF to support the growth of human vascular endothelial cells in culture[20]. Shortly thereafter, an 18 kDa endothelial cell mitogen, from the extracellular matrix deposited in culture by chondrosarcoma cells, was purified by its ability to bind to heparin affinity columns[21]. After these initial reports, successful use of heparin columns to purify both acidic and basic FGF appeared.

Structure of FGFs

The complete amino acid sequence of aFGF from bovine brain[9] is shown in Fig. 1. The two microheterogeneous forms of aFGF seen by SDS gel electrophoresis correspond to the full length 140-residue aFGF-1 (15.9 kDa) and aFGF-2 (15.2 kDa), a form that lacks the six amino terminal residues. The complete 146-residue sequence of bovine pituitary bFGF[22], also listed in Fig. 1, shows 55% identity with the overlapping regions of aFGF-1. The amino terminal sequence of bFGF from bovine brain confirms its identity with the basic pituitary mitogen[23]. This homology between aFGF and bFGF, in addition to the common tissue origins and similarities in sizes and activities, clearly establishes that both mitogens arose by gene duplication and divergence from a common ancestral protein.

A distant sequence homology has been detected between FGFs and interleukin-1s[5,9,10]. As shown in Fig. 1, the carboxyl terminal halves of the precursors for both human IL-1β, and to a lesser extent IL-1α, are similar to the complete

```
AFGF                                              PHE-ASN-      -LEU-PRO-
BFGF   PRO-    -ALA-LEU-PRO-GLU-ASP-GLY-GLY-      SER-GLY-ALA- -PHE-PRO-
IL-1B  VAL-HIS-ASP-ALA-PRO-VAL-ARG-               SER-LEU-ASN- -CYS-THR-
IL-1A  PRO-ARG-SER-ALA-PRO-PHE-SER-PHE-LEU-SER-ASN-VAL-LYS-TYR-ASN-PHE-MET-ARG-


AFGF   -LEU-GLY-ASN-TYR-LYS-        -LYS-PRO-LYS-LEU-LEU-        -TYR-CYS-
BFGF   -PRO-GLY-HIS-PHE-LYS-        -ASP-PRO-LYS-ARG-LEU-        -TYR-CYS-
IL-1B  -LEU-ARG-ASP-SER-GLN-        -GLN-    -LYS-SER-LEU-       -VAL-MET-
IL-1A  -ILE-ILE-LYS-TYR-GLU-PHE-ILE-LEU-ASN-    -ASP-ALA-LEU-ASN-GLN-SER-ILE-ILE-


AFGF   -SER-    -ASN-GLY-GLY-TYR-PHE-    -LEU-ARG-ILE-LEU-PRO-ASP-GLY-THR-VAL-ASP-
BFGF   -LYS-    -ASN-GLY-GLY-PHE-PHE-    -LEU-ARG-ILE-HIS-PRO-ASP-GLY-ARG-VAL-ASP-
IL-1B  -SER-        -GLY-PRO-TYR-GLU-    -LEU-LYS-ALA-LEU-HIS-LEU-GLN-GLY-GLN-ASP-
IL-1A  -ARG-ALA-ASN-ASP-GLN-TYR-LEU-THR-ALA-ALA-ALA-LEU-HIS-ASN-LEU-ASP-GLU-ALA-


AFGF   -GLY-                        -THR-LYS-ASP-ARG-SER-ASP-
BFGF   -GLY-                        -VAL-ARG-GLU-LYS-SER-ASP-
IL-1B  -MET-GLU-GLN-GLN-VAL-VAL-PHE-SER-MET-SER-PHE-VAL-GLN-GLY-GLU-GLU-SER-ASN-
IL-1A  -VAL-LYS-                    -PHE-ASP-MET-GLY-ALA-TYR-LYS-SER-SER-LYS-ASP-ASP-


AFGF   -GLN-HIS-ILE-GLN-LEU-GLN-LEU-CYS-ALA-GLU-SER-ILE-GLY-GLU-VAL-TYR-ILE-
BFGF   -PRO-HIS-ILE-LYS-LEU-GLN-LEU-GLN-ALA-GLU-GLU-ARG-GLY-VAL-VAL-SER-ILE-
IL-1B  -ASP-LYS-ILE-PRO-VAL-ALA-LEU-GLY-LEU-LYS-GLU-    -LYS-ASN-LEU-TYR-LEU-SER-
IL-1A  -ALA-LYS-ILE-THR-VAL-ILE-LEU-ARG-ILE-SER-LYS-    -THR-GLN-LEU-TYR-VAL-THR-


AFGF           -LYS-SER-THR-GLU-THR-GLY-GLN-PHE-LEU-ALA-MET-ASP-THR-ASP-GLY-
BFGF           -LYS-GLY-VAL-CYS-ALA-ASN-ARG-TYR-LEU-ALA-MET-LYS-GLU-ASP-GLY-
IL-1B  -CYS-VAL-LEU-LYS-ASP-ASP-LYS-PRO-THR-LEU-GLN-LEU-GLU-    -SER-VAL-ASP-PRO-
IL-1A      -ALA-GLN-ASP-GLU-ASP-GLN-PRO-VAL-LEU-LEU-LYS-GLU-MET-PRO-GLU-ILE-PRO-


AFGF   -LEU-LEU-TYR-GLY-SER-GLN-THR-PRO-ASN-GLU-GLU-CYS-LEU-PHE-LEU-GLU-ARG-LEU-
BFGF   -ARG-LEU-LEU-ALA-SER-LYS-CYS-VAL-THR-ASP-GLU-CYS-PHE-PHE-PHE-GLU-ARG-LEU-
IL-1B  -LYS-ASN-TYR-PRO-    -LYS-LYS-LYS-MET-GLU-LYS-ARG-PHE-VAL-PHE-ASN-LYS-ILE-
IL-1A  -LYS-THR-ILE-THR-GLY-SER-GLU-THR-ASN-LEU-LEU-    -PHE-PHE-TRP-GLU-THR-HIS-


AFGF   -GLU-GLU-ASN-HIS-TYR-ASN-THR-TYR-ILE-SER-LYS-LYS-HIS-ALA-GLU-LYS-HIS-TRP-
BFGF   -GLU-SER-ASN-ASN-TYR-ASN-THR-TYR-ARG-SER-ARG-LYS-TYR-SER-          -SER-TRP-
IL-1B  -GLU-ILE-ASN-ASN-LYS-LEU-GLU-PHE-GLU-SER-ALA-GLN-PHE-PRO-          -ASN-TRP-
IL-1A  -GLY-THR-LYS-ASN-TYR-    -PHE-    -THR-SER-VAL-ALA-HIS-PRO-         -ASN-LEU-


AFGF   -PHE-VAL-GLY-LEU-LYS-LYS-ASN-GLY-ARG-SER-LYS-    -LEU-GLY-PRO-ARG-THR-
BFGF   -TYR-VAL-ALA-LEU-LYS-ARG-THR-GLY-GLN-TYR-LYS-    -LEU-GLY-PRO-LYS-THR-
IL-1B  -TYR-ILE-SER-THR-SER-GLN-ALA-GLU-ASN-MET-PRO-VAL-PHE-LEU-GLY-GLY-    -THR-
IL-1A  -PHE-ILE-ALA-THR-LYS-GLN-ASP-TYR-TRP-VAL-        -CYS-LEU-ALA-GLY-


AFGF   -HIS-PHE-GLY-GLN-LYS-ALA-ILE-LEU-    -PHE-LEU-PRO-LEU-PRO-VAL-SER-SER-ASP
BFGF   -GLY-PRO-GLY-GLN-LYS-ALA-ILE-LEU-    -PHE-LEU-PRO-MET-SER-ALA-LYS-SER
IL-1B  -LYS-GLY-GLY-GLN-ASP-    -ILE-THR-ASP-PHE-THR-MET-GLN-PHE-VAL-SER-SER
IL-1A          -GLY-PRO-PRO-SER-ILE-THR-ASP-PHE-GLN-ILE-LEU-GLU-ASN-GLN-ALA
```

amino acid sequences of the FGFs. These regions of IL-1s correspond to the biologically active, processed portions of the precursor molecules. Although IL-1β, and presumably IL-1α, are fibroblast mitogens, aFGF does not have IL-1s thymocyte mitogenic activity (bFGF has not been measured for this activity). IL-1s and FGFs appear to have long ago diverged from a common ancestral protein, followed by the split between the two interleukin-1s and finally the emergence of the two FGFs.

Deca- and octapeptides, flanked on both ends by basic dipeptides, are found in both aFGF (102–111) and bFGF (111–118). Since basic dipeptides are proteolytic recognition sites for many active polypeptides to be cleaved from their longer precursor proteins, we compared these sequences to other known bioactive peptides. A similarity was observed between the aFGF decapeptide and active neuropeptides of the tachykinin and bombesin classes. Although peptides of these types have been reported to have mitogenic activity, a synthetic aFGF 102–111 peptide was not mitogenic for Balb/c 3T3 fibroblasts[9]. The activity of this polypeptide, if any, remains to be discovered.

Activities

FGF activity was originally identified and subsequently purified on the basis of the induction of DNA synthesis by Balb/c 3T3 cells in the presence of low serum concentrations in culture. A variety of cells from embryonic mesoderm were found to be stimulated to divide by the partially purified FGF preparations[5]. Since both aFGF and bFGF have been purified from the partially fractionated brain extract, it seems likely that both were present in some or all of these preparations perhaps with varying ratios; other uncharacterized mitogens might also have been present. Numerous types of cells have now been reported to be stimulated to synthesize DNA and divide in response to either pure aFGF or bFGF, including primary fibroblasts, vascular and corneal endothelial cells, chondrocytes, osteoblasts, myoblasts, smooth muscle and glial cells[22,24]. The FGFs, therefore, are very broad spectrum mitogens in culture.

Although bFGF has been claimed to be 30- to 100-fold more active than aFGF[22], this difference is probably the result of partial inactivation of the acidic mitogen. In the presence of heparin, a polyanionic glycosaminoglycan that appears both to stabilize the active conformation of aFGF and to decrease the apparent K_d of binding to its receptor[25], the activity of the mitogen is increased from 3- to greater than 100-fold[12,26]. Heparin has relatively little, if any, effect on the activity of bFGF. Thus in the presence of heparin, both aFGF and bFGF are essentially equally active mitogens[26] with induction of half-maximal DNA synthesis at concentrations of 10–100 pM. The relevance of heparin binding to both FGFs and its effect on the mitogenic activity of aFGF *in vivo* remains to be determined. Endothelial cell surfaces and basement membranes both contain heparin or heparin-like polysaccharides. These could possibly partition free FGFs onto either the cell surface or the basement membranes on which the target cells reside.

Fig. 1. Amino acid sequences of FGFs and homologies with interleukin-1s. The complete amino acid sequences of bovine brain-derived aFGF (AFGF)[9] and pituitary-derived bFGF (BFGF)[22] are aligned with the carboxyl terminal halves of the precursors of both human IL-1β (IL-1B) and IL-1α (IL-1A) beginning at residues 114 and 110, respectively. The amino terminus of IL-1β starts at Ala117. Mature mouse IL-1α starts at a position equivalent to Ser112 in the human protein. Common aligned residues are enclosed in boxes.

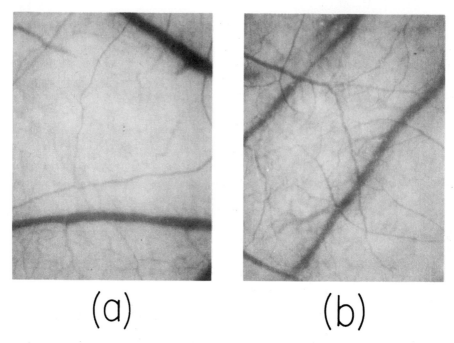

Fig. 2 *The angiogenic activity of aFGF. Agarose pellets containing either (a) control (10μg heparin) or (b) mitogen (1 μg aFGF plus 10 μg heparin) were applied on the extra-embryonic chorioallantoic membrane of a 10-day old chicken egg grown suspended in a pouch made of a thin plastic sheet. After three days the responses were photographed at ×40 magnification[10].*

Considering the many functions[27] and structural heterogeneity of heparin, only a subset of its multiple forms might bind to the FGFs and augment the activity of aFGF. Given the wide variety of target cells of the FGFs, their binding to heparin seems unlikely to be uniquely correlated with their mitogenicity for vascular endothelial cells.

Physiological significance

The presence of two such structurally and functionally similar FGFs is puzzling. It is possible that either they ultimately will be found to have important activity differences *in vivo* or that they differ in their cellular sources or the controls on their synthesis and secretion. Even the relative amounts of these two FGFs are not certain. Although the acidic mitogen is the principal form in the 0.15 M ammonium sulfate extracts of brain[11,18,22], higher salt concentrations have been reported to lead to increased yields of bFGF[11].

Little is known about the normal activities of the FGFs *in vivo*. Both aFGF (Fig. 2) and bFGF are reported to induce blood vessel capillary growth *in vivo*[10,22,28]. However, since FGFs have such a broad spectrum of target cells in culture, it would be quite surprising if angiogenesis was their sole, or perhaps even principal, significant biological function. Under normal conditions it appears more likely that FGFs might be rather general tissue growth factors that stimulate and coordinate mitogenesis of multiple cell types during animal growth, maintenance and tissue repair. In this regard, they are excellent candidates for the therapeutic promotion of wound healing in man.

The FGFs, or FGF-related mitogens, might be associated with various proliferative pathologies such as tumor growth. If either one of the FGFs, or an oncogene equivalent of these mitogens, was abnormally expressed in neoplastically transformed cells, then they could induce the hyperplasia often observed in host tissues surrounding the transformed cells, the autocrine stimulation of tumor cell growth, and tumor angiogenesis. In this regard, the observation of endothelial cell mitogenic proteins with similar masses and pIs to the FGFs found in experimental animal tumors is intriguing[29]. Furthermore, antibodies to bFGF inhibit the growth of a chondrosarcoma used as the source of a mitogen for vascular endothelial cells that has a similar mass and pI to bFGF[30]. If FGF-like mitogens are commonly used by solid tumors to induce and support their vascularization then it might be feasible to inhibit the development or maintenance of this pathological vascularity with antagonists of FGFs. Inhibition of tumor neovascularization by FGFs could then either arrest or reverse the growth of solid tumors.

References

1 Heldin, C.-H. and Westermark, B. (1984) *Cell* 37, 9–20
2 Trowell, O. A., Chir, B. and Willmer, E. N. (1939) *J. Exp. Biol.* 16, 60–70
3 Hoffman, R. S. (1940) *Growth* 4, 361–376
4 Armelin, H. A. (1973) *Proc. Natl Acad. Sci. USA* 70, 2702–2706
5 Gospodarowicz, D., Mescher, A. L. and Birdwell, C. R. (1978) *Natl Cancer Inst. Monogr.* 48, 109–130
6 Thomas, K. A., Riley, M. C., Lemmon, S. K., Baglan, N. C. and Bradshaw, R. A. (1980) *J. Biol. Chem.* 255, 5517–5520
7 Lemmon, S. K., Riley, M. C., Thomas, K. A., Hoover, G. A., Maciag, T. and Bradshaw, R. A. (1982) *J. Cell Biol.* 95, 162–169
8 Thomas, K. A., Rios-Candelore, M. and Fitzpatrick, S. (1984) *Proc. Natl Acad. Sci. USA* 81, 357–361
9 Gimenez-Gallego, G., Rodkey, J., Bennett, C., Rios-Candelore, M. DiSalvo, J. and Thomas, K. (1985) *Science* 230, 1385-1388
10 Thomas, K. A., Rios-Candelore, M., Gimenez-Gallego, G., DiSalvo, J., Bennett, C., Rodkey, J. and Fitzpatrick, S. (1985) *Proc. Natl Acad. Sci. USA* 82, 6409–6413
11 Lobb, R. R. and Fett, J. W. (1984) *Biochemistry* 23, 6295–6299
12 Schreiber, A. B., Kenney, J., Kowalski, J., Thomas, K. A., Gimenez-Gallego, G., Rios-Candelore, M., DiSalvo, J., Barritault, D., Courty, J., Courtois, Y., Moenner, M., Loret, C., Burgess, W. H., Mehlman, T., Friesel, R., Johnson, W. and Maciag, T. (1985) *J. Cell Biol.* 101, 1623–1626
13 D'Amore, P. A. and Klagsbrun, M. (1984) *J. Cell Biol.* 99, 1545–1549
14 Gambarini, A. G. and Armelin, H. A. (1982) *J. Biol. Chem.* 257, 9692–9697
15 Lemmon, S. K. and Bradshaw, R. A. (1983) *J. Cell. Biochem.* 21, 195–208
16 Bohlen, P., Baird, A., Esch, F., Ling, N. and Gospodarowicz, D. (1984) *Proc. Natl Acad. Sci. USA* 81, 5364–5368
17 Gospodarowicz, D., Cheng, J., Ge-Ming, L., Baird, A. and Bohlen, P. (1984) *Proc. Natl Acad. Sci. USA* 81, 6963–6967
18 Maciag, T., Mehlman, T., Freisel, R. and Schreiber, A. (1984) *Science* 225, 932–935
19 Taylor, S. and Folkman, J. (1982) *Nature* 297, 307–312
20 Thornton, S. C., Mueller, S. N. and Levine, E. M. (1983) *Science* 222, 623–625
21 Shing, Y., Folkman. J., Sullivan, R., Butterfield, C., Murray, J. and Klagsbrun, M. (1984) *Science* 223, 1296–1299
22 Esch, F., Baird, A., Ling, N., Ueno, N., Hill, F., Denoroy, L., Klepper, R., Gospodarowicz, D., Bohlen, P. and Guillemin, R. (1985) *Proc. Natl Acad. Sci. USA* 82, 6507–6511
23 Bohlen, P., Esch, F., Baird, A., Jones, K. L. and Gospodarowicz, D. (1985) *FEBS Lett.* 185, 177–181

24 Duo, M-D., Huang, S. S. and Huang, J. S. (1985) *Fed. Proc.* 44, 695
25 Schreiber, A., Kenney, J., Kowalski, W. J., Friesel, R., Mehlman, T. and Maciag, T. (1985) *Proc. Natl Acad. Sci. USA* 82, 6138–6142
26 Gimenez-Gallego, G., Conn, G., Hatcher, V. B. and Thomas, K. A. (1986) *Biochem. Biophys. Res. Commun.* 135, 541–548
27 Dawes, J. (1982) in *Heparin: New Biochemical and Medical Aspects,* pp. 45–67, Walter de Gruyter
28 Lobb, R. R., Alderman, E. M. and Fett, J. W. (1985) *Biochemistry* 24, 4969–4973
29 Vallee, B. L., Riordan, J. F., Lobb, R. R., Higachi, N., Fett, J. W., Crossley, G., Buhler, R., Budzik, G., Breddam, K., Bethune, J. L. and Alderman, E. M. (1985) *Experientia* 41, 1–15
30 Baird, A., Mormede, P. and Bohlen, P. (1985) *J. Cell. Biochem.* 59A, 141

K. A. Thomas and G. Gimenez-Gallego are at the Department of Biochemistry and Molecular Biology, Merck Institute for Therapeutic Research, Merck Sharp and Dohme Research Laboratories, PO Box 2000, Rahway, NJ 07065, USA.

The transforming growth factors

Joan Massagué

Transforming growth factors are hormonally active polypeptides that induce anchorage-independent proliferation of normal cells. Two types of transforming growth factors, TGF-α and TGF-β, from both humans and rodents have recently been purified, characterized and cloned. With the identification of cellular receptors for TGF-α and TGF-β we now have more approaches available to address their mode of action and their role in normal and malignant cell proliferation.

Cellular proliferation is potently stimulated by a family of hormonally active polypeptides, the growth factors. Growth factors have the potential to induce cellular transformation if they act at the wrong time or in the wrong place. The membrane receptors for growth factors, and the intracellular components that mediate their action share this potential. The possibility that these three categories of elements mirror or are indeed the products of known oncogenes has been substantiated by three key findings during the last few years (for a review see Ref. 1). First it was found that one of the two chains of the platelet-derived growth factor (PDGF) is encoded by the *sis* oncogene. The second finding was that *erb*-B, a member of the *src* tyrosine kinase oncogene family, encodes a truncated version of the membrane receptor for epidermal growth factor (EGF), a potent mitogen for many cells in culture. Third, the expression of the normal *myc* and *fos* genes is acutely increased shortly after cellular stimulation with specific mitogens. Thus, *erb*-B, *myc* and *fos* exemplify the oncogenic potential of growth factor receptors and their intracellular targets and *sis* illustrates a situation in which transformation may occur upon expression of, and 'autocrine' stimulation by, an apparently normal growth factor.

In fact, the concept of autocrine stimulation was first proposed a few years ago after it was shown that certain transformed cells produce growth factors which elicit cellular transformation when added to normal, non-neoplastic counterparts[2]. This special class of growth factors was termed the 'transforming growth factors' (TGFs). Fibroblasts and other cell types treated with TGFs behaved like genuinely transformed cells. They no longer required attachment to a solid substratum for proliferation, nor was their growth inhibited by cell-to-cell contact. However, in contrast to genetically transformed cells, cells treated with TGFs returned to their normal pattern of proliferation when TGFs were removed from the medium.

The hormonal nature of TGFs was further suggested by the observation that extracts containing TGFs could interact with cellular receptors for EGF. It seemed that a relative of EGF able to phenotypically transform fibroblasts had been discovered[2]. The results of subsequent efforts to purify TGF secreted by retrovirally-transformed cells suggested a more complicated picture. Thus, after initial chromatography of extracts from culture fluids it was found that the EGF-related factor was no longer a potent transforming agent[3,4]. The strong transforming activity was only recovered when the EGF-related factor or EGF itself were reconstituted with material from a separate chromatographic fraction that was also inactive when assayed alone. These findings set the search for two seemingly synergistic TGFs, one related to EGF and termed TGF-α and the other termed TGF-β.

TGF-α, an EGF analogue from transformed cells

TGF-α (also called EGF-like TGF) has been purified by chromatography of extracts from culture fluids of transformed cells[4-7]. The resulting preparations contain a single polypeptide, 50 amino acids long. N-terminal amino acid sequencing of TGF-α from human tumor-derived cells, and from rat and mouse fibroblasts indicates very little difference (94–100% homology) between TGF-α from these three species. As expected from its ability to interact with EGF receptors but not with anti-EGF antibodies, TGF-α exhibits significant, although limited (33–44%), homology with the amino acid sequences of human and mouse EGFs[4,6,7]. These findings have recently been confirmed by molecular cloning of TGF-α and EGF[8-10]. In addition, analysis of the corresponding cDNAs proved that these two polypeptides are products of separate genes. Mature EGF appears to derive from a large precursor polypeptide that encodes another eight EGF-related sequences[8,9]. Interestingly, none of these EGF-like sequences is as similar to TGF-α as EGF proper is.

The structure of the cDNA for human TGF-α suggests that this polypeptide is synthesized as a 18 kDa precursor that spans a cellular membrane[10]. The peculiar amino acid sequences flanking both ends of the mature, 6 kDa polypeptide imply the involvement of a unique protease in the post-translational processing and/or release of TGF-α. So far, the production of TGF-α has been documented only in tumor-derived or retrovirally transformed cells and embryonic tissues. The chromatographic properties of EGF-like factors in extracts from other transformed sources indicate that they are also TGF-α, not EGF. Thus, TGF-α production appears to be selectively linked to cellular transformation. It is not known how cellular transformation by a variety of otherwise unrelated oncogenes (*fes*, *mos*, *ras*, *abl*, and polyoma middle T) results in the selective induction of TGF-α production.

Components of polypeptide hormone families which share 50–70% of their primary structure (for example, insulin and the insulin-like growth factors, IGFs) exhibit a weak ability to cross-react with each other's receptors. Thus, one might predict that the extensive differences in primary structure between TGF-α and EGF would be reflected in their mode of interaction with cellular receptors. However, available experimental data do not support this prediction.

Table 1. Molecular and biological properties of transforming growth factors and their receptors

	TGF-α (EGF)	TGF-β
Molecular structure	one chain	Disulfide-linked dimer
Molecular mass (kDa)	6	23–25
Membrane receptors structure	170 kDa glycoprotein	280–330 kDa glycoprotein in a disulfide-linked 565–615 kDa complex
Activity	Tyrosine protein kinase	Unknown
ID_{50} (pM)	30–50	1–5

TGF-α and EGF interact equipotently with the same receptor

A wealth of information has been generated in recent years on the structure, biochemistry and dynamics of the EGF receptor[11]. It is a cell surface glycoprotein of 170 kDa with tyrosine protein kinase activity. The ligand acts as an allosteric activator of this enzyme. Upon ligand binding, the ligand–receptor complex is rapidly internalized and degraded in lysosomes inside the cell. As a consequence, sustained exposure of cells to EGF induces a decrease, 'down-regulation', in the total number of cellular receptors for this ligand.

Using pure preparations of TGF-α and EGF, it has been shown that both ligands exhibit equivalent, very high affinity for this receptor type in various intact cell and isolated membrane preparations[12]. TGF-α and EGF are equipotent in activating the receptor-associated tyrosine kinase[13] and inducing receptor down-regulation[12]. The interactions of TGF-α and EGF with this receptor type are equally affected by plant lectins which presumably bind to the receptor's carbohydrate moiety and by phorbol ester tumor promoters[14] which alter the receptor by phosphorylating it at a specific site (Thr 654) in a reaction catalysed by protein kinase C[15]. No other receptor types, besides the EGF receptor, have been found to bind purified TGF-α. Thus, one would expect TGF-α and EGF to elicit the same biological actions with similar potency. Indeed, they are equipotent as mitogens for monolayer cultures of fibroblasts[5,7] and as promoters of the transforming action of TGF-β in cell lines (NRK fibroblasts and others) that require synergistic interaction between TGF-β and EGF analogues to express the transformed phenotype.

If TGF-α plays some normal role in development, why is an apparent duplicity of growth factors, TGF-α and EGF, conserved through the evolution of the mammalian genome? Perhaps the different regulation of the expression and secretion of both factors dictates different physiological roles for EGF and TGF-α. The correlation of TGF-α production with oncogene activation suggests that TGF-α is specific for normal situations requiring autocrine or paracrine stimulation of growth. Two obvious examples of this are embryogenesis and tissue regeneration in which acute expression of cellular proto-oncogenes is known to take place[16,17]. In contrast, EGF secreted by well-organized glandular systems may fulfil an endocrine role not devoted to the induction of extensive cell proliferation.

TGF-β, an ubiquitous growth factor

TGF-β is present in many normal tissues as well as in transformed cells[18]. Blood platelets, in particular, store relatively large amounts of TGF-β (about 1500 molecules of TGF-β per cell), supporting the view that TGF-β has a normal role in wound healing[19]. TGF-β purified to homogeneity from retrovirally transformed rat cells, and from bovine kidney, human placenta and human platelets share the same biological properties and potency, and have similar molecular structure[19,20]. They consist of two 12 kDa polypeptide chains linked by disulfide bonds to form a 23–25 kDa dimer. The presence of a unique N-terminal amino acid sequence in reduced and alkylated TGF-β from normal sources suggests that both chains are identical[19]. The exceedingly small amounts of TGF-β recovered from transformed cells prevented amino acid sequence analysis to determine whether TGF-β from this source differs from TGF-β from normal sources.

Cellular actions of TGF-β

The coordinated action of three types of growth factors, PDGF, EGF and insulin-like growth factor (IGF) can drive normal fibroblasts in culture through the mitogenic cycle[21]. Each one of these three growth factors is also required to induce the transformed phenotype by TGF-β. Initial progress in understanding the biological action of TGF-β was made with the finding that TGF-β acts synergistically with EGF or TGF-α. This fortuitous discovery arose because the indicator fibroblast line (NRK cells) first used in soft-agar assays for TGF happens to have a higher requirement for EGF in semisolid medium than in monolayer culture. Calf serum (10%) contains enough PDGF, EGF and IGF to sustain monolayer growth of NRK cells but insufficient EGF for full stimulation of these cells in soft-agar medium. The need for supplementation of these assays with EGF or TGF-α was the basis for the concept of synergism between EGF analogues and TGF-β.

More recent studies have shown that the action of TGF-β also requires cellular stimulation by PDGF and IGF. Thus, plasma with a low platelet content, and so containing little PDGF, cannot substitute for calf serum in soft-agar assays[22]. Similarly, TGF-β-induced proliferation of NRK cells in soft agar can be inhibited by IGF carrier protein which presumably acts by reducing the concentration of free IGF supplied by calf serum in the assays[23]. Thus, the combination of intracellular signals elicited by receptors for PDGF, EGF and IGF is a prerequisite for the induction of the transformed phenotype by TGF-β (Fig. 1).

In sharp contrast to the transforming response of various fibroblastoid cell lines to TGF-β, this factor has recently been reported to act as a potent growth inhibitor for certain normal and transformed cell types in culture[24,25]. The biochemical basis for this dual behavior is not known but it may have important physiological significance.

TGF-β is very potent in eliciting its cellular actions, with half-maximal effects usually observed at around 1 pM concentration. The high potency of TGF-β and

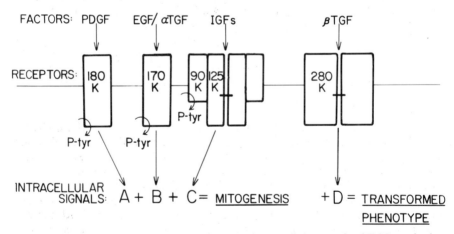

Fig. 1. Interrelationships among the receptors and intracellular signals of TGFs and other growth factors. Normal proliferation of rodent fibroblasts in culture results from concerted stimulation by three types of growth factors, PDGF, EGF and IGFs[21]. The cell surface receptors for these factors are glycoproteins with ligand-activated tyrosine kinase activity[1]. TGF-α is an analogue of EGF. Complementation of the signals elicited by receptors for PDGF, EGF/TGF-α and IGFs, with cellular stimulation by TGF-β results in anchorage-independent cell proliferation, the 'transformed phenotype'. The receptor for TGF-β is a disulfide-linked, oligomeric membrane glycoprotein of 565 kDa containing a 280 kDa binding subunit. (K, kilodalton.)

its lack of affinity for receptors of other growth factors suggested that TGF-β exerts its biological effects by binding with high affinity to a unique type of membrane receptor.

The structure of TGF-β receptors

Predictably ^{125}I-labeled TGF-β binds with high affinity (K_d = 20–120 pM) to receptors which do not recognize other growth factors[26,27]. The number of TGF-β binding sites per cell in the cell lines so far examined varies between 6000 and 40 000, with a few exceptions in which TGF-β receptors are either absent or too low to be detected. The structure of target cell membrane components that have the properties expected from high affinity TGF-β receptors has been revealed by affinity labeling studies using ^{125}I-TGF-β and a crosslinking agent[27,28]. ^{125}I-TGF-β could be covalently linked with a 280 kDa membrane component present in cells from rat, mouse and chick. This component displays high affinity and specificity for TGF-β. In human fibroblasts, ^{125}I-TGF-β labels a receptor species slightly larger (330 kDa) than the receptor in mouse and rat cells, but comparative peptide maps show a strong structural relationship between TGF-β receptors from human and rodent cells.

The affinity-labeled 280–330 kDa receptor species is linked with other subunits via disulfide bonds[28]. Hydrodynamic studies indicate a molecular size of about 565 (mouse) or 615 (human) kDa for the native, nonreduced TGF-β receptor complex in the presence of the ligand. The TGF-β receptor can be solubilized under conditions in which the structural and ligand-binding properties of the native state are retained. TGF-β receptors solubilized from human, mouse and chick cells interact specifically with immobilized lectin columns. These observations picture the major TGF-β receptor type as a disulfide-linked, glycosylated 565–615 kDa complex with a 280–300 kDa subunit that contains the ligand-binding site. The oligomeric structure of the TGF-β receptor does not appear to be induced by receptor occupancy with the ligand.

Unlike the receptors for EGF, PDGF, insulin and IGF-I, the TGF-β receptor does not appear to be subject to acute down-regulation by the ligand[27]. The widespread occurrence of this receptor type in many of the normal cell types examined further supports its participation in normal growth processes.

Perspectives

Much progress has been made in identifying and structurally characterizing TGF-α, TGF-β and their respective receptors since their discovery, only a few years ago. Four directions for future work on TGFs can be identified as especially attractive and challenging. First, more work is needed to understand the physiological roles of TGF-α and TGF-β, and their participation in neoplasia. Second, the mechanisms of expression and release of these factors, their regulation, and their accessibility to activated oncogenes must also be clarified. Third, a better understanding of the mechanism of action of TGF-α and TGF-β at the receptor and postreceptor levels is urgently needed. Particularly encouraging in this respect, are the recent spectacular observations[29,30] on the molecular biology and regulation of the EGF/TGF-α receptor, and the first glimpse of the structure of the TGF-β receptor. Finally, the identification of the biochemical actions of TGF-β is a virgin area.

Further progress will certainly result from the current impetus of research on the growth factor/oncogene interface. The elucidation of the biology of TGFs and TGF receptors should improve our understanding of normal growth processes, and suggest therapeutic strategies against disorders involving aberrant cell proliferation.

Acknowledgements
The work performed by the author and cited in this article was supported by NCI grant CA34610. The author received a Career Development Award from the Juvenile Diabetes Foundation.

References
1   Heldin, C.-H. and Westermark, B. (1984) *Cell* 37, 9–20
2   Sporn, M. B. and Todaro, G. J. (1980) *N. Engl. J. Med.* 303, 878–880
3   Roberts, A. B., Anzano, M. A., Lamb, L. C., Smith, J. M., Frolik, C. A., Marquardt, H., Todaro, G. J. and Sporn, M. B. (1981) *Nature* 295, 417–419
4   Massagué, J. (1983) *J. Biol. Chem.* 258, 13607–13613
5   Marquardt, H. and Todaro, G. J. (1982) *J. Biol. Chem.* 257, 5220–5225
6   Marquardt, H., Hunkapiller, M. W., Hood, L. E., Twardzik, D. R., DeLarco, J. E. and Todaro, G. J. (1983) *Proc. Natl Acad. Sci. USA* 80, 4684–4688
7   Marquardt, H., Hunkapiller, M. J., Hood, L. E. and Todaro, G. J. (1984) *Science* 223, 1079–1082
8   Gray, A., Dull, T. J. and Ullrich, A. (1983) *Nature* 303, 722–725
9   Scott, J., Urdea, M., Quiroga, M., Sanchez-Pescador, R., Fong, N., Selby, M., Rutter, W. J. and Bell, G. I. (1983) *Science* 221, 236–240
10 Derynck, R., Roberts, A. B., Winkler, M. E., Chen, E. Y. and Goeddle, D. V. (1984) *Cell* 38, 287–289
11 Carpenter, G. (1984) *Cell* 37, 357–358
12 Massagué, J. (1983) *J. Biol. Chem.* 258, 13614–13620
13 Pike, L. J., Marquardt, H., Todaro, G. J., Gallis, B., Casnellie, J., Bornstein, P. and Krebs, E. G. (1982) *J. Biol. Chem.* 257, 14628–14631
14 Davis, R., Like, B. and Massagué, J. (1985) *J. Cell. Biochem.* 27, 23–30
15 Hunter, T., Ling, N. and Cooper, J. A. (1984) *Nature* 311, 480–483
16 Muller, R., Verma, I. M. and Adamson, E. D. (1983) *EMBO J.* 2, 679–684
17 Goyette, M., Petropoulos, C. J., Shank, P. R. and Fausto, N. (1983) *Science* 219, 510–512
18 Roberts, A. B., Anzano, M. A., Lamb, L. C. and Sporn, M. B. (1981) *Proc. Natl Acad. Sci. USA* 78, 5339–5343
19 Assoian, R. K., Komoriya, A., Meyers, C. A., Miller, D. M. and Sporn, M. B. (1983) *J. Biol. Chem.* 258, 7155–7160
20 Massagué, J. (1984) *J. Biol. Chem.* 259, 9756–9761
21 Stiles, C. D., Pledger, W. J., Tucker, R. W., Martin, R. G. and Scher, C. D. (1980) *J. Supramol. Struct. Cell Biochem.* 13, 489–499
22 Assoian, R. K., Grotendorst, G. R., Miller, D. M. and Sporn, M. B. (1984) *Nature* 309, 804–806
23 Massagué, J., Kelly, B. and Mottda, C. (1985) *J. Biol. Chem.* 260, 4551–4556
24 Tucker, R. F., Shipley, G. D., Moses, H. L. and Holley, R. W. (1984) *Science* 226, 705–707
25 Roberts, A. B., Anzano, M. A., Wakefield, L. M., Roche, N. S., Stein, D. F. and Sporn, M. B. (1985) *Proc. Natl Acad. Sci. USA* 82, 119–123
26 Frolik, C. A., Wakefield, L. M., Smith, D. M. and Sporn, M. B. (1984) *J. Biol. Chem.* 259, 10995–11000
27 Massagué, J. and Like, B. (1985) *J. Biol. Chem.* 260, 2636–2645
28 Massagué, J. (1985) *J. Biol. Chem.* 260, 7059–7066
29 Ulrich, A., Coussens, L., Hayflick, J. S. *et al.* (1984) *Nature* 309, 418–425
30 Hunter, T., Ling, N. and Cooper, J. A. (1984) *Nature* 311, 480–483

J. Massagué is at the Department of Biochemistry, University of Massachusetts Medical Center, 55 Lake Avenue North, Worcester, MA 01605, USA.

Addendum – *Joan Massagué*

Significant progress has been made recently in understanding the biological properties of TGF-β and related polypeptides. Analysis of molecularly cloned cDNAs has shown a significant degree of amino acid sequence homology between TGF-β[31] and the newly isolated polypeptides inhibin/activin[33,34] and müllerian inhibiting substance (MIS)[34]. Inhibin is a gonadal protein that inhibits the secretion of pituitary follicle-stimulating hormone (FSH). Two forms of inhibin have been found, each one consisting of an identical α-subunit and a distinct but related β-subunit that shows homology to TGF-β. The two types of inhibin β-subunits can independently form a dimer which, quite surprisingly, is an activator of FSH secretion[33]. MIS, a protein of gonadal origin, produced during male embryonic development causes the regression of the müllerian duct, which in the female embryo develops into the uterus, vagina and fallopian tubes[34]. Thus, TGF-β is the prototype of a newly discovered family of polypeptide hormones whose members display a vast array of biological activities. TGF-β itself is now recognized as a potent regulator of the expression of various phenotypes. TGF-β regulates processes of adipogenesis[35], myogenesis[36], osteogenesis[37] and epithelial differentiation[38]. The biochemical basis of these multiple cellular actions has been proposed to be due, at least in part, to the ability of TGF-β to alter the architecture of extracellular matrices[39]. Interestingly, it has recently been noted that TGF-β can interact with the distinct 85 kDa and 65 kDa receptor forms present in many cell types in addition to the oligomeric receptor type described above[40]. It is possible that the family of TGP-β-related polypeptides elicits the varied biological actions through crossreactions with a family of receptor structures in target cells.

References
31 Derynck, R., Jarret, J. A., Chen, Y., Eaton, D. H., Bell, J. R., Assoian, R. K., Roberts, A. B., Sporn, M. B. and Goeddle, D. V. (1985) *Nature* 316, 701–705
32 Mason, A. J., Hayflick, J. S., Ling, N., Esch, F., Ueno, N., Ying, S-Y., Guillemin, R., Niall, H. and Seeburg, P. H. (1986) *Nature* 318, 659–663
33 Ling, N., Ying, S-Y., Ueno, N., Shimasaki, S., Esch, F., Hotta, M. and Guillemin, R. (1986) *Nature* 321, 779–782
34 Cate, R. L., Mattaliano, R. J., Hession, C., Tizard, R., Farber, N. M., Cheung, A., Ninfa, E. G., Frey, A. Z., Gash, D. J., Chow, E. P., Fisher, R. A., Bertonis, J. M., Torres, G., Wallner, B. P., Ramachandran, K. L., Ragin, R. C., Manganaro, T. F., MacLaughlin, D. T. and Donahue, P. K. (1986) *Cell* 45, 685–698
35 Ignotz, R. A. and Massagué, J. (1985) *Proc. Natl Acad. Sci. USA* 82, 8530–8534
36 Massagué, J., Cheifetz, S., Endo, T. and Nadal-Ginard, B. *Proc. Natl Acad. Sci. USA* (in press)
37 Seydin, S. M., Thompson, A. Y., Bentz, H., Rosen, D. M., McPherson, J. M., Conti, A., Siegel, N. R., Galluppi, G. R. and Piez, K. A. (1986) *J. Biol. Chem.* 261, 5693–5695
38 Masui, T., Wakefield, L. M., Lechner, J. F., LaVeck, M. A., Sporn, M. B. and Harris, C. C. (1986) *Proc. Natl Acad. Sci. USA* 83, 2438–2442
39 Ignotz, R. A. and Massagué, J. (1986) *J. Biol. Chem.* 261, 4337–4345
40 Cheifetz, S., Like, B. and Massagué, J. *J. Biol. Chem.* (in press)

Hemopoietic colony-stimulating factors

Nicos A. Nicola and Mathew Vadas

Hemopoietic colony-stimulating factors (CSFs) are glycoprotein growth factors produced by many tissues in the body; they are essential for the survival, growth and differentiation of hemopoietic progenitor cells in vitro. *This chapter discusses the classes of CSF that have now been purified (M-CSF, GM-CSF, G-CSF and Multi-CSF). Each is active* in vitro *at picomolar concentrations, but each can be distinguished from the others by its unique molecular properties and unique spectrum of biological activity. In addition to their proliferative effects, these regulators also appear able to stimulate functional activities in mature hemopoietic cells.*

Since the advent of semi-solid culture systems which allow the proliferation and differentiation of hemopoietic progenitor cells to occur *in vitro*[1,2], it has become apparent that hemopoietic cell proliferation is under the absolute control of a family of regulators called colony-stimulating factors (CSFs). These regulators are active at extremely low concentrations (10^{-11}–10^{-13} M) and are assayed by their ability to stimulate the development of colonies of differentiated cells from committed progenitor cells (colony-forming cells). It is now possible to grow hemopoietic colonies from nearly all the different types of committed progenitor cells[3].

Functionally distinct members of the CSF family

Since CSFs can be obtained from a multitude of sources including serum, urine, nearly all tissues and several cell lines, and since they exhibit multiple biological activities, it has not been simple to determine how many distinct members of the family exist. Moreover, determination of the molecular properties of a particular CSF has not always been helpful in determining the class to which it belongs since many CSFs apparently interact with other molecules in crude conditioned media and, as a consequence of their glycosylated nature, can exist in several forms of different size and charge.

Nevertheless, it is now possible to clearly distinguish on both molecular and functional grounds four different classes of murine CSF (see Table 1), each of which has been purified to homogeneity or near-homogeneity[4-7]. They can all stimulate granulocyte and/or macrophage colony formation in semi-solid cultures of murine bone marrow and are all remarkably stable glycoproteins requiring intact disulfide bonds for full activity. Each is active *in vitro* at low concentrations of 10^{-11}–10^{-13} M.

M-CSF has been purified from L cell-conditioned medium and is a 70 000 molecular weight glycoprotein consisting of two disulfide-bonded subunits[5]. The subunits are biologically inactive and after removal of the carbohydrate chains have a molecular weight of 15 000 each[8]. M-CSF stimulates predominantly[9] or exclusively[10] macrophage colonies from murine bone marrow; this specificity has been confirmed by the binding of radiolabeled derivatives of M-CSF to various tissues. Antisera specific to M-CSF have been described which do not cross-react at all with the other three species of CSF[11]. So far, no M-CSF derived from normal murine

Table 1. Molecular properties of the different colony-stimulating factors (CSFs)[a]

CSF	Other names	Molecular weight	Subunits	Attached carbo-hydrate	Isoelectric point	Elution from RP-HPLC (% acetonitrile)	Con A binding
M-CSF	MGF, CSF-1, MGI-1M	70 000	2	+	4.0–5.0	55	+
GM-CSF	MGI-1G	23 000	1	+	3.5–4.5	41	+
G-CSF	MGI-2, DF	25 000	1	+	5.0–7.0	51	–
Multi-CSF	BPA, IL3, PSF, MCGF, HCGF	24 000	1	+	4.5–8.0	35	+

[a]MGF, macrophage growth factor; MGI, macrophage/granulocyte inducer; BPA, burst promoting activity; DF, differentiation factor; IL3, interleukin 3; MCGF, mast cell growth factor; HCGF, hemopoietic cell growth factor; PSF, P-cell stimulating factor; RP-HPLC, reverse-phase high-performance liquid chromatography; Con A, concanavalin A.

tissues has been described that has the same molecular properties as M-CSF derived from L cells, but antibodies to the L cell-derived M-CSF do react with some CSFs from murine serum and tissues[11]. It may be that the L cell-derived M-CSF is glycosylated or processed differently to M-CSF in normal murine tissues.

GM-CSF has been purified from endotoxin-injected mouse lung-conditioned medium[4] and is a 23 000 molecular weight glycoprotein which contains no disulfide-bonded subunits. It differs from M-CSF in that it stimulates colony formation from both granulocyte and macrophage progenitor cells as well as from bipotential granulocyte/macrophage progenitor cells. The major species of CSF in serum and CSF produced by various tissues have molecular and biological properties that are identical to GM-CSF[12].

G-CSF has also been purified from endotoxin-injected mouse lung-conditioned medium[6] and is a 25 000 molecular weight glycoprotein which contains internal disulfide bonds but no subunits. At low concentrations, G-CSF stimulates exclusively a subset of granulocyte colony-forming cells, but at higher concentrations it also stimulates mixed granulocyte/macrophage colony-forming cells[13].

Multi-CSF has been highly purified from medium conditioned by WEHI-3B cells[7] and has a reported molecular weight of between 23 000 and 28 000. It can stimulate a wide range of colony-forming cells and consequently has been given several names. It now appears that burst promoting activity (BPA)[14], interleukin 3 (IL3)[7], P-cell stimulating factor (PSF)[15], mast cell growth factor (MCGF)[16], hemopoietic cell growth factor (HCGF)[17], and erythroid, megakaryocyte and eosinophil colony-stimulating factors (E-CSF, MEG-CSF, EO-CSF)[18] all are Multi-CSF. Multi-CSF also stimulates granulocyte, macrophage and mixed granulocyte/macrophage colony formation.

All four CSFs show considerable heterogeneity in charge and sometimes in size. This appears to be due predominantly to heterogeneity in the attached carbohydrate since both size and charge heterogeneity can be reduced by removing the carbohydrate, especially sialic acid. In addition, some CSFs display a tendency to aggregate or associate with other proteins in crude conditioned media, giving misleading apparent molecular weights. At least for M-CSF[8] and G-CSF (N. A. Nicola, unpublished observations), a considerable fraction (up to 50%) of the apparent molecular weight is contributed by carbohydrate. The four CSFs are clearly distinguishable by their molecular properties (Table 1). GM-CSF and G-CSF commonly occur together in various tissue-conditioned media[12,19], in lung-conditioned medium[40], and in serum from mice injected with endotoxin[20,21]. They can be resolved completely by using differences in salting-out characteristics and hydrophobicity on phenyl-Sepharose or reverse-phase high-performance liquid chromatographic columns[6]. Similarly, GM-CSF and Multi-CSF commonly occur together in spleen cell-conditioned media or media conditioned by cloned T cells but these can be completely resolved by separative techniques utilizing differences in charge and hydrophobicity (especially reverse-phase columns) (R. L. Cutler, unpublished observations). M-CSF can be resolved most easily from other CSFs by using specific antisera[11].

Biological actions of different CSFs

The four classes of CSF have in common four separate but possibly interrelated types of action. (1) They are required for the survival *in vitro* of responsive progenitor cells. In the absence of CSFs, colony-forming cells die at the rate of 5–10% per hour[22]. (2) They are required continuously for every cell division originating from a colony-forming cell. Upon withdrawal of GM-CSF from cultures, cell division ceases and the rate of progression through the cell cycle is dependent on the concentration of GM-CSF[23]. (3) They are required for the production of differentiated progeny cells. In cultures of normal hemopoietic cells it is difficult to determine if CSF induces differentiation directly or whether this is an inevitable consequence of cell proliferation. However, in the case of myeloid leukemic cell lines, G-CSF acts as a genuine differentiation inducer unrelated to the proliferative status of the cells[24]. (4) They act as pleiotropic stimuli for mature post-mitotic hemopoietic cells of the appropriate specificity and, in some cases, stimulate important biological functional activities of mature cells. This will be dealt with in more detail in a later section.

Despite these common actions the four CSFs are easily distinguished by a unique spectrum of activities. The predominant types of colony stimulated to develop by the different CSFs are indicated by the prefix used for the CSF as described in the previous section. Multi-CSF and GM-CSF appear to stimulate all available granulocyte and macrophage colony-forming cells, but M-CSF and G-CSF stimulate only a subset of these cells with virtually no overlap with each other's subset. GM-CSF shows an interesting concentration dependence in the types of colony it stimulates: at low concentrations it stimulates predominantly macrophage colony formation but at higher concentrations it also stimulates granulocyte and mixed granulocyte/macrophage colony formation[25]. This is partly due to selective stimulation of colony-forming cell subsets at low GM-CSF concentrations[3] but the concentration of GM-CSF may also determine the direction of differentiation taken by bipotential progenitor cells[26]. G-CSF shows the reverse concentration dependence to GM-CSF, selectively stimulating a subset of granulocytic progenitor cells at low concentrations[6,13].

Multi-CSF is the only CSF supporting the survival, proliferation and differentiation of multipotential stem cells (CFU-S or pre-CFC)[27,28], and the only one stimulating colony formation from early erythroid progenitor cells (BFU-E) and eosinophil, megakaryocyte and mast cell progenitor cells[14-16,18]. However, both GM-CSF and G-CSF can stimulate the first few proliferative divisions in most of these cell lineages[13,19], although they do not result in colony formation with differentiated cells in the colonies (except for the granulocyte/macrophage cell lineage). This has been determined by initiating clones in GM-CSF or G-CSF and then adding Multi-CSF two days later (delayed-addition experiments) or transferring proliferating clones initiated in GM-CSF or G-CSF to cultures containing Multi-CSF (clone-transfer experiments)[13,29]. These studies have indicated that GM-CSF and G-CSF have a much broader specificity than is indicated by their prefix but they lack the ability to support terminal proliferative and differentiative events in cell lineages other than the granulocyte macrophage lineage. M-CSF cannot support the survival or early proliferative divisions in any cell lineages except the macrophage lineage.

G-CSF is unique among the CSF classes in its very potent differentiation-inducing activity on myeloid leukemic cell lines. It is capable of inducing complete terminal differentiation in some lines of WEHI-3B cells and complete suppression of the leukemic stem cell line[24,30]. M-CSF and Multi-CSF have no detectable differentiation-inducing activity on WEHI-3B cells, and GM-CSF has detectable but weak activity[31]. A summary of the distinguishing biological activities of the four CSF classes is shown in Table II.

As yet it is difficult to understand how this pattern of overlapping and unique biological specificities are co-ordinated to result in the regulated production of the

Table 2. Biological properties of the different colony-stimulating factors (CSFs) [a]

CSF	Colony types[b]	Initiation of multiple colony types	Maintenance of factor-dependent cell lines	Induced differentiation of myeloid leukemic line (WEHI-3B)	Stem cell maintenance and differentiation	Mature cell activation
M-CSF	M>>GM	−				Macrophages
GM-CSF	G,M,GM	+ +	−	−/+	−	Granulocytes, macrophages
G-CSF	G>>GM	+	−	+ + +	−	Granulocytes
Multi-CSF	G,M,GM,EO, MEG,E,Mast, Mixed	+ + +	+ +	−	+ +	?

[b]M, macrophage; G, granulocyte; EO, eosinophil; MEG, megakaryocyte; E, erythroid.
[a]Shaded properties are those most easily distinguishing one CSF class from the others.

differentiated hemopoietic cells. It is apparent, however, that hemopoietic cell lineages must acquire and lose specific receptors for the different CSFs during their differentiation, and some activities of the CSFs may reflect cross-reactivity at the receptor level. Determination of the distribution of specific receptors on hemopoietic cells during their differentiation, the cross-reactivity of CSFs with different receptors, and the sites, times and signals for the production of the different CSFs should help to resolve these issues.

Human CSFs have been less well characterized than the murine CSFs: most sources of human CSF contain GM-CSF, EO-CSF and probably E-CSF activities but it is not clear how many different molecular species of CSF exist. Unlike mouse CSFs, which show very little activity on human progenitor cells, most sources of human CSF do have activity on murine progenitor cells. However, the molecular characteristics of murine-active CSFs from human sources are different from those of human-active CSFs from the same source[32]; surprisingly, these murine-active species have relatively little capacity to stimulate human progenitor cells. At least one murine-active human CSF, that from urine, has been shown to stimulate accessory adherent cells in human bone marrow to secrete human-active CSF[33]. This may mean that the receptor for such CSFs has been retained on the progenitor cells in mice but that during the course of evolution this receptor has been lost on human progenitor cells but retained on macrophages to signal functional activation. A similar situation may exist with murine G-CSF which cannot stimulate human progenitor cell proliferation but which can stimulate functional activation of human granulocytes[59].

The human-active CSFs are all probably glycoproteins of molecular weight about 30 000. Two types of CSF activity have been separated on the basis of their relative hydrophobicity[35]. The first activity, termed CSFα, contains GM-CSF, EO-CSF and probably E-CSF activities. Further characterization is required to determine if CSFα is the human equivalent of the murine Multi-CSF activity. The second activity is termed CSFβ and its molecular and biological characteristics appear to be very similar to the murine G-CSF. A similar separation of such activities has been reported with conditioned medium from the GCT cell line[36].

Production of CSFs

Unlike most 'classical' hormones which have a unique site or organ of production and multiple target-cell specificities, the CSFs can be produced by most organs and tissues but appear to show a unique specificity for subsets of hemopoietic cells. Most murine organs and tissues have the capacity to synthesize and secrete GM-CSF with indistinguishable molecular and biological properties regardless of the tissue of origin[12]. This is probably because cells common to all tissues (fibroblasts, activated T cells, endothelial cells in man, and possibly macrophages) can produce GM-CSF. Similarly, most murine tissues can synthesize and secrete G-CSF with its unique molecular and biological properties[19]. It is not clear which cells synthesize this factor although it is known that T cells do not and that macrophages probably do (D. Metcalf and N. A. Nicola, unpublished observations). M-CSF is certainly produced by murine fetal tissues (whole embryo, uterus, yolk sac[37,38]) but the only adult tissues known to produce it are fibroblasts[39]. Multi-CSF is produced only by activated T cells, probably with help from macrophages, so that lectin-stimulated spleen cells are the predominant source of this factor[40]. The only other known Multi-CSF-producing cell is the myeloid leukemic cell line WEHI-3B[15-17].

In the mouse only GM-CSF, G-CSF and M-CSF have been detected in serum. The levels of GM-CSF and G-CSF in serum and their production by isolated tissues *in vitro* are both dramatically elevated by injection of bacterial endotoxin into the animal[41,42]. Bacterial infection thus appears to be the major signal *in vivo* for CSF production although repeated injection of endotoxin does eventually result in a state of tolerance. Interestingly, retrovirus infection of fibroblasts increases their rate of production of GM-CSF[43], and treatment of epidermis and dermis with the tumor-promoter tetradecanoyl phorbol acetate (TPA) results in the production of GM-CSF[44]. It is probable that in these circumstances the elevated production of GM-CSF and elevated levels of serum GM-CSF occur not to signal increased production of mature cells in the marrow but to signal activation of tissue granulocytes and monocytes for functional activities associated with bacterial killing and tissue repair. Indeed it is not clear to what extent the marrow hemopoietic progenitor cells respond to circulating CSF levels, and there is some evidence from the microanatomy of the bone marrow and long-term bone-marrow cultures[45] that CSF action may be local in nature and very short-range, possibly involving cell–cell contact. Nevertheless, circulating levels of CSF may also play an important role in marrow hemopoiesis as evidenced by the cyclic fluctuations in serum CSF levels in cyclic neutropenia[46].

In man, CSFs can also be produced by many tissues *in vitro* such as placenta, spleen, lung, peripheral blood cells and bone-marrow stroma. Again this appears to be due to production of CSFs by common tissue cells (activated lymphocytes, fibroblasts and endothelial cells), and most tissues appear to be able to synthesize GM-CSFα, GM-CSFβ and EO-CSF. Although most early evidence indicated that macrophages were important for CSF production there is now some evidence that their role may be indirect. Macrophages may be stimulated in several ways to secrete a factor which, in turn, stimulates endothelial or fibroblastic cells to secrete CSFs[47]. Lactoferrin, a granulocyte product, appears to act on macrophages to inhibit production of the macrophage-stimulating factor[48].

It should be emphasized, however, that most of the data described in this review have been obtained *in vitro* and very little is known about the action of CSF *in vivo* or of the sites of CSF production or control of CSF production *in vivo*. It is hoped that the availability of larger amounts of pure CSFs anticipated from gene-cloning work and the generation of monoclonal antibodies will help to rectify this situation.

Actions of CSFs on mature cells

Although defined primarily by their ability to stimulate hemopoietic colony formation, it has now become apparent that CSFs stimulate important functional activities of mature cells. In this context 'mature cell' denotes the differentiated progeny within a cell lineage, found in the blood or tissues. In most cases these cells are post-mitotic but there is evidence that cells with the morphological appearance of macrophages[49] or mast cells[50] can be induced to divide by M-CSF or Multi-CSF, respectively.

Murine M-CSF has been shown to stimulate not only the proliferation of macrophages[49] but also RNA and protein synthesis[25], the production and release of interleukin 1 (IL1)[51], prostaglandin[52] and plasminogen activator[53], and the ability of macrophages to kill tumor cells[54]. GM-CSF can also stimulate some of these functions as well as the ability of macrophages to kill intracellular parasites of *Leishmania tropica*[55].

Some functions of mature granulocytes have also been shown to be stimulated by CSF-containing materials. These effects include the prolongation of *in-vitro* survival[56], stimulation of *in-vitro* RNA and protein synthesis[56], and enhancement of antibody-dependent killing of tumor cells[57] or parasite[58] targets. The evidence that CSF (an operationally defined molecule) is responsible for these effects rests mainly on two lines of evidence.

(a) Co-purification

In the human system, the capacities to enhance tumor-cell killing and stimulate colonies co-purify both on gel filtration and hydrophobic chromatography with either placental[56] or mononuclear cell-conditioned media (Ref. 34 and M. Vadas and N. A. Nicola, unpublished observations). In mice, the evidence is stronger since 'pure' G-CSF and GM-CSF stimulate neutrophil killing capacity[59] as well as the capacity of neutrophils to phagocytose bacteria (I. J. Stanley and D. Metcalf, unpublished observations).

(b) Lineage specificity

This phenomenon is striking. Only G-CSF and GM-CSF (not M-CSF) stimulate neutrophils[59] and, in a similar way, human eosinophils are stimulated only by CSFs containing eosinophilopoietic activity (CSFα), whilst CSF-β which contains only GM-CSF activity has no effect on eosinophils but is active on neutrophils[57].

The stimulatory effect of CSFs described above is a strong one, and one that gives rise to a number of important questions.

(i) What is the source of CSFs in the periphery?

In man a monocyte-like cell in blood has been shown to produce large quantities of granulocyte stimulators[34] that co-purify with CSF. There is evidence, however, that T-lymphocyte products can also stimulate granulocytes[60]. The relative importance of these two cells in the regulation of granulocyte function remains to be determined.

(ii) Why do two different CSFs stimulate neutrophils?

In man, both a GM-CSF in CSFα and another GM-CSF in CSFβ, and in the mouse, both G-CSF and GM-CSF stimulate neutrophil function. The effects of these substances seem to be additive[59]. There are two interesting possible reasons for this apparent redundancy. First, there may exist subsets of neutrophils that are defined by their CSF receptors or, secondly, the CSFs may stimulate a different set of functions in the cell.

(iii) Do CSFs and other granulocyte regulators interact functionally?

There is evidence that bacterial lipopolysaccharides, chemotactic peptides and complement components can stimulate activities associated with granulocyte function. It will be interesting to determine whether these activation pathways are independent of those stimulated by CSFs or whether the effects of such stimulators are additive.

Conclusions

There have now been clearly demonstrated many more important biological effects of CSFs on hemopoietic cells than simply the induced proliferation of progenitor cells that formed the first assay for such regulators. It is also clear now that several distinct but probably related CSFs can each act on one or several hemopoietic cell lineages. The precise details of how these CSFs interact in concert to produce regulated cell growth and function, how they signal information to responsive cells, and how their production and action is regulated *in vivo* remain to be determined. It is hoped that such knowledge may lead to therapeutic use of this important class of growth regulators.

References

1 Bradley, T. R. and Metcalf, D. (1966) *Aust. J. Exp. Biol. Med. Sci.* 44, 287–299
2 Ichikawa, Y., Pluznik, D. H. and Sachs, L. (1966) *Proc. Natl Acad. Sci USA* 56, 488–495
3 Metcalf, D. (1977) *Hemopoietic Colonies,* Springer-Verlag, Berlin
4 Burgess, A. W., Camakaris, J. and Metcalf, D. (1977) *J. Biol. Chem.* 252, 1998–2003
5 Stanley, E. R. and Heard, P. M. (1977) *J. Biol. Chem.* 252, 4305–4312
6 Nicola, N. A., Metcalf, D., Matsumoto, M. and Johnson, G. R. (1983) *J. Biol. Chem.* 258, 9017–9021
7 Ihle, J. N., Keller, J., Henderson, L. *et al.* (1982) *J. Immunol.* 129, 2431–2436
8 Das, S. K. and Stanley, E. R. (1982) *J. Biol. Chem.* 257, 13679–13684
9 Byrne, P. V., Guilbert, L. J. and Stanley, E. R. (1981) *J. Cell. Biol.* 91, 848–853
10 Shadduck, R. K., Pigoli, G. and Waheed, A. (1980) *J. Supramol. Struct. Suppl.* 4, 116
11 Stanley, E. R. (1979) *Proc. Natl Acad. Sci. USA* 76, 2969–2973
12 Nicola, N. A., Burgess, A. W. and Metcalf, D. (1979) *J. Biol. Chem.* 254, 5290–5299
13 Metcalf, D. and Nicola, N. A. (1983) *J. Cell. Physiol.* 116, 198–206
14 Iscove, N. N., Roitsch, C. A., Williams, N. and Guilbert, L. J. (1982) *J. Cell. Physiol., Suppl.* 1, 65–78
15 Clark-Lewis, I. and Schrader, J. W. (1981) *J. Immunol.* 127, 1941–1947
16 Yung, Y.-P., Eger, R., Tertian, G. and Moore, M. A. S. (1981) *J. Immunol.* 127, 794–799
17 Bazill, G. W., Haynes, M., Garland, J. and Dexter, T. M. (1983) *Biochem. J.* 210, 747–759
18 Burgess, A. W., Metcalf, D., Russell, S. H. M. and Nicola, N. A. (1980) *Biochem. J.* 185, 301–314
19 Nicola, N. A. and Metcalf, D. (1981) *J. Cell. Physiol.* 109, 253–264
20 Burgess, A. W. and Metcalf, D. (1980) *Int. J. Cancer* 26, 647–654
21 Lotem, J., Lipton, J. H. and Sachs, L. (1980) *Int. J. Cancer* 25, 763–771
22 Metcalf, D. and Merchav, S. (1982) *J. Cell. Physiol.* 112, 411–418
23 Metcalf, D. (1970) *J. Cell. Physiol.* 76, 89–100
24 Metcalf, D. and Nicola, N. A. (1982) *Int. J. Cancer* 30, 773–780
25 Burgess, A. W. and Metcalf, D. (1977) in *Experimental Hematology Today* (Baum, S. J. and Ledney, G. D., eds), pp. 135–139, Springer-Verlag, New York
26 Metcalf, D. (1980) *Proc. Natl Acad. Sci. USA* 77, 5327–5330
27 Schrader, J. W. and Clark-Lewis, I. (1982) *J. Immunol.* 129, 30–35
28 Nicola, N. A. and Johnson, G. R. (1982) *Blood* 60, 1019–1029
29 Metcalf, D., Johnson, G. R. and Burgess, A. W. (1980) *Blood* 55, 138–147
30 Metcalf, D. (1980) *Int. J. Cancer* 25, 225–233
31 Metcalf, D. (1979) *Int. J. Cancer* 24, 616–623
32 Wu, M.-C. and Yunis, A. A. (1980) *J. Clin. Invest.* 65, 772–775
33 Motoyoshi, K., Suda, T., Kusumoto, K. *et al.* (1982) *Blood* 60, 1378–1391
34 Veith, M. C. and Butterworth, A. E. (1983) *J. Exp. Med.* 157, 1828–1843
35 Nicola, N. A., Metcalf, D., Johnson, G. R. and Burgess, A. W. (1979) *Blood* 54, 614–627
36 Abboud, C. N., Brennan, J. K., Barlow, G. H. and Lichtman, M. A. (1981) *Blood* 58, 1148–1154
37 Bradley, T. R., Stanley, E. R. and Sumner, M. A. (1971) *Aust. J. Exp. Biol. Med. Sci.* 49, 595–603
38 Johnson, G. R. and Metcalf, D. (1978) *Exp. Hematol.* 6, 327–335
39 Tushinski, R. J., Oliver, I. T., Guilbert, L. J. *et al.* (1982) *Cell* 28, 171–181
40 Johnson, G. R. and Metcalf, D. (1977) *Proc. Natl Acad. Sci. USA* 74, 3879–3882
41 Metcalf, D. (1971) *Immunology* 21, 427–436

42 Sheridan, J. W. and Metcalf, D. (1972) *J. Cell. Physiol.* 80, 129–140
43 Koury, M. J. and Pragnell, I. B. (1982) *Nature (London)* 299, 638–640
44 Koury, M. J., Balmain, A. and Pragnell, I. B. (1983) *EMBO J.* 2, 1877–1882
45 Dexter, T. M., Allen, T. D. and Lajtha, L. G. (1977) *J. Cell. Physiol.* 91, 335–344
46 Lange, R. D. (1983) *Exp. Hematol.* 11, 435–451
47 Bagby, G. C., Jr, McCall, E., Bergshorn, K. A. and Burger, D. (1983) *Blood* 62, 663–668
48 Broxmeyer, H. E., De Sousa, M., Smithyman, A. *et al.* (1980) *Blood* 55, 324–336
49 Stanley, E. R., Cifone, M., Heard, P. M. and Defendi, V. (1976) *J. Exp. Med.* 143, 631–647
50 Schrader, J. W., Lewis, S. J., Clark-Lewis, I. and Culvenor, J. G. (1981) *Proc. Natl Acad. Sci USA* 78, 323–327
51 Moore, R. N., Oppenheim, J. J., Farrar, J. J. *et al.* (1982) *J. Immunol.* 125, 1302–1306
52 Kurland, J. I., Pelus, L. M., Ralph, P. *et al.* (1979) *Proc. Natl Acad. Sci USA* 76, 2326–2330
53 Hamilton, J. A., Stanley, E. R., Burgess, A. W. and Shadduck, R. K. (1980) *J. Physiol.* 103, 435–445
54 Wing, E. J., Waheed, A., Shadduck, R. and Nagle, L. (1982) *J. Clin. Invest.* 69, 270–276
55 Handman, E. and Burgess, A. W. (1979) *J. Immunol.* 122, 1134–1138
56 Vadas, M. A., Varigos, G., Nicola, N. *et al.* (1983) *Blood* 61, 1232–1241
57 Vadas, M. A., Nicola, N. and Metcalf, D. (1983) *J. Immunol.* 130, 795–799
58 Dessein, A., Vadas, M. A., Nicola, N. *et al.* (1982) *J. Exp. Med.* 156, 960–968
59 Lopez, A., Nicola, N., Burgess, A. W. *et al.* (1983) *J. Immunol.* 131, 2983–2988
60 Vadas, M. A. (1983) in *Immunobiology of the Eosinophil* (Yoshida, T. Y. and Terisu, M., ed.), pp. 369–382, Elsevier/North-Holland, Amsterdam

N. A. Nicola is at the Cancer Research Unit and M. Vadas is at the Experimental Allergy Laboratory of the Clinical Research Unit, Walter and Eliza Hall Institute of Medical Research, PO Royal Melbourne Hospital, Parkville, 3050, Victoria, Australia. The present address of M. A. Vadas is Division of Human Immunology, Institute of Medical and Veterinary Science, PO Box 14, Rundle Male, Adelaide South Australia, 5000.

Addendum – *Nicola and Vadas*

The field of hemopoietic colony-stimulating factors has moved forward extremely quickly since publication of this article. cDNA clones for both murine GM-CSF[61] and Multi-CSF (interleukin 3)[62,63] have now been obtained and the expressed products (both glycosylated and non-glycosylated) shown to possess all the biological activities ascribed to the purified factors[64-68]. The genes for these two factors have also been sequenced[69-72] and shown to be single copy genes with a typical exon/intron structure. The human analogues of murine GM-CSF and M-CSF have now also been cloned, both as cDNA and genomic clones, and sequenced[73-76]. It has been definitively established that human CSFα and CSFβ are the equivalents of murine GM-CSF and G-CSF, respectively[77,78]. Human and murine G-CSFs show complete species cross-reactivity while human and murine GM-CSFs do not. However, the actions of human GM-CSF expressed from a cDNA clone have confirmed all the biological activities previously ascribed to CSFα, including its action in activating mature blood neutrophils and eosinophils[77,79].

Extensive binding studies have been performed with all four murine CSFs[78,80-85]. Each CSF binds to a unique receptor (M_r ~150 000 for G-CSF and M-CSF, M_r ~60 000 for Multi-CSF and GM-CSF) which shows no direct cross-reactivity with other CSFs or other growth factors. The distribution of these receptors on bone marrow cells exactly matches the known biological specificity of each CSF on both immature and mature cells. Two special features of CSF binding are that in all cases it is nearly irreversible, even at 4°C, and that at 37°C the CSFs show a specific pattern of indirect receptor down-modulation. This specific hierarchical pattern of receptor down-modulation has suggested a model of CSF biological cross-reactivity based on the ability of each CSF to down-modulate lineage-specific receptors[85].

Several observations of special relevance to oncogenes have been made recently. The *fms* oncogene product has been shown to be closely related or identical to the M-CSF receptor on macrophages[86] showing a possible parallelism to the relationship between the *erb* oncogene and epidermal growth factor receptor[87]. Factor-dependent hemopoietic cell lines have been made tumorigenic by transformation with Abelson virus without any evidence of autocrine mechanisms[88-90]. On the other hand, retroviruses containing expressible GM-CSF cDNA were also able to transform factor-dependent hemopoietic cell lines, rendering them factor independent and tumorigenic, the evidence favouring an autocrine mechanism[91]. Some spontaneous autonomous mutant cell lines acquire tumorigenicity concomitantly with the ability to produce and secrete Multi-CSF[92]. Similarly, the WEHI-3B leukemic cell line constitutively produces Multi-CSF and has a specific rearrangement of the Multi-CSF gene involving insertion of a viral-like element[93] while factor-dependent avian myeloid cell lines super-infected with *src*-related oncogenes concomitantly acquire factor independence and secrete growth factor[94]. These data suggest that in some, but not all, cases autocrine production of a CSF or an activated CSF receptor may play a part in leukemogenesis.

References

61 Gough, N. M., Gough, J., Metcalf, D., Kelso, A., Grail, D., Nicola, N. A., Burgess, A. W. and Dunn, A. R. (1984). *Nature*, 309, 763–768

62 Fung, M. C., Hapel, A. J., Ymer, S., Cohen, D. R., Johnson, R. M., Campbell, H. D. and Young, I. G. (1984). *Nature* 307, 233–237

63 Yokota, T., Lee, F., Rennick, D., Hall, C., Arai, N., Mosmann, T., Nabel, G., Cantor, H. and Arai, K. (1984) *Proc. Natl Acad. Sci. USA* 81, 1070–1074

64 DeLamarter, J. F., Mermod, J. J., Liang, C-M., Eliason, J. F. and Thatcher, D. (1985) *EMBO J.* 4, 2575–2583

65 Hapel, A. J., Fung, M. C., Johnson, R. M., Young, I. J., Johnson, G. R. and Metcalf, D. (1985) *Blood* 65, 1453–1459

66 Kindler, V., Thorens, B., Dekossodo, S., Allet, B., Eliason, J. F., Thatcher, D. and Vassalli, P. (1985) *Proc. Natl Acad. Sci. USA* 83, 1001–1005

67 Greenberger, J. S., Humphries, R. K., Messner, H., Reid, D. M. and Sakakeeny, M. A. (1985) *Exp. Hematol.* 13, 249–260

68 Rennick, D. M., Lee, F. D., Yokota, T., Arai, K-I., Cantor, H. and Nabel, G. K. (1985) *J. Immunol.* 134, 910–914

69 Miyatake, S., Otsuka, T., Yokota, T., Lee, F. and Arai, K. (1985) *EMBO J.* 4, 2561–2568

70 Campbell, H. D., Ymer, S., Fung, M. C. and Young, I. G. (1985) *Eur. J. Biochem.* 150, 297–304

71 Stanley, E., Metcalf, D., Sobieszczuk, P., Gough, N. M. and Dunn, A. R. (1985). *EMBO J.* 4, 2569–2573

72 Miyatake, S., Yokota, T., Lee, F. and Arai, K-I. (1985) *Proc. Natl Acad. Sci. USA* 82, 316–320

73 Wong, G. G., Wilek, J., Temple, P. A., Wilkens, K. M., Leary, A. C., Luxenberg, D. P., Jones, S. S., Brown, E. L., Kay, R. M., Orr, E. C., Shoemaker, C., Golde, D. W., Kaufman, R. J., Hewick, R. M., Wang, E. A. and Clark, S. C. (1985) *Science* 228, 810–815

74 Lee, F., Yokota, T., Otsuka, T., Genamell, L., Larson, N., Luh, J., Arai, K. and Rennick, D. (1985). *Proc. Natl Acad Sci. USA* 82, 4360–4365

75 Cantrell, M. A., Anderson, D., Cerretti, D. P., Price, V., McKereghan, K., Tushinski, R. J., Mochizuki, D. Y., Larsen, A., Grabstein, K., Gillis, S. and Cosman, D. (1985) *Proc. Natl Acad. Sci. USA* 82, 6250–6254

76 Kawasaki, E. S., Ladner, M. B., Wang, A. M., Van Arsdell, J., Warren, M. K., Coyne, M. Y., Schneichardt, V. L., Lee, M-T., Wilson, K. J., Boosman, A., Stanley, E. R., Ralph, P. and Mark, D. F. (1985) *Science* 230, 291–296

77 Metcalf, D., Begley, C. G., Johnson, G. R., Nicola, N. A., Vadas, M. A., Lopez, A. F., Williamson, D. J., Wong, G. G., Clark, S. C. and Wang, E. A. (1986) *Blood* 67, 37–45

78 Nicola, N. A., Begley, C. G. and Metcalf, D. (1985) *Nature* 314, 625–628

79 Begley, C. G., Lopez, A. F., Nicola, N. A., Warren, D. J., Vadas, M. A., Sanderson, C. J. and Metcalf, D. (1986) *Blood* 68, 162–166

80 Stanley, E. R. (1981). *J. Immunol. Methods* 42, 253–284

81 Nicola, N. A. and Metcalf, D. (1985) *Proc. Natl Acad. Sci. USA* 81, 3765–3769

82 Palaszynski, E. W. and Ihle, J. N. (1984) *J. Immunol.* 132, 1872–1878

83 Walker, F. and Burgess, A. W. (1985) *EMBO J.* 4, 933–939

84 Nicola, N. A. and Metcalf, D. (1985) *J. Cell Physiol.* 124, 313–321

85 Walker, F., Nicola, N. A., Metcalf, D. and Burgess, A. W. (1985) Cell 43, 269–276

86 Scherr, C. J., Rettenmier, C. W., Sacca, R., Roussel, M. F., Look, A. T. and Stanley, E. R. (1985) *Cell* 41, 665–676

87 Downward, J., Yarden, Y., Mayes, E., Scrace, G., Totty, N., Stockwell, P., Ullrich, A., Schlessinger, J. and Waterfield, M. D. (1984) *Nature* 307, 521–527

88 Cook, W. D., Metcalf, D., Nicola, N. A., Burgess, A. W. and Walker, F. (1985) *Cell* 41, 677–683

89 Pierce, J. H., Ditiore, P. P., Aaronson, S. A., Potter, M., Pumphrey, J., Scott, A. and Ihle, J. N. (1985) *Cell* 41, 685–693

90 Oliff, A., Agranousky, O., McKinney, M. D., Murty, V. V. V. S. and Bauchwitz, R. (1985) *Proc. Natl Acad. Sci. USA* 82, 3306–3310

91 Lang, R. A., Metcalf, D., Gough, N. M., Dunn, A. R. and Gonda, T. J. (1985) *Cell* 43, 531–542

92 Schrader, J. W. and Crapper, R. M. (1983) *Proc. Natl Acad. Sci. USA* 80, 6892–6896

93 Ymer, S., Tucker, W. Q. J., Sanderson, C. J., Hapel, A. J., Campbell, H. D. and Young, I. G. (1985) *Nature* 317, 255–258

94 Adkins, B., Leutz, A. and Graf, T. (1984) *Cell* 39, 439–445

Pre-adipose cell replication and differentiation

Daniel A. K. Roncari

Pre-adipose cells in culture have been valuable in studies of replication and adipose differentiation, processes influenced by growth factors and hormones from the anterior pituitary and other glands. Clones of pre-adipose cells have also revealed excessive replication and differentiation in human massive obesity.

Pre-adipose cells in culture have facilitated the recent acquisition of appreciable new knowledge about factors influencing their replication, differentiation, and role *in vivo* (see Refs 1–12; 7, 11 and 12 are reviews). Green and co-workers[2,6–9] have conducted elegant studies using sublines of the fibroblast-like 3T3 cells (originally derived from mouse fetuses) that undergo adipose differentiation at high frequency. Adipocyte precursors from post-natal human adipose tissue (original isolation and culture of pre-adipose cells was from adults) and rat adipose tissue have also provided valuable information[1,3–5,10–12].

Pre-adipose cells probably derive from a pluripotent mesenchymal progenitor. It may be pertinent that 5-azacytidine, which decreases DNA methylation, induces differentiation of cultured Chinese hamster embryo fibroblasts along several possible pathways, leading to adipose cells, chondroblasts or myoblasts[13]. Factors mitogenic on some of these mesenchymal cells will now be described.

Growth factors and hormones influencing cell number

Since adipose cells do not replicate[2,12], their number can only be influenced when they are (relatively) undifferentiated and non-confluent (i.e. still able to spread on the culture plate).

Anterior pituitary fibroblast growth factor(s) and a newly recognized class of pituitary 'adipocyte growth factors' (at least five acidic and basic proteins, $M_r \sim 8200$–55 000) stimulate the replication of adipocyte precursors[14,15]. Cells cultured from human and rat adipose tissue have been the main test systems. In addition to acting on adipocyte precursors, these proteins are mitogenic for cultured skin fibroblasts and chondrocytes. Indeed, the 'adipocyte growth factors', as well as fibroblast and chondrocyte growth factors, are probably interrelated and might be termed collectively 'mesenchymal growth factors'. Verification *in vivo* is required to demonstrate that any of these factors has physiological significance. An increased number of adipocyte precursors would, after differentiation, increase both adipose tissue mass and function.

Of the 'classic hormones', only 17β-estradiol is mitogenic on cultured human adipocyte precursors at concentrations approaching physiological levels[16]. Clinical correlations, including changes in adipose cellularity and configuration in girls during puberty, suggest that the findings *in vitro* reflect events *in vivo*. Since adipocyte precursors actively convert androgens to estrogens, the latter might act in fat tissue by paracrine or autocrine mechanisms*, in addition to

---

*Paracrine mechanism: substances released by cells into surrounding interstidial fluids modify the biological activity (e.g. growth) of neighbouring cells. Autocrine mechanism: substances act directly on their cells of origin or after release and re-uptake by these cells.

gaining access to adipose depots via the blood circulation.

Fat tissue elements of developing and adult mammals, particularly differentiated adipocytes, release proteins mitogenic on cultured adipocyte precursors[17]. These substances might influence adipose tissue mass by acting as paracrine growth factors.

In contrast to the mitogenic substances, pancreatic polypeptide suppresses the replication of cultured human adipocyte precursors[14]. This potentially critical function of pancreatic polypeptide requires confirmation *in vivo*.

Hormones inducing or promoting adipose differentiation

Committed, quiescent pre-adipose cells can undergo adipose differentiation 'spontaneously' or when induced by certain 'adipogenic' substances. This conversion to adipocytes is characterized by a change from fibroblast-like to spherical shapes, specific alterations in gene expression, and triacylglycerol accumulation, the extent of this accumulation depending on the availability of substrates and promoting factors. This review will only describe those hormones whose induction or promotion of differentiation in culture seems to be consistent with their role *in vivo*.

Growth hormone

Pursuant to studies indicating that pituitary substances are involved in the growth of adipose tissue *in vivo* and of human adipocyte precursors in culture[12,14], Green and co-workers[18] demonstrated that growth hormone (somatotropin) from the pituitary gland of different species (including the human hormone synthesized in *E. coli*), at concentrations similar to those found in plasma, induced adipose differentiation in susceptible 3T3 cells in the presence of the promoting hormones, insulin and triiodothyronine. No other pituitary hormone had this effect. Should this action of growth hormone reflect an effect *in vivo*, it would signify that the brain may regulate the number of differentiated cells in adipose tissue through hypothalamic control of growth hormone secretion.

Since plasma from hypophysectomized rats can induce differentiation and since certain sera have a more potent effect on differentiation than growth hormone, a number of complementary factors may be necessary for adipose differentiation[18].

Insulin

Insulin has a critical role in every phase of those characteristic processes of fat tissue that promote synthesis and storage of triacylglycerol[12]. Thus, insulin plays a prominent role during the expression of adipose differentiation. As expected, therefore, the number of insulin receptors increases during differentiation[7,19]. The developing post-receptor mechanisms, as manifested by specific biological effects of insulin, are even more characteristic of adipose differentiation since they are hardly expressed at all in pre-adipose cells[19].

Is insulin in fact a 'commitment factor' for adipose differentiation? That the answer is 'no' is indicated by studies of Steinberg and Brownstein[20] who found that insulin had no influence during exponential growth, a stage when commitment of pre-adipose 3T3 cells occurred at constant probability. Insulin enhanced such features of differentiation as synthesis and storage of triacylglycerol only in committed, quiescent cells. Thus, insulin is neither a commitment factor nor, in contrast to growth hormone, an inducer of differentiation, but it is critical for the phenotypic manifestation of adipocytes.

Biochemistry of adipose differentiation

Glucose uptake and metabolism

While pre-adipose cells bind insulin to a certain extent, the acute stimulation by insulin of glucose transport and metabolism only occurs after the cells enter the differentiation program[19]. In addition to this acute effect, pre-incubation of adipose 3T3 cells with insulin leads to persistent enhancement of glucose transport[19]. This confirms previous findings with isolated, mature adipocytes and *in vivo* after prolonged insulin administration.

Derived from glycolysis, dihydroxyacetone phosphate is reduced to *sn*-glycero-3-phosphate (glycerophosphate) by cytosolic glycerophosphate dehydrogenases, which provide a critical link between glucose and lipid metabolism. Indeed, glycerophosphate is the source of the glycerol backbone of triacylglycerols formed in adipose cells[12]. The physiological importance of this glucose–lipid link is indicated by the spectacular increment in the specific activity of the thermostable isoenzyme of cytosolic glycerophosphate dehydrogenase during adipose differentiation of 3T3 cells[8].

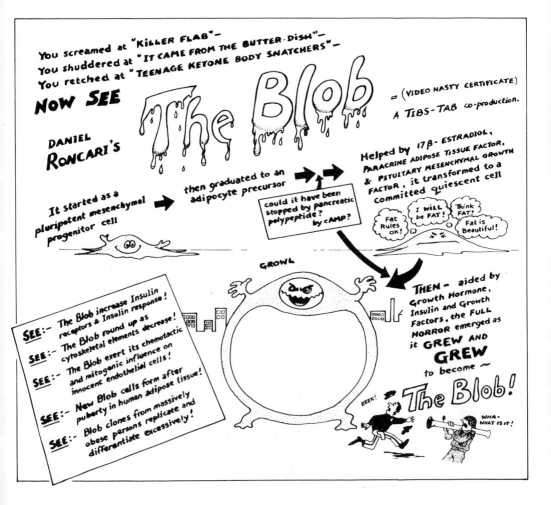

Lipoprotein lipase

This enzyme, which catalyses the hydrolysis of lipoprotein-triacylglycerols so that the freed fatty acids can be taken up by adipose cells, is also an excellent marker of adipose differentiation[3,6,7,21]. From very low or negligible levels in pre-adipose cells, the content and releasable activity of lipoprotein lipase rise considerably in differentiating 3T3 sublines and adipocyte precursors. Insulin promotes both the synthesis of the enzyme and the extent of its release[21].

De novo *fatty acid synthesis*

During adipose differentiation, the activities of the enzymes involved in *de novo* fatty acid synthesis increase substantially, as reflected by the augmented incorporation of acetyl-CoA into long-chain fatty acids[7,11]. As is probably the case for the other enzymes (and hormone receptor and post-receptor machineries) involved in triacylglycerol metabolism, the increased activity is due to enhanced synthesis and also in some instances to activation (e.g. stimulation of dephosphorylation of pyruvate dehydrogenase); both processes are promoted by insulin.

Differentiating 3T3 sublines have provided the opportunity to study the relative quantitative importance of *de novo* fatty acid synthesis vs uptake from circulating lipoprotein-triacylglycerols (or triacylglycerol emulsified in the culture medium) in supplying the acyl chains of stored triacylglycerols[6]. When biotin is removed from the culture medium to interrupt fatty acid synthesis, only minute quantities of triacylglycerol accumulate if external supplies are at limiting concentration[6]. However, when external concentration is adequate, lipid assimilation mediated by lipoprotein lipase accounts for most of the fatty acids required for triacylglycerol accretion. This probably represents the usual situation *in vivo,* but *de novo* fatty acid synthesis in adipocytes may afford an effective accessory mechanism under some conditions and may explain the normal triacylglycerol content in adipocytes of patients with genetic forms of severely depressed lipoprotein lipase activity.

Triacylglycerol synthesis and hydrolysis

The specific activity of the enzymes catalysing triacylglycerol synthesis from glycerophosphate and fatty acids rises several-fold in differentiating 3T3 cells and adipocyte precursors[7,11,22]. As is the case with many expressions of adipose differentiation, the peak of activity is attained 6–13 days after onset of this process, followed by a decline which probably results from regulatory processes.

Along with the expression of mechanisms for triacylglycerol synthesis, the 'lipolytic cascade' from specific receptors for lipolytic hormones to hydrolysis of stored triacylglycerols (catalysed by hormone-stimulated lipase) is expressed in the differentiating cells[7,11,23,24]. In 3T3-L1 cells, most of the increase in cyclic AMP-dependent protein kinase activity is due to expression of the Type I isoenzyme[24].

Expression of some processes decreases during differentiation

In contrast to the dramatic expression related to triacylglycerol metabolism, some processes are abrogated during adipose differentiation. At very early stages of this process, and preceding the expression of functions related to lipid metabolism, the synthesis of cytoskeletal proteins such as actins, vimentin, and tubulins decreases substantially[25]. This depressed expression of cytoskeletal elements contributes to the conversion of a fusiform, motile (fibroblast-like) cell to a spherical cell specialized in triacylglycerol storage.

Molecular biology of differentiation

Green and co-workers[6,9,26] have conducted penetrating studies on the mechanisms subtending the expression of adipose differentiation. Triacylglycerol accretion in differentiating 3T3 cells is mainly prevented by raising cyclic-AMP concentration or by omitting biotin from the medium[2,6]. This only represents phenotypic modulation since the fundamental features of differentiation persist, i.e. a spherical shape with marked alterations in the content of translatable mRNA for many (but not all) characteristic proteins, such as glycerophosphate dehydrogenase[26]. Thus, once differentiation is induced its basic program is transacted even in the absence of triacylglycerol accumulation.

Spiegelman *et al.*[9] have constructed a recombinant DNA library in *E. coli* of cDNA prepared from mRNA of differentiated 3T3 cells. From this library, they isolated DNA sequences complementary to mRNAs encoding four proteins whose expression is altered substantially during differentiation; these include glycerophosphate dehydrogenase, a $M_r \sim 13\ 000$ protein (which may be the fatty acid-binding or Z protein) and actin. Characterization of these recombinants, along with translation studies of the corresponding mRNAs confirmed that the alterations in protein content result from changes in the quantities of translatable mRNA. Further, the rise in mRNA of three of the proteins (actin mRNA decreased) varied temporally and quantitatively[9]. Thus, while the expression of enzymes of one pathway (such as triacylglycerol synthesis) may be coordinated, several proteins are expressed at distinct stages of differentiation.

Adipose–endothelial cell interactions

In contrast to adipose cell cultures, adipose tissue *in vivo* requires profuse vascular supply and innervation. The studies in culture suggest that adipose cells play an important role in the development of adipose tissue by securing a profuse vascular network through the production of substances mitogenic and chemotactic on endothelial cells[27,28].

Significance of adipocyte precursors

The isolation of adipocyte precursors from fat tissue of adult humans and rats suggested that, contrary to prevailing beliefs, new fat cells could be formed during adulthood[1,3,12]. This concept is now widely accepted and confirmed by studies *in vivo*[12]. Further, studies of precursors from different adipose regions have indicated that fat depots vary not only in their metabolic characteristics (e.g. contrasting responses to glucocorticoids) but also their growth characteristics[10]. Even within a single region, precursor clones vary in their potential for proliferation and differentiation[10].

When compared to cells from lean or moderately obese persons, omental adipocyte precursors from subjects with massive obesity (both childhood- and adult-onset), proliferate excessively, an effect perpetuated in successive subcultures and in cloned cells[29]. Some omental† clones also display an unusual propensity to differentiation[29]. As is the case for massively obese rodents, some adipose regions display much greater growth responses than others; for example, human omental precursors have much greater proliferative potential than subcutaneous cells whose replication in culture is only slightly greater than normal[29]. Further, paracrine factors mitogenic on adipocyte precursors seem to be more abundant in fat tissue of massively obese than normal subjects[17]. Such a

---

†The omentum is a fold of the peritoneum connecting the stomach to other viscera.

paracrine mechanism might contribute to the excessive number of enlarged adipocytes characteristic of massive obesity. Studies just beginning on the gene expression and biochemistry related to massive obesity are providing promising results.

Conclusion

Growth factors and hormones from the anterior pituitary and other glands influence the replication of pre-adipose cells, and in committed, quiescent pre-adipose cells, certain hormones affect differentiation. This process is characterized by early decreases in translatable mRNA for cytoskeletal proteins (contributing to cell rounding) and increases in mRNA for proteins related to triacylglycerol accretion (insulin-dependent) and hydrolysis, the specialized functions of adipocytes. Studies on adipocyte precursors have suggested that replication and differentiation can occur throughout adulthood. In the extreme situation, clones from massively obese humans replicate and differentiate excessively, probably accounting for the adipocyte hyperplasia present *in vivo*.

Acknowledgements

Studies in the author's laboratory have been supported by the Medical Research Council of Canada, the Canadian (Ontario and Alberta) Heart Foundation, and the Alberta Heritage Foundation for Medical Research.

References

1 Poznanski, W. J., Waheed, I. and Van, R. (1973) *Lab. Invest.* 29, 570–576
2 Green, H. and Kehinde, O. (1974) *Cell* 1, 113–116
3 Van, R. L. R., Bayliss, C. E. and Roncari, D. A. K. (1976) *J. Clin. Invest.* 58, 699–704
4 Van, R. L. R. and Roncari, D. A. K. (1978) *Cell Tissue Res.* 195, 317–329
5 Björntorp, P., Karlsson, M., Gustafsson, L., Smith, U., Sjöström, L., Cigolini, M., Storck, G. and Pettersson, P. (1979) *J. Lipid Res.* 20, 97–106
6 Kuri-Haruch, W., Wise, L. S. and Green, H. (1978) *Cell* 14, 53–59
7 Green, H. (1978) in *10th Miami Winter Symposium on Differentiation and Development*, pp. 13–36, Academic Press, New York
8 Pairault, J. and Green, H. (1979) *Proc. Natl Acad. Sci. USA* 76, 5138–5142
9 Spiegelman, B. M., Frank, M. and Green, H. (1983) *J. Biol. Chem.* 258, 10083–10089
10 Djian, P., Roncari, D. A. K. and Hollenberg, C. H. (1983) *J. Clin. Invest.* 72, 1200–1208
11 Cryer, A. (1980) *Trends Biochem. Sci.* 5, 196–198
12 Roncari, D. A. K. (1983) in *Clinical Medicine* (Spittell, J. A., Jr and Volpé, R., eds), Vol. 9, pp. 1–46, Harper and Row, Philadelphia
13 Sager, R. and Kovac, P. (1982) *Proc. Natl Acad. Sci. USA* 79, 480–484
14 Roncari, D. A. K. (1981) *Int. J. Obesity* 5, 547–552
15 Lau, D. C. W., Roncari, D. A. K., Yip, D. J., Kindler, S. and Nilsen, S. G. E. (1983) *FEBS Lett.* 153, 395–398
16 Roncari, D. A. K. and Van, R. L. R. (1978) *J. Clin. Invest.* 62, 503–508
17 Lau, D. C. W., Hollenberg, C. H. and Roncari, D. A. K. (1984) *Proc. 7th Intern. Congress Endocr.*, p. 866, Excerpta Medica, Amsterdam
18 Morikawa, M., Nixon, T. and Green, H. (1982) *Cell* 29, 783–789
19 Rosen, O. M., Smith, C. J., Fung, C. and Rubin, C. S. (1978) *J. Biol. Chem.* 253, 7579–7583
20 Steinberg, M. M. and Brownstein, B. L. (1982) *J. Cell Physiol.* 113, 359–364
21 Eckel, R. H., Fujimoto, W. Y. and Brunzell, J. D. (1977) *Biochem. Biophys. Res. Commun.* 78, 288–293

22 Roncari, D. A. K., Mack, E. Y. W. and Yip, D. K. (1979) *Can. J. Biochem.* 57, 573–577
23 Roncari, D. A. K., Wang, H. and Desai, K. S. (1980) *Can. J. Biochem.* 58, 201–205
24 Liu, A. Y.-C. (1982) *J. Biol. Chem.* 257, 298–306
25 Spiegelman, B. M. and Farmer, S. R. (1982) *Cell* 29, 53–60
26 Spiegelman, B. M. and Green, H. (1980) *J. Biol. Chem.* 255, 8811–8818
27 Castellot, J. J., Jr, Karnovsky, M. J. and Spiegelman, B. M. (1982) *Proc. Natl Acad. Sci., USA* 79, 5597–5601
28 Björntorp, P. (1983) *Exp. Cell Res.* 149, 277–287
29 Roncari, D. A. K., Lau, D. C. W., Djian, P., Kindler, S. and Yip, D. K. (1983) in *The Adipocyte and Obesity: Cellular and Molecular Mechanisms* (Angel, A., Hollenberg, C. H. and Roncari, D. A. K., eds), pp. 65–73, Raven Press, New York

Daniel Roncari is at the Departments of Medicine and Medical Biochemistry and at the Diabetes Research Unit, Faculty of Medicine, The University of Calgary, Health Sciences Centre, 3330 Hospital Drive, Calgary, Alberta T2N 4N1, Canada.

Growth factors which affect bone

Ellen Simpson

The coupled processes of bone resorption and bone formation occur throughout life. New research suggests that some well-characterized growth factors affect bone and that transforming growth factors and tumor-derived growth factors may also influence bone growth and remodeling.

Dramatic changes in skeletal mass and bone modeling occur during fetal life and in adolescence. Bone is continuously being broken down (resorption) and formed and imbalances in the linked processes of resorption and formation result in bone growth early in life and in the progressive loss of bone which occurs shortly after maximal bone mass is reached (in the third decade of life for humans). How these changes in bone mass take place is not known but clearly the interaction of several skeletal growth factors (which are still not well defined) is involved. Some of these growth factors, such as insulin-like growth factor (IGF-1)[1], stimulate new bone formation, while others, notably epidermal growth factor (EGF), stimulate breakdown of bone[2]. It should be emphasized, however, that in most situations bone resorption is a prerequisite for new bone formation and so growth factors may be viewed as modulators of bone remodeling. Thus, certain factors stimulate or inhibit bone resorbing cells (osteoclasts), while others act mainly on bone-forming cells (osteoblasts). The role of growth factors in both bone resorption and formation is reviewed here and their possible involvement in normal bone remodeling is discussed.

Normal development and structure of bone

Bone is a complex connective tissue composed of a mineralized matrix and a wide assortment of cells, including osteoblasts, osteoclasts and a myriad of other cells located in the marrow. Also, its composition and structure vary with age, bone type, and disease state. Thus the study of the normal development and structure of bone is particularly complicated.

Embryonic bone formation includes a well defined sequence of events which are analogous to bone remodeling in the mature individual. Bone formation during embryogenesis proceeds by one of two modes: either mesenchymal cells present in the skull bones directly differentiate into osteoblasts, which lay down matrix which is subsequently mineralized into bone, or mesenchymal cells migrate into a calcified cartilage matrix containing hypertrophic chondrocytes, leading to longitudinal growth in long bones. This is followed by simultaneous osteoclastic resorption and osteoblastic deposition of true bone matrix[3]. The coupling of bone deposition and bone resorption occurs in embryonic bone formation, in adult bone remodeling and in various disease states and is one of the most intriguing aspects of bone physiology. The known involvement of migration and induction of mesenchymal cells in bone formation and resorption may hold further clues to the regulation of these processes by growth factors. Bone remodeling in the adult skeleton proceeds linearly in space and time via (1) an activation phase in which precursor cells are somehow induced to form osteoclasts; (2) a resorptive phase in which osteoclasts secrete degradative enzymes and acidify their environment, leading to release of bone mineral and destruction of bone matrix; (3) a reversal phase in which mononuclear cells enter the resorbed area and (4) a formative phase in which osteoblasts appear and osteoid (non-mineralized matrix) is laid down and subsequently mineralized[4].

Assay of bone formation and resorption

The examination of factors which affect bone development and remodeling has been hindered by unsatisfactory parameters for assessing bone formation *in vitro*. Bone formation has been investigated by methods ranging from the overall induction of increased mass or increased calcium incorporation in an intact animal to increasing collagen synthesis in bone organ cultures or increasing mRNA for collagen in isolated osteosarcoma cells. Similarly, bone resorption has been assayed by release of previously incorporated ^{45}Ca from rodent bone organ cultures, by histomorphometry of bone *in vivo* and by the appearance of bone-specific proteins in the serum, such as alkaline phosphatase and a bone protein containing γ-carboxy glutamate (bone Gla protein)[5]. As with other complex developmental systems, the most practical approach may be to examine the effect of a given factor in as simple a system as possible. Thus one could test the ability of a given factor to stimulate or depress synthesis of a given protein or mRNA in an isolated cell system, and concomitantly determine its effect *in vivo* or in an organ culture, preferably of the same species as the factor. For example, the effect of tumor-conditioned medium on calcium release by isolated calvaria could be examined. As always in growth factor studies, time-course and dose-response data are crucial because many factors which are stimulatory at one concentration or time period in bone cell studies (such as 1,25-dihydroxyvitamin D) are inhibitory or have no effect at another[6]. Note that a given factor may not possess more than one of these activities, and more than one agent may be needed to elicit a given response. For example, platelet-derived growth factor (PDGF) may be required to prepare cells for progression through the cell cycle before such cells can respond to an additional stimulatory agent[7].

Growth factors which enhance bone formation

Several growth factors whose effects on other systems are well characterized have recently been found to affect bone formation also. These include insulin and IGF-1. Insulin directly affects bone by increasing collagen synthesis in osteoblasts[8]. Growth hormone mediates its effects on bone formation indirectly through somatomedin C (or IGF-1)[9,10].

In addition to these well-characterized peptide growth factors several new factors which stimulate bone formation have been reported recently. These fall into two groups: (1) bone-derived, which are presumably local factors; and (2) tumor-derived, which may be systemic as well as local factors.

Bone-derived factors that activate osteoblasts have been described by several groups. Baylink *et al.*[11] isolated a protein of M_r 83 000, termed skeletal growth factor, from human bone. This protein increases DNA synthesis in cultured chick calvarial cells and also enhances dry-weight accumulation and ^{3}H-proline incorporation in cultured chick tibiae and femurs. Similarly, Urist *et al.*[12] isolated a protein of M_r 18 000 from bovine bone, termed bone morphogenetic protein, which stimulates new bone formation by inducing *in vivo* differentiation of mesenchymal cells into cartilage and woven bone. Finally, Canalis[13] has identified two proteins in bone, termed 'bone-derived growth factors 1 and 2' (BDGF). BDGF-1 has a M_r of 10 000 and appears to have properties similar to somatomedin C. BDGF-2 is larger (M_r 25 000–30 000) and has properties more characteristic of PDGF.

Tumors such as metastatic prostate and breast cancer are often associated with new bone formation. Previous work concentrated on identifying the protein responsible for this phenomenon. Jacobs et al.[14] reported that extracts of a well-differentiated prostatic carcinoma stimulated incorporation of ³H-thymidine into fibroblasts, as did extracts of benign prostatic hyperplasia. Preliminary character-ization of the protein factor released from the prostatic carcinoma indicated that it was a protein of M_r 67 000 or more. Harrod et al.[15] found that a human prostatic cancer cell line derived from a bone metastasis[16], produced an osteoblast-stimulating factor which is sensitive to heat and protease and has a M_r of approximately 20 000. This protein stimulates the incorporation of ³H-thymidine and increases the alkaline phosphatase concentration in osteoblast-like bone-forming cells. Nevertheless, preliminary evidence indicates that con-ditioned media harvested from prostatic cancer cells stimulate incorporation of ³H-proline into collagenase-digestible protein, a commonly used assay for bone collagen synthesis (E. Simpson, unpublished results). The relationship of factors affecting bone formation to each other and to previously characterized hormones will have to await the purification and structural characterization of these factors. Several growth factors will probably be found to be involved in the regulation and timing of cellular events which lead to the coupled processes of resorption and subsequent formation.

Table 1. *Agents which affect bone formation or resorption*

	Bone formation
Humoral factors	*Mechanisms of Action*
Somatomedin C (IGF-1)	Collagen synthesis
Platelet-derived growth factor	Progression in cell cycle
Insulin	Collagen synthesis
Growth hormone	Indirect: mediated by somatomedin-C or IGF-1
Parathyroid hormone	*In vivo:* possibly mediated by coupling factor
Bone-derived factors	
Skeletal growth factor	Cell division, collagen synthesis
Bone morphogenetic protein	*In vivo* bone formation and mineralization
Bone-derived growth factor-1	Somatomedin C-like
Bone-derived growth factor-2	PDGF-like
Tumor-derived factors	
Prostatic hyperplasia (Ref. 14)	³H-thymidine incorporation
Prostatic carcinoma (Ref. 15)	³H-thymidine incorporation, alkaline phosphatase

	Bone resorption
Parathyroid hormone	Decreased formation, acts directly on osteoblast
Epidermal growth factor	Decreased formation/increased resorption
Platelet-derived growth factor	Resorption mediated by prostaglandins
Transforming growth factors	Increased resorption

Growth factors which enhance bone resorption

The classic example of a protein which enhances bone resorption is para-thyroid hormone (PTH), the most important regulator of extracellular calcium concentration *in vivo*. PTH is active in all of the currently available *in vitro* systems for assaying bone resorption and appears to act directly on osteoblasts to decrease bone formation, resulting in high net resorption as osteoclasts continue to resorb bone. However, *in vivo* administration of PTH may cause increased bone formation in some patients[17]. One explanation for this effect is that PTH causes synthesis of an osteoblast stimulating factor(s) (a so-called coupling factor) at the site of resorption which attracts osteoblasts to the resorption site and stimulates them to lay down new bone[18].

Several other well characterized growth factors have recently been found to affect bone resorption. Among these are EGF, PDGF and the transforming growth factors (TGFs).

EGF, a peptide of M_r 6 000 first described in the salivary glands of mice, has attracted considerable interest because of its capacity to stimulate the division of mesenchymal cells and to accelerate developmental processes[19]. Although its precise physiological role is unknown, it has been used as a prototype for the tumor-derived TGFs, one class of which requires the EGF receptor to exert its biological effects. The binding of EGF to its cell surface receptor is associated with enhanced phosphorylation of tyrosine residues catalysed by the protein kinase activity of the receptor. A similar mechanism of action of EGF may be envisaged to operate in bone cells. Indeed, antibodies to the EGF receptor block the bone-resorbing activities of EGF *in vitro*[20].

EGF causes decreased bone formation *in vitro*[2] and may increase bone resorp-tion in organ cultures of neonatal mouse calvarial cells via a prostaglandin-mediated mechanism[21]. The EGF dose needed for bone resorption in this system is 10^{-9} M. However, in a similar bone resorption assay which uses fetal rat forearm bones, bone resorption is independent of prostaglandin and the resorp-tive action of EGF is evident only after a 5-day incubation (versus 2 days with PTH).

EGF is a powerful stimulator of osteoclastic bone resorption and tumors produce a family of polypeptide stimulators of cell growth and replication (the TGFs) which have some biological and chemical properties in common with EGF. These observations prompted an examination of tumors associated with hypercalcemia of malignancy to determine if one or more of the TGFs produced by these tumors induced the observed bone resorption.

TGFs occur in a variety of tissues, including fresh human and animal tumors, virus-transformed cells and certain normal tissues. There are two main types: one type inhibits binding of ^{125}I-EGF to its receptors while the other is dependent on EGF (or TGF-I) for its biological activity but does not bind to the EGF receptor. All TGFs stimulate normal mesenchymal indicator cells to form colonies in soft agar, and this is the activity which corresponds best to their ability to maintain the transformed phenotype. TGF-I has been described in a variety of tumors but its production by normal tissue still remains uncertain. In contrast, TGF-II has been purified from platelets, placenta and kidney and has also been found in a number of tumors. TGF-II stimulates fibroblast collagen synthesis and has been proposed as a potential wound healing factor *in vivo*[22]. Recently, TGF-II and PDGF have been shown to work in concert to stimulate soft-agar formation of indicator cells[23]. This may be a very important phenomenon since platelets accumulate at sites of injury such as fracture sites and are also present in the marrow cavity. Factors which have a synergistic effect at a fracture site or site of bone remodeling may promote collagen synthesis, callus formation or remodeling of bone.

The hypothesis that a TGF can resorb bone has been tested in two animal models of malignant hypercalcemia and in a patient with lung cancer and hypercalcemia. In these tumors, bone resorbing activity and TGF activity, as assessed by capacity to stimulate colony growth of indicator cells in soft agar and EGF radioreceptor assays, co-purify[24]. Moreover, in one of the animal models antibodies to the EGF receptor which inhibit TGF-I activity also block bone resorbing activity[20]. Since normal tissues as well as transformed tissues produce TGFs it is exciting to speculate that these growth factors represent a new class of bone-active agents that act at very low concentrations to affect bone remodeling.

As already mentioned, another factor reported to stimulate bone resorption is PDGF, the major circulating growth factor for cells of mesenchymal origin[7]. It is contained within the alpha granules of circulating blood platelets and is released during clotting. Unlike EGF, PDGF appears to prepare cells for progression through the cell cycle; other factors, such as the somatomedins, also mediate progression through the cell cycle. Tashjian et al.[25] found that PDGF stimulates bone resorption in mouse calvaria in a similar manner to EGF. Stimulation of bone resorption by PDGF was dependent on prostaglandin synthesis, and was inhibited by indomethacin.

Much recent interest has been generated in PDGF because of its close structural relationship to the oncogene encoded by the Simian sarcoma virus[23,26]. This is the first demonstration that the product of an oncogene may be a protein with known physiological effects in normal cells. As PDGF may be a bone-resorbing factor, it is of interest that tumors associated with malignant hypercalcemia could be expressing and secreting a viral or cellular product related to this growth factor. Expression of the *sis* oncogene commonly occurs in osteosarcomas, which are usually associated with bone resorption but not with hypercalcemia. In tumors which are not expressing the *sis* oncogene, expression of other oncogenes may stimulate tumor cells to produce growth factors that act directly on bones. For example, activation and expression of *ras* oncogenes appears to be associated with transforming growth factor-like activity in tumor cells[27]. Thus, oncogenes may be involved in the production of bone-resorbing factors by malignant cells. It is attractive to speculate that the normal cellular counterparts of the *sis* or *ras* oncogenes somehow affect normal bone remodeling.

Future directions

The coupled processes of bone formation and bone resorption in fetal tissue and in the adult skeleton are subject to control by local and systemic growth factors. The nature of the coupling factor or factors which initiate bone formation following a wave of resorption remains to be elucidated. Whether the same factors which act to recruit osteoblast precursors in fetal tissue are active in adult bone is also unclear, although the involvement of the process of differentiation of mesenchymal cells in both cases suggests that these factors are operative throughout life.

Evidence is accumulating that factors expressed in malignancy, such as oncogene products and TGFs, are also produced in normal tissues and play a role in normal cellular physiology. As this review shows, several tumor-derived products are extremely active in stimulating both bone formation and resorption. It remains to be seen whether these same tumor factors are expressed in a regulated and concerted manner by normal tissues to bring about the tightly coupled processes of formation and resorption seen in bone remodeling.

Acknowledgements

This work was supported by NIH grants AM30668 and CA29537. I thank Greg Mundy and John Jacobs for helpful advice on this manuscript.

References

1   Canalis, E. (1980) *J. Clin. Invest.* 66, 709–719
2   Canalis, E. and Raisz, L. G. (1979) *Endocrinology* 104, 862–869
3   Reddi, A. H. (1982) in *Biochemical Development of the Fetus and Neonate* (Jones, C. T., ed.), pp. 163–184, Elsevier Biomedical Press
4   Baron, R., Vignery, A. and Horowitz, M. (1984) in *Bone and Mineral Research* (Peck, W. A., ed.), Vol. 2, pp. 175–243, Elsevier Science Publishers
5   Stern, P. H. and Raisz, L. G. (1979) in *Skeletal Research: An Experimental Approach* (Simmons, D. J. and Kunin, A. S., eds), pp. 22–59, Academic Press
6   Rodan, G. A., Majeska, R. J., Wiren, K. M. and Rodan, S. B. (1984) in *Endocrine Control of Bone and Calcium Metabolism* (Cohn, D. V., Fujita, T., Potts, J. T. Jr, and Talmadge, R. V., eds), Vol. 8A, pp. 117–124, Elsevier Science Publishers B.V.
7   Stiles, C. D. (1983) *Cell* 33, 653–655
8   Canalis, E. M., Dietrich, J. W., Mania, D. M. and Raisz, L. G. (1977) *Endocrinology* 100, 668–674
9   Canalis, E. M., Hintz, R. L., Dietrich, J. W., Mania, D. M. and Raisz, L. G. (1977) *Metabolism* 26, 1079–1087
10 Canalis, E. (1980) *J. Clin. Invest.* 66, 709–719
11 Farley, J. R. and Baylink, D. J. (1982) *Biochemistry* 21, 3502–3507
12 Urist, M. R., Huo, Y. K., Brownell, A. G., Hohl, W. M., Buyske, J., Lietze, A., Tempst, P., Hunkapiller, M. and DeLange, R. J. (1984) *Proc. Natl Acad. Sci. USA* 81, 371–375
13 Canalis, E. (1983) *Endocrine Reviews* 4, 62–77
14 Jacobs, S. C., Pikna, D. and Lawson R. K. (1979) *Invest. Urol.* 17, 195–198
15 Harrod, J., D'Souza, S., Bertolini, D., Ibbotson, K., Smith, D. and Mundy, G. (1983) *Calcif. Tissue Intl* 35, Suppl. 671
16 Kaighn, M. E., Narayan, K. S., Ohnuki, Y., Lechner, J. F. and Jon, L. W. (1979) *Invest. Urol.* 17, 16–23
17 Tam, C. S., Heersche, J. N. M., Murray, T. M. and Parsons, J. A. (1982) *Endocrinology* 110, 506–512
18 Howard, G. A., Bottemiller, B. L., Turner, R. T., Rader, J. I. and Baylink D. J. (1981) *Proc. Natl Acad. Sci. USA* 78, 3204–3208
19 Cohen, S. (1983) *Cancer* 51, 1787
20 D'Souza, S. M., Ibbotson, K. J., Carpenter, G. and Mundy, G. R. (1984) *Calcif. Tissue Intl* 36, Suppl. A31
21 Raisz, L. G., Simmons, H. A., Sandberg, A. L. and Canalis, E. (1980) *Endocrinology* 107, 270–273
22 Sporn, M. B., Roberts, A. B., Shull, J. H., Smith, J. M. and Ward, J. M. (1983) *Science* 219, 1329–1331
23 Waterfield, M. D., Scrace, G. T., Whittle, N., Stroobant, P., Johnsson, A., Wasteson, A., Westermark, B., Heldin, C.-H., Huang, J. S. and Deuel, T. F. (1983) *Nature* 304, 35–39
24 Ibbotson, K. J., D'Souza, S. M., Ng, K. W., Osborne, C. K., Niall, M., Martin, T. J. and Mundy, G. R. (1983) *Science* 221, 1292–1294
25 Tashjian, A. H., Hohmann, E. L., Antoniades, H. N. and Levine, L. (1982) *Endocrinology* 111, 118–124
26 Doolittle, R. F., Hunkapiller, M. W., Hood, L. E., Devare, S. G., Robbins, K. C., Aaronson, S. A. and Antoniades, H. N. (1983) *Science* 221, 275–277
27 Assoian, R. K., Grotendorst, G. R., Miller, D. M. and Sporn, M. B. (1984) *Nature* 309, 804–806

E. Simpson is at the Division of Endocrinology and Metabolism, Dept of Medicine, University of Texas Health Science Center, San Antonio, Texas 78284, USA.

Protease nexins: cell-secreted proteins which regulate extracellular serine proteases

Daniel J. Knauer and Dennis D. Cunningham

Cultured normal human fibroblasts release three different proteins called protease nexins into their medium which selectively form covalent linkages with certain serine proteases. These protease–protease nexin complexes then bind to cells, are internalized and degraded. For the protease thrombin, it has been shown that this process modulates its mitogenic action on the cells.

Proteases and biological control

Specific proteolytic enzymes play central roles in the activation of many biological processes, including blood coagulation, platelet aggregation and release, fibrinolysis, complement activation, hormone processing and cell division (Refs 1–4 contain many reviews on this). The key event in these activation processes is limited proteolysis by proteases that are usually very specific in their actions. The activation step itself is essentially irreversible since proteolysis is an exergonic reaction and, under normal physiological conditions, there are no simple biological mechanisms to repair a broken peptide bond. An important feature of most biological events which are reglulated by proteolysis is the possibility for modulation by certain protease inhibitors. By their ability to limit the extent, duration and site of protease action, they provide added specificity to the regulatory systems[5]. In this review, we will describe what is known about the three recently-described protease nexins (PN-I, PN-II and PN-III) and their ability to inhibit and thus modulate the actions of certain regulatory serine proteases.

General properties of protease nexins

Before considering the individual protease nexins (PN) we will first describe the general properties common to all of them[6–11]. Figure 1 summarizes many of these features. Each PN is released into serum-free culture medium by normal human fibroblasts as well as a number of other cultured cells. If the appropriate protease is present in the extracellular environment, it forms a covalent linkage with the PN. The resulting complex between the protease and the PN can be detected by sodium dodecyl sulfate polyacrylamide gel electrophoresis, although it should be emphasized that the complexes are not stable at high pH in the presence of primary amine buffers and are more effectively detected using gel systems run at a lower pH with other buffers[6,8].

It appears that the protease and PN in the complexes are stabilized by an acyl linkage, as judged by the ability of hydroxylamine and high pH to dissociate them. This suggests that the complexes are stable intermediates of a reaction in which the protease cleaves a fragment from the PN, similar to complexes between thrombin and antithrombin III (ATIII), a prominent inhibitor of thrombin in plasma[12]. In fact, Baker and his colleagues[11] have recently shown this directly in studies using purified PN-I and thrombin. They demonstrated that the molecular weight of PN-I was reduced after complex formation and that a peptide was released during the process. Consistent with these results is the finding that if proteases are derivitized at their catalytic site serine with a diisopropylphospho- (DIP-) group they will not form linkages with the PNs[6,10].

Thus, all available evidence indicates that the complexes between proteases and PNs result from initial cleavage of a fragment from the PN and that the complex itself is an acyl intermediate involving the serine residue in the catalytic site of the protease. Although the PNs are substrates for the proteases they link, they apparently differ from 'normal' substrates in their capacity to strongly interact with the protease during and after formation of the acyl-linked complex. These interactions probably also include electrostatic and hydrophobic interactions which stabilize the acyl linkage in the complex.

Another feature common to the three PNs is that protease–PN complexes readily bind to the cells that secrete the PNs[6-9]. The binding has been studied mostly with normal human fibroblasts although it has been seen with several other types of cells also. Binding was observed before any purification of the PNs simply by adding the appropriate ^{125}I-labeled protease to cells cultured in serum-free conditioned medium. Under these conditions, ^{125}I-protease–PN complexes were found in the medium and it was shown that they could bind to cells. As illustrated in Fig. 1, the available evidence indicates that the complexes bind to cells via the PN portion of the complexes. However, it should be emphasized that definitive studies on the mechanism of this binding must await purification of each of the PNs. Among the important questions to be answered are whether there are distinct binding sites on cells for each of the protease–PN complexes and whether 'free' unclipped PNs specifically bind to cells.

For each of the PNs it has been shown that, following binding of protease–PN complexes to cells, the complexes are rapidly internalized and degraded[7-10]. This conclusion comes from studies on complexes in which the protease was labeled with ^{125}I and shown to be internalized and degraded to ^{125}I-tyrosine. The fate of the PN portion of internalized protease–PN complexes is unknown; it may also be degraded or, perhaps, recycled. Recycling seems less likely since PN is cleaved during complex formation. The answer to this question must await the use of radiolabeled purified PNs to follow their fate directly.

The PNs can account for most of the specific cellular binding of proteases which become linked to a PN; however, it appears that some of these proteases have distinct binding sites on the cell surface. This conclusion is depicted in Fig. 1, and came from experiments on the binding of thrombin[13] and the gamma subunit of nerve growth factor (NGF-γ)[9] as well as the DIP-derivatives of these two proteases. As noted above, DIP-proteases are not linked by PN and thus are not bound to cells by this mechanism. However, certain cells specifically bind DIP-thrombin and DIP-NGF-γ and the underivatized proteases compete for this binding, indicating the presence of binding sites for the unlinked protease.

Properties of the individual PNs

Table I summarizes some of the features of the PNs. The molecular weights refer to the PNs in the linked complexes; since each PN is apparently cleaved during complex formation, the unlinked PNs are probably larger. Of a number of proteases tested PN-I binds all arginine-specific serine proteases examined: thrombin, urokinase[6], trypsin[14], NGF-γ[9] and plasmin[15]. It does not bind chymotrypsin or pancreatic elastase[11]. Studies with purified PN-I have demonstrated that bound proteases are inactive[11,15,16]. One property of PN-I that is not

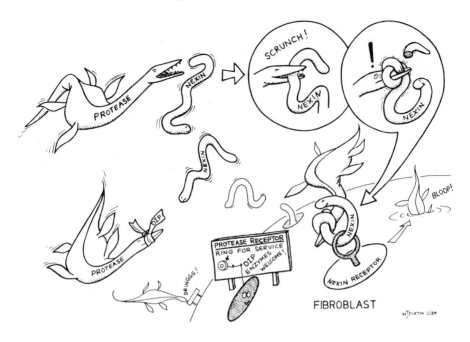

Fig. 1. Interactions of a protease (P) and its protease nexin (PN) with cells.

shared by PN-II or PN-III is that its protease linkage and cellular binding are strongly modulated by heparin. Heparin markedly accelerates the rate of linkage between thrombin and PN-I although it inhibits the binding of protease-PN-I complexes to cells. These results prompted experiments which showed that PN-I binds heparin[6]; this property was exploited during the purification of PN-I[11]. Purified PN-I has a molecular weight of about 43 000; it exhibits all of the known properties attributed to PN-I in culture medium[11].

Although PN-II and PN-III are quite different in size in their linked complexes with proteases (Table 1), they share the property of linking proteases which are binding proteins for growth factors. PN-II links the binding protein for epidermal growth factor (EGF)[8], while PN-III links NGF-γ[9]. As with other protease–PN complexes, these complexes also bind to cells. The complexes are subsequently internalized and the protease moiety is degraded. Unlike PN-I, the protease linkage by PN-II and PN-III and the subsequent cellular binding of the complexes are not markedly affected by heparin. Although the protease specificity of PN-II and PN-III have not been examined extensively, it appears that they are more selective in their linkage than PN-I. This is illustrated by the findings that PN-II will not link NGF-γ and PN-III will not link the binding protein for EGF even though these two proteases show extensive homology[17]. As shown in Table 1, NGF-γ displays cross-reactivity for EGF binding protein in competitive cellular binding assays with PN-II, and, likewise, the EGF binding protein shows cross-reactivity for NGF-γ in similar assays with PN-III[10]. However, this appears to result from the ability of the cross-reacting protease to weakly bind to the other PN and not from the ability to link to it.

Table 1. Summary of the protease nexins thus far indentified and comparison of their properties

Nexin	$\sim M_r$	Proteases linked	Cross-reactivity in competitive cellular binding assays	Protease linkage or cellular binding strongly augmented by heparin
Protease nexin-I (PN-I)	38000	Thrombin, urokinase, trypsin, NGF-γ, plasmin	NGF-γ	Yes
Protease nexin-II (PN-II)	95000	EGF-binding protein	NGF-γ	No
Protease nexin-III (PN-III)	31000	NGF-γ subunit	EGF binding protein	No

Biological roles of the PNs

Although studies on possible physiological functions of the PNs are only at a very early stage, it is possible to make reasonable predictions based on the knowledge that the activity of proteases in the linked complexes is blocked and that the PNs enable cells to remove certain proteases from their extracellular environment. Several possibilities have been explored. For example, advantage has been taken of the observation that heparin blocks the binding of thrombin-PN-I complexes to cells. Experiments have shown that added heparin does not shift the dose–response curve for thrombin-simulated cell division, indicating that the binding of thrombin–PN-I complexes to cells neither mediates nor inhibits the mitogenic signal produced by thrombin[18]. In contrast, added PN-I shifts the dose–response curve to higher concentrations of thrombin, indicating that PN-I probably modulates the mitogenic action of thrombin[19]. This is consistent with previous findings that the proteolytic activity of thrombin is required for its mitogenic action[13]. Of course, these results do not demonstrate that PN-I negatively regulates this action of thrombin in vivo, but it does provide interesting leads.

PN-I may function as an inhibitor of urokinase activity. It is the primary urokinase inhibitor released by human fibroblasts[14]; these cells secrete urokinase as a proenzyme[16]. PN-I also inhibits plasmin[15], the most potent known activator of urokinase proenzyme[16,20]. The possibility that PN-I functions to regulate endogenous urokinase is further suggested by the finding that phorbol ester, EGF and thrombin, which stimulate urokinase proenzyme secretion, also stimulate PN-I secretion, but not total protein secretion[15].

Studies have not yet been conducted to examine the possible roles of PN-II or PN-III. However, in view of their ability to selectively link binding proteins for EGF and NGF, it seems possible that they could control the ratio of free growth factor to growth factor bound by binding protein and thus possibly the delivery of these factors to cells.

Similarities of PNs to serum protease inhibitors

Circulating blood contains a number of potent protease inhibitors (e.g. alpha$_1$-antitrypsin, alpha$_2$-antiplasmin, ATIII, CI-inactivator, alpha$_2$-macroglobulin, heparin cofactor II) which are continually present at high concentrations and appear to bring about a constant control in this very large compartment of the body[21]. Of these, ATIII and heparin cofactor II appear similar to PN-I, although their molecular weights are different, and antibodies to ATIII do not cross-react with PN-I[6]. Perfusion studies have indicated that thrombin-ATIII complexes bind to hepatocytes[22], although direct binding studies on cells have not yet been reported. In general, the PNs appear not to be major protease inhibitors in plasma, and may be mainly involved in proteolytic control processes in interstitial fluid at the cellular or tissue level. Additional studies will be required to clarify the distinctions and relationships between proteolytic control mechanisms in plasma and interstitial fluid.

References

1 Reich, E., Rifkin, D. and Shaw, E. (eds) (1975) *Proteases and Biological Control*, Cold Spring Harbor Laboratory
2 Ribbons, D. and Brew, K. (eds) (1976) *Proteolysis and Physiological Regulation*, Academic Press
3 Agarwal, M. (ed.) (1979) *Proteases and Hormones*, Elsevier/North-Holland
4 Walz, D. and McCoy, L. (eds) (1981) *Contributions to Hemostasis*, The New York Academy of Sciences
5 Neurath, H. and Walsh, K. (1976) *Proc. Natl Acad. Sci. USA* 73, 3825–3832
6 Baker, J., Low, D., Simmer, R. and Cunningham, D. (1980) *Cell* 21, 37–45
7 Low, D., Baker, J., Koonce, W. and Cunningham, D. (1981) *Proc. Natl Acad. Sci. USA* 78, 2340–2344
8 Knauer, D. and Cunningham, D. (1982) *Proc. Natl Acad. Sci. USA* 79, 3210–3214
9 Knauer, D. and Cunningham, D. (1982) *J. Biol. Chem.* 257, 15098–15104
10 Knauer, D., Thompson, J. and Cunningham, D. (1983) *J. Cell Physiol.* 117, 385–396
11 Scott, R. and Baker, J. (1983) *J. Biol. Chem.* 258, 10439–10444
12 Rosenberg, R. and Damus, D. (1973) *J. Biol. Chem.* 248, 6490–6505
13 Glenn, K., Carney, D., Fenton, J., II and Cunningham, D. (1980) *J. Biol. Chem.* 255, 6609–6615
14 Low, D., Cunningham, D., Scott, R. and Baker, J. (1981) in *Receptor-Mediated Binding and Internalization of Toxins and Hormones* (Middlebrook, J. and Kohn, L., eds), pp. 259–270, Academic Press
15 Eaton, D. and Baker, J. (1983) *J. Cell Biol.* 97, 323–328
16 Scott, R., Eaton, D., Duran, N. and Baker, J. (1983) *J. Biol. Chem.* 258, 4397–4403
17 Lazure, C., Seidah, N., Thibault, G., Boucher, R., Genest, J. and Chretien, M. (1981) *Nature* 292, 383–384
18 Baker, J., Low, D., Eaton, D. and Cunningham, D. (1982) *J. Cell Physiol.* 112, 291–297
19 Low, D., Scott, R., Baker, J. and Cunningham, D. (1982) *Nature* 298, 476–478
20 Wun, T.-C., Ossowski, L. and Reich, E. (1982) *J. Biol. Chem.* 257, 7262–7268
21 Collen, D., Wiman, B. and Verstraete, M. (eds) (1979) *The Physiological Inhibitors of Blood Coagulation and Fibrinolysis*, Elsevier/North-Holland
22 Shifman, M. and Pizzo, S. (1982) *J. Biol. Chem.* 257, 3243–3248

D. J. Knauer, is at the Department of Developmental and Cell Biology, School of Biological Sciences, and D. D. Cunningham is at the Department of Microbiology, College of Medicine, University of California, Irvine, California 92717, USA.

Negative regulators of cell growth
John L. Wang and Yen–Ming Hsu

Endogenous inhibitors of cell proliferation have been purified from several sources, including normal tissues and conditioned medium from epithelial and fibroblast cell lines. Structural and functional studies on these molecules and their receptors will provide new insights into the significance of growth inhibitors in cellular homeostasis.

Cellular homeostasis, the delicate balance between cell production and cell removal in various tissues, depends to a large extent on two alternative modes of existence of most animal cells: the quiescent and the proliferative. The growth and division of normal cells is usually well regulated by the action of various endogenous stimulators and inhibitors. Thus, one of the fundamental challenges in the study of growth control is to determine the biochemical nature and sites of action of agents that can shift cells from one state to the other.

Over the past decade, much progress has been made in our understanding of the structure and activities of polypeptide growth factors and their specific receptors on the cell surface (for review see Ref. 1). In contrast, much less progress has been made in the study of endogenous growth inhibitors that may function in cellular homeostasis. The existence of endogenous inhibitors of cell division was first suggested by studies on epidermal wound healing and carcinogenesis (for reviews see Refs 2 and 3). The term 'chalone' was given to this putative class of molecules that acted as inhibitory growth regulators. The distinguishing characteristics of these chalones were postulated as: (1) complete tissue specificity, (2) lack of species-specificity, and (3) reversibility. A major difficulty in developing the chalone concept experimentally has been the formidable problem of isolation and chemical characterization of these molecules.

More recently, two independent lines of research have provided a firm experimental basis for the notion of negative regulators of cell growth. First, endogenous inhibitors of cell proliferation have been successfully purified from several sources, including normal tissues[4,5] and conditioned medium from epithelial[6] and fibroblast cell lines[7] (see Table 1). Second, comparative molecular and functional analyses of type β transforming growth factor (TGF-β) and a growth inhibitor purified from the kidney epithelial cell line BSC-1 suggest that these molecules are either identical or closely related[8].

TGF-β and growth inhibitor from conditioned medium of BSC-1 cells

Transforming growth factors (TGFs) are a family of polypeptides that reversibly induce non-neoplastic cells to express the transformed phenotype; this is measured by loss of density-dependent inhibition of growth and acquisition of anchorage-independent growth (for a review of TGFs, see p. 157).

Two distinct sets of TGFs have been purified to homogeneity. TGF-α is a single chain polypeptide (M_r 5700) that shares sequence homology with epidermal growth factor (EGF); TGF-α and EGF both bind to the EGF receptor and have indistinguishable biological activities *in vitro*. TGF-β consists of two identical polypeptide chains (M_r 12 500) linked by disulfide bonds[4,9]; the activity of the native molecule (M_r 25 000) is destroyed upon reduction of the disulfide groups (Table 1). TGF-β is a ubiquitous molecule; it has been found in many normal

Table 1. Properties of some negative regulators of cell growth

Source	Nomenclature	Target (indicator cells)	Native molecular weight	SDS gels (reducing conditions)	Refs
Various tissues, cells, and conditioned medium	Transforming growth factor-β (TGF-β)	NRK cells AKR-2B cells	25 000	12 500	4, 9
BSC-1 conditioned medium	BSC-1 growth inhibitor	BSC-1 cells CCL 64 mink lung cells	25 000	12 500	6,13
Human fibroblasts	Interferon-β	HeLa cells	28 000–35 000	18 000	28
3T3 conditioned medium	Fibroblast growth regulator (FGR-s (13 K))	3T3 cells	13 000	13 000	7,19
Mouse embryo fibroblast concitioned medium	—	Mouse embryo fibroblasts	10 000–15 000	11 000–14 000	21
Rat liver	Hepatic proliferation inhibitor (HPI)	Rat hepatocytes	26 000	26 000	5, 18
Bovine mammary gland	—	Ehrlich ascites mammary cells	13 000	13 000	22,23
Bovine cerebral cortex cells	Bovine glycopeptide inhibitor (BCSG)	Mouse fibroblasts (3T3, LM), BHK-21	45 000	16 000–18 000	24
	Sialoglycopeptide inhibitor	3T3, BHK-21	18 000	18 000	31

tissues as well as in serum-free conditioned medium of normal and transformed cells[9]. TGF-β binds to unique cell-surface receptors in responsive cells[10,11]. Affinity labelling studies indicate that the TGF-β receptor is composed of a disulfide-bonded, glycosylated complex (M_r 560 000–620 000) containing a ligand-binding subunit of M_r 280 000–300 000 (Ref. 12).

Holley and co-workers have isolated a growth inhibitor from medium conditioned by BSC-1 cells, derived from African green monkey kidney epithelial cells[6,13]. This growth inhibitor yielded a native molecular weight of 25 000 and a polypeptide of M_r 12 500 after gel electrophoresis in the presence of sodium dodecyl sulfate and reducing agents (Table 1). The action of this BSC-1 growth inhibitor is apparently autocrine (it is produced by the same cells on which it acts). One early response of target cells treated with this BSC-1 growth inhibitor is the appearance of an 'inhibitor-induced' protein (M_r 48 000) that is secreted into the medium[14].

Recently, it has been shown that TGF-β and the growth inhibitor of BSC-1 cells have identical biological activities[8]: (1) stimulation of the growth of AKR-2B cells in soft agar; (2) inhibition of DNA synthesis in AKR-2B, BSC-1 and CCL-64 (mink lung) cells; and (3) binding to TGF-β specific receptors on the cell surface. Therefore, TGF-β and the BSC-1 growth inhibitor are either identical or closely related[8]. In corroboration of these results, Roberts *et al.*[15] have reported that TGF-β can either stimulate or inhibit growth. The expression of these two activities is modulated by other growth factors and is not solely dependent on cell type or conditions of anchorage-dependent versus anchorage-independent growth.

TGF-β now stands as a paradigm for several important features of growth regulation: (1) it is one of the first peptide growth inhibitors purified to homogeneity and its amino acid sequence has been determined[16]; (2) it is a negative growth regulator that may function in the autocrine pathway[17]; and (3) it is bifunctional (stimulatory and inhibitory growth regulatory activities)[15].

Hepatic proliferation inhibitor

An inhibitor of hepatocyte proliferation has been purified from rat liver[5]. This hepatic proliferation inhibitor (HPI) migrates as a polypeptide (M_r 26 000) in sodium dodecyl sulfate gels under reducing conditions (Table 1); its isoelectric point is 4.65. This protein reversibly inhibits the proliferation of non-malignant rat liver cells in culture; it exerts no effect on the proliferation of hepatoma cells. Polyclonal rabbit antisera directed against HPI bound to parenchymal liver cells, but not to endothelial and connective tissue cells[18]. Little, if any, immunoreactive staining could be observed in hepatocellular carcinoma cells.

Fibroblast growth regulator

A growth inhibitory factor has also been isolated from medium conditioned by exposure to density-inhibited 3T3 cells[7,19]. This factor consists of a single polypeptide (M_r 13 000) and is designated FGR-s (13K), for fibroblast growth regulator secreted or shed in a soluble form (Table 1). It is an endogenous 3T3 cell product. The dose–response curve of growth inhibition showed that 50% inhibition of cell proliferation was achieved at a concentration of $\sim$ 3 ng ml^{-1}, corresponding to $\sim$ 0.23 nM. It is not cytotoxic and its effects on target cells are reversible.

A rat monoclonal antibody, designated 2A4, specifically bound FGR-s (13K). The activity of FGR-s (13K) was depleted by passing the material over an affinity column containing Antibody 2A4. Antibody 2A4 also neutralized the growth inhibitory effect of FGR-s (13K) in a concentration-dependent fashion[20]. Particularly striking was the observation that DNA synthesis is enhanced when Antibody 2A4 is added to cultures of 3T3 cells in the absence of any exogenously added FGR-s (13K)[20]. A control monoclonal antibody, which binds to 3T3 cells but is unreactive with FGR-s (13K), did not have the same effect. These results suggest that Antibody 2A4 may be neutralizing the activity of FGR-s (13K) molecules endogenous to the culture and reversing the effect of density inhibition. Therefore, it is inferred that FGR-s (13K) may play a role in the normal mechanism of density-dependent inhibition of growth in 3T3 cells. This negative action of FGR-s (13K) on the growth of cells in 3T3 cultures is autocrine.

Using procedures similar to those reported above, it has been shown that secondary mouse embryo fibroblasts release into the medium a growth inhibitor whose physicochemical behavior closely parallels that of FGR-s (13K). The molecular weights of the polypeptides in the active fractions were 11 000 and 14 000 (Ref. 21). (Note that growth inhibitory fractions from 3T3 cells, both soluble and associated with the plasma membrane, have been reported. The molecular properties of these active fractions and their relationship to FGR-s (13K) are not yet known.)

Growth inhibitor for mammary cells

A growth inhibitor for Ehrlich ascites mammary carcinoma cells *in vitro* has been purified from bovine mammary gland[22,23]. The active preparation consisted mainly of a single polypeptide (M_r 13 000) (Table 1). An antiserum raised in mice specifically bound the bovine mammary gland polypeptide (M_r 13 000) and neutralized the inhibitory activity of the preparation. Using this antiserum to analyse the tissue distribution of the inhibitor showed a high concentration of the protein in lactating (but not non-lactating) bovine mammary glands. Milk fat globule membranes and lung tissue also showed reactivity. Finally, the growth inhibitory effect on Ehrlich ascites mammary cells could be abolished by epidermal growth factor and insulin.

Cerebral cortex cell surface glycopeptides

Two distinct growth inhibitory polypeptides have been isolated from bovine cerebral cortex cells (Table 1). One is a glycopeptide preparation ($M_r \sim 18\ 000$) that inhibits protein synthesis and cell growth of normal but not transformed cells[24]. More recently, a sialoglycopeptide ($M_r \sim 18\ 000$) has also been purified from the same source[31]. Although these two glycopeptide inhibitors exhibit very similar biological properties, they appear to be distinct molecules on the basis of isoelectric point differences, lectin binding differences, and lack of cross-reactivity, when tested with an antiserum directed against the sialoglycopeptide.

Other systems

Three other growth inhibitors, partially purified and characterized, deserve a mention: (1) growth inhibiting factor(s) ($M_r \sim 10\ 000$–16 000), derived from conditioned medium of the human rhadomyosarcoma cell line A673, that acts on human tumor cells[32]; (2) a heparin-like molecule, produced by cultured endothelial cells, that inhibits the growth of smooth muscle cells[25,26]; and (3) a lipid molecule on the plasma membrane of lymphoid cells that inhibits the growth of normal lymphocytes and lymphoid tumor cells[27].

In addition, growth inhibitory activity has been shown for two other families of molecules: the interferons[28] and the mating factors, α and **a**, in yeasts[29]. Although these families of molecules have not been studied with cell growth and proliferation directly in mind, they must be considered as bona fide negative regulators of cell growth.

Perspectives

Despite recent successes in purifying endogenous inhibitors of cell proliferation, several key issues remain as challenges for future investigations:

Structure

The amino acid sequence of TGF-β has been determined by molecular cloning techniques[16]. Together with the structures of interferon and the yeast mating factors, this information provides reference structures against which future comparisons will be based. Clearly, structural information would facilitate our understanding at several levels: (1) The relationship between the growth inhibitors and known protein products, protein kinases, or oncogenes, as demonstrated strikingly for growth factors (for a review, see p. 135). (2) The relationship between TGF-β , FGR-s (13K) and other growth inhibitors. It is striking that the constituent polypeptide chains of several growth inhibitors have molecular weights of 13 000 or 26 000 (see Table 1). A family of growth inhibitors might be defined and perhaps a more informative system of nomenclature might be agreed upon by all workers in the field.

Identification and characterization of receptors for growth inhibitors

Both TGF-β and FGR-s (13K) have been shown to bind to cell surface receptors. The molecular identity of the TGF-β receptor has recently been elucidated[12]; however, possible enzymatic activities of the receptor remain to be determined. A survey of the distribution of receptors (number and/or affinity differences) in normal and neoplastic cells, cells of different tissues etc., might provide clues about the specificity of action of the inhibitors on target cells. Tissue specificity in terms of target cell responsiveness was perhaps the most attractive feature of the original 'chalone' hypothesis that prompted an enormous amount of research on growth inhibitors[2,3]. Now that a few inhibitors of cell growth have been purified, this notion can be rigorously tested.

Associated with this issue is the fate of the inhibitor–receptor complex and a mechanism of growth inhibition. One possible mechanism envisages the growth inhibitor acting like a hormone, with the binding of the inhibitor to its cell surface receptor triggering an intracellular signal that regulates the initiation of DNA synthesis and cell division. Alternatively, the growth inhibitor may modulate/counteract the mitogenic action of growth factors by altering the concentration of free growth factor available for interaction with its specific growth factor receptor. One clear example of this type of negative control is the action of protease nexins (for a review, see p. 189) in antagonizing the mitogenic effects of thrombin.

Effects of transformation

The ability of tumor cells to produce and to respond to their own growth factors provided a central concept linking oncogene and growth factor research. The 'autocrine hypothesis' states that oncogenes confer growth factor autonomy on cells not only by coding directly for peptide growth factors or their receptors (enzyme activities) but also by amplifying the mitogenic signals generated by a growth factor at its receptor. The 'autocrine hypothesis' may now be extended to include the concept that malignant transformation may be the result not only of excessive production, expression, and action of positive autocrine growth factors, but also of the failure to express or respond to specific negative regulators of cell growth[17]. This general concept has been championed for a number of years[30] but the recent developments on endogenous growth inhibitors have given it a firm experimental basis.

Associated with this issue is the question of whether tumor cells can be categorized in terms of their responsiveness to negative growth regulators? Are they unresponsive to inhibitors (compared to normal counterparts)? Although TGF-β appears to inhibit both neoplastic and non-neoplastic cells[15], there is evidence that normal cells are more responsive to other inhibitors[5,24]. If tumor cells indeed show less sensitivity, can we restore this responsiveness or take advantage of the unresponsiveness? If tumor cells are less susceptible to growth inhibitors, could they be made the selective targets of anti-proliferative agents while the normal cells are held in a resting state? The protection of normal cells by growth inhibitors might greatly enhance the effectiveness and specificity of chemotherapeutic techniques.

Physiological activity of growth inhibitors in vivo
Practically all the studies cited in this review were carried out in tissue culture systems, where the effects of inhibitor addition could be manipulated and rigorously studied. It remains to be seen whether the knowledge about the properties of the growth inhibitors gained *in vitro* can now be applied to *in-vitro* systems.

Acknowledgements
The work performed in the authors' laboratory and cited in this article was supported by grant GM 27203 from the National Institutes of Health and by Faculty Research Award FRA-221 from the American Cancer Society.

References
1 James, R. and Bradshaw, R. A. (1984) *Annu. Rev. Biochem.* 53, 259–292
2 Bullough, W. S. (1975) *Biol. Rev.* 50, 99–127
3 Iversen, O. H. (1981) in *Handbook of Experimental Pharmacology* (Baserga, R., ed.), Vol. 57, pp. 491–550 Springer-Verlag
4 Assoian, R. K., Kamoriya, A., Meyers, C. A., Miller, D. M. and Sporn, M. B. (1983) *J. Biol. Chem.* 258, 7155–7160
5 McMahon, J. B., Farrelly, J. G. and Iype, P. T. (1982) *Proc. Natl Acad. Sci USA* 79, 456–460
6 Holley, R. W., Bohlen, P., Fava, R., Baldwin, J. H., Kleeman, G. and Armour, R. (1980) *Proc. Natl Acad. Sci. USA* 77, 5989–5992
7 Hsu, Y–M. and Wang, J. L. (1986) *J. Cell Biol.* 102, 362–369
8 Tucker, R. F., Shipley, G. D., Moses, H. L. and Holley, R. W. (1984) *Science* 226, 705–707
9 Roberts, A. B., Frolik, C. A., Anzano, M. A. and Sporn, M. B. (1983) *Fed. Proc. Fed. Am. Soc. Exp. Biol.* 42, 2621–2626
10 Tucker, R. F., Branum, E. L., Shipley, G. D., Ryan, R. J. and Moses, H. L. (1984) *Proc. Natl Acad. Sci. USA* 81, 6757–6761
11 Frolik, C. A., Wakefield, L. M., Smith, D. M. and Sporn, M. B. (1984) *J. Biol. Chem.* 259, 10995–11000
12 Massagué, J. and Like, B. (1985) *J. Biol. Chem.* 260, 2636–2645
13 Holley, R. W., Armour, R., Baldwin, J. H. and Greenfield, S. (1983) *Cell Biol. Int. Rep.* 7, 141–147
14 Nilsen-Hamilton, M. and Holley, R. (1983) *Proc. Natl Acad. Sci. USA* 80, 5636–5640

15 Roberts, A. B., Anzano, M. A., Wakefield, L. M., Roche, N. S., Stern, D. F. and Sporn, M. B. (1985) *Proc. Natl Acad. Sci USA* 82, 119–123
16 Dernyck, R., Jarrett, J. A., Chen, E. Y., Eaton, D. H., Bell, J. R., Assoian, R. K., Roberts, A. B., Sporn, M. B. and Goeddel. D. V. (1985) *Nature* 316, 701–705
17 Sporn, M. B. and Roberts, A. B. (1985) *Nature* 313, 745–747
18 McMahon, J. B., Malan-Shibley, L. and Iype, P. T. (1984) *J. Biol. Chem.* 259, 1803–1806
19 Steck, P. A., Blenis, J., Voss, P. G. and Wang, J. L. (1982) *J. Cell Biol.* 92, 523–530
20 Hsu, Y.–M., Barry, J. M. and Wang, J. L. (1984) *Proc. Natl Acad. Sci. USA* 81, 2107–2111
21 Wells, V. and Mallucci, L. (1983) *J. Cell. Physiol.* 117, 148–154
22 Böhmer, F. D., Lehmann, W., Schmidt, H. E., Langen, P. and Grosse, R. (1984) *Exp. Cell Res.* 150, 466–476
23 Böhmer, F. D., Lehmann, W., Noll, F., Samtleben, R., Langen, P. and Grosse, R. (1985) *Biochim. Biophys. Acta* 846, 145–154
24 Kinders, R. J. and Johnson, T. C. (1982) *Biochem. J.* 206, 527–534
25 Castellot, J. J., Addonizio, M. L., Rosenberg, R. and Karnovsky, M. J. (1981) *J. Cell Biol.* 90, 372–379
26 Willems, Ch., Astaldi, G. C. B., DeGroot, Ph. G., Janssen, M. C., Gonsalvez, M. D., Zeijlemakerr, W. P., Van Mourik, J. A. and Van Aken, W. G. (1982) *Exp. Cell Res.* 139, 191–197
27 Stallcup, K. C., Dawson, A. and Mescher, M. F. (1984) *J. Cell Biol.* 99, 1221–1226
28 Stewart, W. E. (1979) *The Interferon System*, Springer-Verlag
29 Hartwell, L. H. (1978) *J. Cell Biol.* 77, 627–637
30 Potter, V. R. (1983) *Prog. Nucleic Acid Res. Mol. Biol.* 29, 161–173
31 Sharifi, B. G., Johnson, T. C., Khurana, V. K., Bascom, C. C., Fleenor, T. J. and Chou, H. -H. (1986) *J. Neurochem.* 46, 461–469
32 Iwata, K. K., Fryling, C. M., Knott, W. B. and Todaro, G. J. (1985) *Cancer Res.* 45, 2689–2694

John L. Wang and Yen–Ming Hsu are at the Department of Biochemistry, Michigan State University, East Lansing, MI 48824, USA.

Receptors and second messengers

Receptors and recognition: from ligand binding to gene structure

A. D. Strosberg

The concept of recognition of extracellular messengers by membrane-bound or internal molecules which translate ligand binding into cell activation, has in the last decade led to striking new insights into the structure and function of receptors. It is beyond the scope of this article to list all the successes which have been attained in the isolation of receptors and the characterization of their structure and function. Instead I shall summarize the general facts about molecular recognition which are now established and list some of the questions that remain to be answered.

'Receptors are proteins typically composed of several domains. They contain, by definition, at least one binding site specific for natural ligand. Receptors interact with one or several of a variety of effector systems for which they must also possess recognition sites. A single effector system may connect with various receptors. The information for activating the effector system is entirely contained in the membrane receptor; the ligand, or specific anti-receptor antibodies, only act as triggers of receptor-mediated effects, often initiated by receptor change in conformation micro-aggregation, redistribution, internalization or chemical modification.'

This 'consensus-statement' results from observations made on a large variety of systems. Here, some of the facts, with the methods which helped to establish the data, are presented.

Initially, the use of radiolabeled synthetic compounds to demonstrate ligand binding sites generated extensive controversy about variations in agonist and antagonist binding properties, effects of the environment, and the number of receptor classes in the same or in different types of cells. However, agreement has now been reached for a number of systems. Most investigators now agree, for example, on the existence of α_1, α_2, β_1 and β_2 adrenergic receptors; H_1 and H_2 histamine receptors; μ, δ, κ and σ opiates' receptors. The more simple nicotinic acetylcholine receptor from the electric organ of *Torpedo* fish is presently accepted as an accurate model for the study of the mammalian synapse. Nevertheless, discussions continue, for example, on the number of classes among the muscarinic acetylcholine receptors, or on the definition of D_1, D_2, D_3 and D_4 types of dopamine receptors.

The discovery of the endorphins (the endogenous ligands for the morphine receptor), gave a powerful boost to the search for natural counterparts of numerous other drugs, including the cardiac glycoside ouabain, the tricyclic antidepressants such as imipramine, and – last but not least – the benzodiazepines.

The molecular characterization of a number of membrane receptor systems was initiated by the development of efficient solubilization procedures. Affinity chromatography provided the tool for receptor purification using the insolubilized natural ligand, e.g. insulin, epidermal growth factor (EGF); synthetic analogs of the α- and β-adrenergic antagonists; specific toxins such as α-bungarotoxin, for the isolation of the nicotinic acetylcholine receptor; monoclonal antibodies specific for the transferrin and the EGF receptor. Amino acid micro sequencing was initiated on minute amounts of the isolated receptor polypeptide chains.

Affinity labeling of the binding sites by the use of ligand analogs containing photoactivable or chemically reactive groups permitted the determination of the molecular weight and subunit structure of a number of receptors. This approach is expected in the near future to pinpoint the amino acid residues involved in ligand recognition.

Cloning and sequencing of the genes coding, for instance, for the four different subunits of the nicotinic acetylcholine receptor were accomplished by a number of groups[1]. Similarly, recent reports described the isolation of cDNA clones encoding the receptors for human transferrin[2] and bovine low density lipoprotein[3].

Electron microscopic studies of the nicotinic acetylcholine receptor have unambiguously established the ring-like organization of its subunits and strongly support the idea that the ion channel is constituted by the receptor itself (Fig. 1). But the exact location within the α or other subunits of the binding sites for acetylcholine, α-bungarotoxin and local anaesthetics remain unknown. This is so despite the detailed prediction of the secondary structure based on the amino acid sequence and notwithstanding the assignment of the sulfhydryls.

Biochemical studies of receptor expression and effector function are being pursued with equal enthusiasm. Binding of insulin, EGF or low density lipoprotein to the cell surface has been shown to lead to the clustering of their respective receptors and subsequent internalization into vesicles by what is probably an energy driven process. The vesiculated receptors are either destroyed by association with lysosomes or recycled back to the plasma membrane. The loss of receptors from the plasma membrane by internalization may be one of the mechanisms of 'down regulation' induced by prolonged exposure of the cell to the ligand and may constitute a route for signalling to the cell interior. Recent findings furthermore suggest that one mechanism for this 'down regulation' may involve feedback regulation by the mRNA coding for the receptor[3].

Formation of the receptor–ligand complex is followed by specific responses

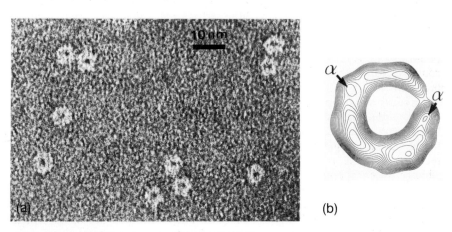

Fig. 1. The nicotinic Ach receptor from Torpedo. *(a) High magnification picture of a purified preparation of receptor molecules reincorporated into phospholipidic vesicles. The two forms of the receptor, light (95) and heavy (135), appear respectively as monomers and dimers (×800 000, negative staining; 1% uranyl acetate)[4]. (b) Reconstructed image of a rosette of receptor computed from 132 individual rosettes. Five domains are observed in the molecule. The arrows point to the two α-bungarotoxin binding sites which probably represent the two α subunits[5].*

such as regulation of enzyme activities through release of secondary chemical messengers (cAMP, cGMP) opening or closing of ion channels, methylation, phosphorylation or increased DNA synthesis.

Recent years have seen an accumulation of information concerning the mechanism by which the signal induced by ligand binding is transmitted to effector systems. Thus, the guanidine triphosphate (GTP) binding regulatory subunits intervening in hormone-induced adenylate cyclase stimulation (N_s) or inhibition (N_i) were isolated and thoroughly studied with the help of cholera toxin for N_s and pertussis toxin for N_i. A third GTP binding protein, transducin, was shown to cause the photoreceptor rhodopsin to stimulate a high affinity cyclic GMP phosphodiesterase upon photoactivation in the rod cell from the vertebrate retina. N_s and N_i contain two different subunits (α and β), and transducin contains three (α, β and γ). The β subunit is apparently an identical polypeptide of 35 000 mol. wt. The α subunits which bind GTP are very different, although they play a similar role: in both N_s and transducin the biological effect (adenylate cyclase activation and photoactivation, respectively) results from the release of the α subunit from the regulatory complex after receptor occupation (reviewed in Ref. 6). The α subunit from transducin has actually been reported to activate adenylate cyclase, in response to the binding of hormones, in various membrane systems unrelated to the retina complex. This finding further supports the hypothesis that receptors, transducers and effector systems may – in analogy to antibodies – share 'constant regions' responsible for the interactions between the various components and 'variable regions', each of which contains a binding site specific for a particular ligand[7,8].

Both the EGF and the insulin receptors express kinase activity: the EGF receptor acts upon target proteins which include the receptor itself by specifically transferring phosphate groups on to tyrosine residues. Similarly, the detergent-solubilized insulin receptor is auto-phosphorylated at tyrosine residues of its β-subunit after exposure to either insulin or anti-insulin receptor antibodies. Yet, in the intact cell, the more usual serine rather than tyrosine residues are phosphorylated. The EGF kinase does not phosphorylate the insulin receptor and vice versa.

It was recently shown that the insertion of pure β-adrenergic receptors into phospholipid vesicles, followed by their fusion with receptor-deficient cells, conveys β-adrenergic responsiveness to the adenylate cyclase system of the recipient cell[9]. When purified effector components, including the elusive adenylate cyclase, also become available, reconstitution experiments should help elucidate the role of carbohydrates and phospholipids in the functioning of hormone- and neurotransmitter-sensitive systems. It is already clear, however, that various components of the cytoskeleton play an essential role in merging the receptor, effector and amplifier systems into transmembrane configurations which ensure signal transmission between extra- and intracellular space.

A number of pathological conditions have been described in which specific receptors are either inactive, severely depleted or absent from the patient's tissues. Symptoms of both myasthenia gravis and a rare form of insulin-resistant diabetes are due to auto-immune reactions in which auto-antibodies bind to the receptors and probably induce their internalization and destruction. Antibodies to the thyroid stimulating hormone (TSH) may block binding of the ligand to the receptor and stimulate TSH-specific adenylate cyclase, thus provoking the symptoms of hyperthyroidism seen in Graves' disease. One form of familial hyperlipidemia may be explained by the absence of active low density lipo-protein receptor.

These few examples have spurred an intense search for other diseases in which receptor status is altered and it is likely that the 200th issue of *TIBS* will report considerable progress in this field. In the mean time, practical applications of research on receptors have emerged. For example, it is now well established that 50–65% of women with breast tumors having estrogen receptors will respond to endocrine therapy, whereas the likelihood of response is at best 10% in women lacking such receptors; cancer cells are recognized as targets by virtue of their receptors. As end products of estrogen action, progesterone receptors seem even better indicators of the efficacy of hormonal therapy: the correlation between presence of progesterone receptors on tumor cells and effect of estrogen is close to 80%[10].

The discovery of diseases associated with an anti-receptor auto-immune reaction has led investigators to produce anti-receptor antibodies by direct immunization. While conventional polyclonal antibodies appeared to be quite useful for functional studies, the technology of somatic cell fusion applied to lymphoid cells has permitted the production of monospecific monoclonal antibodies. Indeed, such antibodies have emerged as remarkable reagents for the analysis of receptor structure and function. Hundreds of different monoclonal antibodies have been raised against the nicotinic acetylcholine receptors, to map the various subunits at the cell surface[11]. Topological studies have also been performed for numerous other systems. A monoclonal antibody against the muscarinic acetylcholine receptor has been shown to induce contractions of the uterus and other agonist-like responses, some of which are blocked by atropine, a powerful antagonist[12]. Monoclonal antibodies against IgE receptor on mast cells have been shown to cause degranulation and histamine release. Similarly, EGF-triggered responses such as receptor clustering and internalization prior to EGF degradation, receptor phosphorylation, alterations in membrane transport and changes in cell morphology as well as in the cycloskeleton, may also be mimicked by monoclonal antibodies to the EGF receptor.

Anti-idiotypic antibodies, raised against the binding site of anti-hormone antibodies, may react with the hormone receptor, either through cross reaction between the two macromolecules recognizing the same ligand, or through mimicry of the ligand by the anti-antibody (Fig. 2). In the first case, the anti-idiotypic antibodies would recognize similar antigenic determinants on the binding sites of anti-hormone antibodies and of the receptor. In the second case, they would actually act as a hormone-like structure recognized by the anti-ligand antibody or by the receptor. The anti-idiotypic itself induces the production of neutralizing anti-anti-idiotypic antibody.

Anti-idiotypes may thus bind to receptors for insulin, β-adrenergic ligands, thyrotropin or acetylcholine, and displace the corresponding ligands. Insulin-like stimulation of 2-deoxyglucose uptake, or activation of catecholamine-sensitive adenylate cyclase by anti-idiotypes, confirm the specificity of the interaction between receptor and antibody. Most impressively, an anti-idiotype recognizing the acetylcholine receptor may even cause the symptoms of experimental myasthenia gravis, otherwise induced by antibody specifically raised against the receptors (reviewed in Ref. 13). Since autoanti-idiotypic antibodies have indeed been found in myasthenia patients[14], future investigations may uncover new explanations of auto-immune diseases involving idiotypic reactions against anti-ligand antibodies.

A directly related question concerns the degree of similarity between macromolecules which bind the same ligand. Structural similarities exist among the

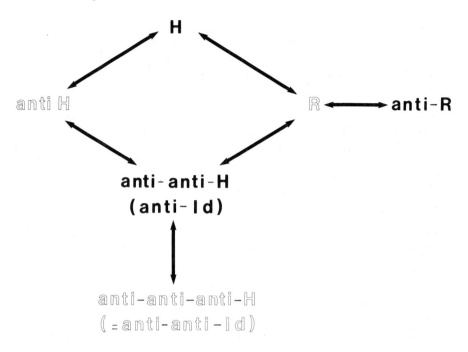

Fig. 2. A network of immunological interactions involving a hormone and its specific receptor and antibodies. The symmetrical positions of the anti-hormone antibodies (anti-H) and the receptor (R) around the hormone (H) are mirrored by those of the anti-R and anti-anti-H antibodies around R. The network of interactions is extended by the emergence of anti-anti-anti-H antibodies which are anti-idiotypic (anti-Id) towards the anti-anti-H immunoglobulins.

variable regions of antibodies which recognize the same antigenic determinant. Does an anti-catecholamine antibody share more than a few residues in the ligand specific site with the binding sites for this hormonal antigen on T lymphocytes or with a catecholamine β-adrenergic receptor? Do anti-idiotypic antibodies truly identify homologous cross-reactive regions? Or do they rather behave as 'internal images' of the ligand? (A crucial point not only if one wants to use antibodies as models for receptors but also if one examines the relationship of molecules involved in recognition.) The question of whether secreted antibodies are merely B-lymphocyte receptors which have exchanged their carboxy-terminal transmembrane hydrophobic anchoring region for a hydrophilic segment has recently gained additional interest through the concept of the 'sacrificial' IgA receptor[15]. This molecule releases, with IgA, a fragment ('secretory component') which protects the IgA against degradation and assists its persistence in the mucosa. Somewhat analogous is the finding that a transforming protein of avian erythroblastosis virus may correspond to a truncated EGF receptor (or closely related protein). This shortened sequence would lack the external EGF-binding domain but would retain the transmembrane domain and the domain involved in stimulating cell proliferation. This suggests that transformation of cells by virus may partially result from the introduction of an altered EGF receptor from the oncogene[16].

New insights are now being gained into the relationships between hormone or neurotransmitter receptors, antibodies, T lymphocyte antigen receptors and histocompatibility antigens. Present immunochemical evidence suggests that a single, two-chain, T cell receptor is responsible for antigen specificity, genetic restriction of lymphocyte recognition and cross reaction with alloantigens from the major histocompatibility complex (reviewed in Ref. 17). Both subunits appear to contain variable and constant portions. cDNA probes prepared from mRNA of T cells detect, in other T cell tumors and hybridomas, a gene which is systematically rearranged in DNA from thymocytes and not from other types of cells. Again evidence for variable and constant regions was obtained. The amino acid sequence predicted from the nucleotides suggests limited homology with immunoglobulins, especially around four cysteine residues that define Ig domains. The molecular characterization of the elusive T cell receptor may thus be realized in the near future.

Conclusion

The past decade has established solid bases for the molecular characterization of a number of receptor systems and has outlined the general properties of molecular recognition which would involve binding of the ligand, change of receptor conformation and redistribution of the complex. The future investigations should lead to the molecular analysis of the steps which follow redistribution, i.e. interaction with effector systems, with cytoskeleton elements, with nuclear elements and intracellular signalling. Covalent alterations consequent to ligand-induced physiological or pathological events may uncover new roles for the modified receptors, and will undoubtedly be the focus of tomorrow's research.

Reading list

Lamble, J. W. (ed.) (1981) Towards Understanding Receptors, *Current Reviews in Biomedicine*, Vol. 1, Elsevier
Lamble, J. W. (ed.) (1982) More about Receptors, *Current Reviews in Biomedicine*, Vol. 2, Elsevier
Cuatrecasas, P. and Greaves, M. F. (eds) *Receptors and Recognition series*, Chapman and Hall

References

A short reference list is a requirement for *TIBS*; I therefore apologize to authors of any papers which have been omitted.
1 Noda, M., Takahashi, H., Tanabe, T., Toyosato, M., Kikyotani, S., Furutani, Y., Hirose, T., Takashima, H., Inayama, S., Miyata, T. and Numa, S. (1983) *Nature* 302, 528–532
2 Schneider, C., Kurkinen, M. and Greaves, M. (1983) *EMBO J.* 2, 2259–2263
3 Russel, D. W., Yamamoto, T., Schneider, W. J., Slaughter, C. J., Brown, M. S. and Goldstein, J. C. (1983) *Proc. Natl Acad. Sci. USA* 80, 7501–7505
4 Cartaud, J., Popot, J. L. and Changeux, J. P. (1980) *FEBS Lett.* 121, 327–332
5 Bon, F., Lebrun, E., Gomel, J., van Rappenbusch, R., Cartaud, J., Popot, J. L. and Changeux, J. P. (1984) *J. Mol. Biol.* 176, 425–430
6 Houslay, M. D. (1984) *Trends Biochem. Sci.* 9, 39–40
7 Strosberg, A. D., Couraud, P. O. and Schreiber, A. B. (1981) *Immunol. Today* 10, 75–79
8 Hollenberg, M. (1981) *Trends Pharmacol. Sci.* 2, 320–322
9 Cerione, R. A., Strulovici, B., Benovic, J. L., Lefkowitz, R. J. and Caron, M. G. (1983) *Nature* 306, 562–566

10   Manni, A. (1983) *New Engl. J. Med.* 309, 1383–1385
11   Tzartos, S. J. (1984) *Trends Biochem. Sci.* 9, 63–67
12   Leiber, D., Harbon, S., Guillet, J. G., Andre, C. and Strosberg, A. D. (1984) *Proc. Natl Acad. Sci. USA* 81, 4331–4334
13   Strosberg, A. D. (1983) *Springer Seminars in Immunopathology* 6, 67–78
14   Dwyer, D., Bradley, R. J., Urquhart, C. K. and Kearny, J. F. (1983) *Nature* 301, 611–614
15   Kuhn, L. C. and Kraehenbuhl, J. P. (1982) *Trends Biochem. Sci.* 7, 299–302
16   Dawnward, J., Yarden, Y., Mayos, E., Scrace, G., Tohy, N., Stockwell, P., Ullrich, A., Schlessinger, J. and Waterfield, M. D. (1984) *Nature* 304, 521–527
17   Williams, A. F. (1984) *Nature* 308, 108–109 (and three research articles in the same issue)

A. D. Strosberg was at the Laboratory of Molecular Immunology, Institut Jacques Monod, CNRS – University Paris VII, 2, Place Jussieu, 75251 Paris Cedex 05, France; he is now at the Department of Biotechnology, Institute Pasteur, 28 rue du Docteur Roux, 75724 Paris Cedex 15, France.

Addendum – *A. D. Strosberg*

It is a true reflection on the present state of art of molecular biology that in the 18 months that went by since the publication of the anniversary issue of *TIBS*, we have learnt more about receptor structure than in the preceding ten years. An update of our review might therefore easily double or triple its size. However, principles underlying receptor structure and function were apparently stated correctly and the dramatic increase in information on structure has not drastically changed our understanding of function. We will briefly summarize here some of the most exciting new findings with their implications on new directions of research.

The receptors of EGF, Insulin and Insulin-like growth factor I share ligand-inducible protein kinase activity, which is likely to constitute the mechanism by which these receptors mediate signal transduction across the plasma membranes of target cells. The complete amino acid sequences of these receptors have now been deduced from the sequence of the complementary DNA[16,18]. The striking similarities in the organization of these membrane proteins have been summarized (Fig. 3).

The human low-density lipoprotein (LDL) receptor also displays an organization in extracellular, transmembrane and cytoplasmic domains[20]: next to the N-terminal cystein-rich LDL binding domain is a domain highly homologous to the EGF precursor, again suggestive of common evolutionary pathways between a number of growth factors and membrane receptors.

The structure of the glucocorticosteroid receptor has also been elucidated[21] and should soon allow the study of the interaction of the DNA binding domain of this regulatory protein with its target gene. As with several other receptors mentioned in this review, the glucocorticoid receptor has a domain structure related to that of the V-*erb*-A oncogene product of avian erythroblastosis virus (AEV), suggesting that oncogenicity by AEV may result in part from the inappropriate activity of a truncated steroid receptor or a related regulatory protein encoded by V-*erb*-A (Ref. 22). It is likely that other steroid receptor structures will soon complete the picture of these eukaryotic transcriptional regulatory proteins.

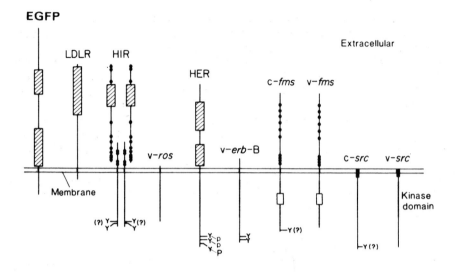

Fig. 3. Schematic comparison of structural features of cell-surface receptors and tyrosine-kinase family oncogene products. Regions of high cysteine concentration are shown as hatched boxes and single cysteine residues as filled circles. The open box in v-fms and c-fms represents a 70-amino acid substitution in the tyrosine-kinase domain. The position of carboxy-terminal tyrosine residues is shown. EGFP, epidermal growth factor precursor; LDLR, low-density lipoprotein receptor; HIR, human insulin receptor; HER, human epidermal growth factor receptor. Transforming genes of oncogenes: ros, UR2 avian sarcoma virus; fms, feline sarcoma virus; v-erb-B, avian erythroblastosis virus; src, Rous sarcoma virus. Reproduced, with permission, from Ref. 19.

Excellent progress has also been made on receptors for neurotransmitters; the structure of mammalian nicotinic acetylcholine receptors has been described, suggesting that organ-specific differences might exist. Current studies of the brain glycin and GABA (gamma amino butyric acid) receptors at the protein and DNA level should again yield striking information[23,24].

The amino acid sequence of human interleukin-2 receptor has been predicted from the cDNA cloned and sequenced by two different groups[25,26]. This receptor is much smaller ($\approx$ 55 kDa) than those described for other growth factors or hormones. Another striking difference is the separation into two domains by a putative transmembrane region.

Finally, the T lymphocyte receptors for antigen have been characterized extensively[27]. Quite a variety of findings were discussed: the existence of the α-, β- and unexpected non-glycosylated γ-chain, and the occurrence and variation during the immune response of $\alpha\beta$ and possibly $\gamma\beta$-receptors. As with anti-bodies, the diversity of the T-cell receptors appears to be generated through rearrangement of variable regions (20 V_β, many more V_α have been identified so far), diversity segments (two D_β, no D_α) and joining regions (12 J_β, many J_α). Somatic mutations and flexible joining add to the T-cell receptor diversity and may compensate the limited variability of the V_α, V_β and V_γ genes. The direct molecular interaction of T-cell receptors with antigen or/and with histocom-patibility genes has still not been demonstrated conclusively.

To conclude this addendum, one should mention the progress on the studies of the effector mechanisms. GTP binding proteins have been purified from several sources and the cDNA corresponding to α-subunit of one of these, transducin, has been sequenced completely[28]. Composed of three chains α, β and γ, transducin certainly is homologous to other GTP binding proteins. Adenylate cyclase has been finally purified[29] and is being analysed at the molecular level currently. The various components of the phosphoinositol metabolic chain have been identified. C-Kinase has been sequenced and its structure should soon become available.

This breathtaking update reflects the pace of progress now set by the molecular biologists: sometimes only a few months separate the moment at which protein sequence data is obtained suitable for the synthesis of an oligonucleotide probe from the complete elucidation of the corresponding cDNA. The functional studies remain the most complex part, but will be greatly facilitated by *in vitro* mutagenesis, as the elegant studies on the acetylcholine receptor by Numa's group have already shown.

References

18 Ullrich, A., Bell, J. R., Chen, E. Y., Herrera, R., Petruzelli, L. M., Dull, T. J., Gray, A., Coussens, L., Liao, Y. C., Tsubokawa, M., Mason, A., Seeburg, P. H., Grunfeld, C., Rosen, O. M. and Ramachandran, J. (1985) *Nature* 313, 756–761

19 Coussens, L., Van Beveren, C., Smith, D., Chen, E., Michell, R. L., Isacke, C. M., Verma, I. M. and Ullrich, A. (1986) *Nature* 320, 277–280

20 Goldstein, J-L., Brown, M. S., Anderson, R. G. W., Russell, D. W. and Schneider, W. J. (1985) *Annu. Rev. Cell. Bio.* 1, 1–39

21 Hollenberg, S. M., Weinberger, C., Ong, E. S., Cerelli, G., Oro, A., Thompson, E. B., Rosenfeld, M. G. and Evans, R. M. (1985) *Nature* 318, 635–641

22 Weinberger, C., Hollenberg, S. M., Rosenfeld, M. G. and Evans, R. M. (1985) *Nature* 318, 670–672

23 Graham, D., Pfeiffer, F., Simler, R. and Betz, H. (1985) *Biochemistry* 24, 990–994.

24 Sigel, E. and Barnard, E. A. (1984) *J. Biol. Chem.* 259, 7219–7223

25 Leonard, W. J., Depper, J. M. Crabtree, G. R., Rudikoff, S., Pumphrey, J., Robb, R. J., Kronke, M., Svetlik, P. B., Peffer, N. J., Waldmann, T. A. and Greene, W. C. (1984) *Nature* 311, 626–631

26 Nikaido, T., Shimizu, A., Ishida, N., Sabe, H., Teshigawara, K., Maeda, M., Uchiyama, T., Yodoi, J. and Honjo, T. (1984) *Nature* 311, 631–635

27 Davies, M. (1985) *Annu. Rev. Immunol.* 3, 537–560

28 Lochrie, M. A., Hurley, J. B. and Simon, M. I. (1985) *Science* 228, 96–99

29 Pfeuffer, E., Dreher, R. M., Metzger, H. and Pfeuffer, T. (1985) *Proc. Natl Acad. Sci. USA* 82, 3086–3090

Insulin: in search of a mechanism

Miles D. Houslay and Clare M. Heyworth

It is somewhat ironic that although insulin is a household name, notably because of diabetes, the molecular mechanism of action of this hormone has proved elusive[1]. This is despite a wealth of observations of its gross physiological effects and detailed knowledge of its ability to regulate both cellular metabolism and development. Generally, insulin promotes anabolic functions as well as slowing down degradative pathways. It is, then, the very wealth and breadth of effects exerted by insulin that demands explanation.

Although a myriad of suggestions for a second messenger of insulin's action have been put forward over the years, none have proved able to explain all of the various effects that insulin exerts on target cells[1]. Indeed, until recently the inability to express any effects of insulin in a broken membrane system has thwarted attempts to identify the molecular events occurring at the plasma membrane as a result of insulin's occupancy of its receptor. However, over the past few years our knowledge of both the structure of the insulin receptor[2,3] and closely associated molecular events has increased dramatically.

Insulin receptors are mobile

What happens when insulin binds to its receptor at the cell surface? One event that immediately ensues is that the receptors cluster and are subsequently internalized into vesicles by an energy driven process. At this point at least two choices appear to present themselves: either the vesiculated receptors can be destroyed by association with lysosomes or they can be recycled back to the plasma membrane[4]. Certainly prolonged challenge with insulin leads to a net loss of receptors from the plasma membrane (down regulation). This dynamic movement of receptors triggered by hormone may provide an important route of signalling to the cell interior and of stimulating specific events. Support for such a contention has come from using anti-insulin receptor antibodies (see Ref. 5). Bivalent antibodies, and not their univalent fragments, mimic a variety of insulin's actions in adipocytes. It may be then that receptor clustering or internalization initiates a signal or that the bivalent antibodies *per se* provoke a conformational change in the receptor, complementary to that elicited by insulin.

The insulin receptor is a protein kinase.

Receptors for epidermal growth factor (EGF) express an unusual kinase activity, acting upon target proteins which include the receptor itself (see Ref. 5). The EGF kinase, however, specifically transfers phosphate groups onto tyrosine residues of its target proteins rather than onto serine or threonine residues as do other protein kinases. Attention was drawn[5] to the fact that there were many similarities between the dynamic properties of insulin receptors and EGF receptors. Subsequently it was demonstrated[6] that the insulin receptor could be phosphorylated on its β-subunit after exposure to either insulin or anti-insulin receptor antibodies. Importantly, phosphorylation of the receptor was observed using a detergent-solubilized receptor preparation. Under such conditions phosphotyrosine was produced exclusively and receptor phosphorylation was clearly shown not to involve the more common cyclic AMP-dependent kinases[7]. However, in the intact cell phosphorylation of serine residues[6], rather than tyrosine in the β-subunit predominated.

Recent evidence[8] has demonstrated that it is the transmembrane β-subunit of the insulin receptor itself which actually expresses this kinase activity, making it analogous to the EGF receptor-kinase system. Both of these receptor kinases, thus, undergo autophosphorylation, as well as being able to act on other substrates. However, the EGF kinase does not phosphorylate the insulin receptor and vice-versa, implying that they have rather distinct substrate specificities[9]. It is tempting to speculate that the physiological relevance of this kinase activity might be associated with the long-term growth-promoting properties of insulin rather than the immediate, short-term metabolic effects which can occur within seconds. The reasons for suggesting this are twofold. Firstly, by analogy with the EGF-kinase and the transforming proteins of RNA tumour viruses (see Ref. 5). These all express a unique tyrosine kinase activity and all express growth promoting or transforming properties. Secondly, the concentration of insulin which elicits half-maximal incorporation of phosphate into the β-receptor is of the order of 2–8 nM. This is considerably higher than values for insulin's action on metabolic processes and circulating insulin concentrations. It may even be that phosphorylation acts as a signal to promote the endocytosis of the receptor (see Ref. 5).

Is there an insulin mediator?

It has been suggested[2,10] that insulin can produce a second messenger by direct addition of insulin to isolated plasma membranes. This has been claimed to be a peptide or 'peptide-like' material released from plasma membranes upon exposure to insulin. Such material appears to exert insulin-like effects on a variety of enzymes which influence, or are influenced by, phosphorylation–dephosphorylation reactions.

In particular, it appears to elicit the activation of mitochondrial pyruvate dehydrogenase (PDH) through what is believed to be the stimulation of a specific phosphatase acting on the α-subunit of this enzyme. The suggestion has been made[2] that this 'mediator' is released from the insulin receptor itself by the activation of an arginine-specific protease. Although if this was to occur then one might expect receptors to become rapidly inactivated, which does not appear to happen. Such a model has obvious attractions in that if it regulates the activity of phosphatases and kinases it could affect a variety of processes by altering the phosphorylation state of target proteins. One of the most disturbing facets of this work is, however, the high-speed supernatants from plasma membranes have been shown to produce substances which exert both inhibitory and activating effects on pyruvate dehydrogenase, independent of whether insulin is present or not. Nevertheless, insulin does appear to cause a small increase in the release of a particular molecular weight fraction, exerting a small stimulatory effect on PDH activity, measured under conditions far removed from those experienced physiologically. The mediator is unlikely to be a simple peptide as it has eluded even simple characterization for a number of years. The latest views about it suggest that it may have lipid and carbohydrate components; even that a family of mediators are produced[10]. Clearly this is a provocative hypothesis which has aroused considerable interest. However, there are serious anomalies, not the least of which is the contention that the liberation of such a mediator would not give rise to a sufficient amplification of the hormonal response within the cell (see Ref. 1).

Is a specific guanine nucleotide regulatory protein involved?

Insulin, in a broken membrane preparation, has been shown to activate a high affinity cyclic AMP phosphodiesterase associated with liver plasma membranes. This was achieved through the cyclic AMP-dependent phosphorylation of the enzyme[11]. Activation of this enzyme occurs at physiological concentrations (10^{-10} M) of insulin and cyclic AMP (10^{-6} M), and has also been demonstrated in intact hepatocytes[12]. If, however, the cells were pre-treated with glucagon prior to exposure to insulin, then insulin's activation of this phosphodiesterase appeared to be completely abolished[12]. This intriguing phenomenon displayed the same time dependence, and the same unusual concentration dependence upon glucagon, as did the glucagon desensitization of adenylate cyclase (see Ref. 12). Now, glucagon normally activates adenylate cyclase in liver plasma membranes by interaction with its receptor, which subsequently exerts its effects on catalytic unit of adenylate cyclase via a specific, stimulatory (N_s) guanine nucleotide regulatory protein (see Ref. 13). During desensitization some modification, which leads to a loss in function, of this regulatory protein appears to be elicited by a small fraction of high affinity glucagon receptors[14]. We therefore proposed[12] that a specific species of guanine nucleotide regulatory protein might mediate the effect of insulin on the plasma membrane kinase and phosphodiesterase. This would obviously have to be very different from the species through which glucagon activates adenylate cyclase, as glucagon does not activate the phosphodiesterase. Nevertheless, the activation of such a regulatory protein was presumed to be terminated by the process by which glucagon desensitized the stimulatory regulatory protein in intact cells. Observations supporting the involvement of such a regulatory protein came from using cholera toxin, which causes the ADP-ribosylation of certain guanine nucleotide regulatory proteins including N_s. In hepatocytes it actually activated the plasma membrane phosphodiesterase, after which insulin failed to elicit further activation, which would be expected if they shared a common pathway. Furthermore, guanine nucleotides also activated the phosphodiesterase in a broken membrane system through an ATP-requiring process[15].

The sensitivity of this regulatory protein to either GTP or its non-hydrolysable analogues was, however, entirely different from that of the regulatory protein exerting simulatory effects on adenylate cyclase. Indeed, at high physiological GTP concentrations, insulin can actually inhibit adenylate cyclase[16]. This effect is blocked by either glucagon-desensitization or cholera toxin treatment of hepatocytes in an analogous fashion to the effects on cyclic AMP phosphodiesterase[12]. The guanine nucleotide dependence of these effects closely resembles that of a genetically distinct guanine nucleotide regulatory protein (N_i) which mediates the action of hormones exerting inhibitory effects on adenylate cyclase (see Ref. 13). N_i is, however, unlikely to be identical with the putative regulatory protein involved in insulin action as cholera toxin appears to 'turn-on' this protein, whilst having no effect on N_i. Furthermore, pertussis toxin which blocks the action of N_i (see Ref. 13) does not block insulin's activation of the phosphodiesterase.

A 'multi-pathway' mechanism for insulin's action

Insulin elicits both the phosphorylation and dephosphorylation of many proteins in target tissues (see Refs 1 and 5). It has been proposed[1,5] that by determining the activity of plasma membrane-bound cyclic AMP-dependent and independent kinases, insulin could exert a controlling influence on a wide variety of cellular processes. Indeed this would show special flexibility if it also led to an

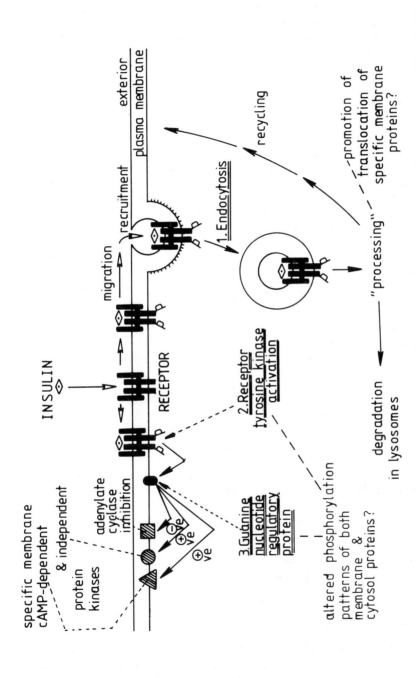

Fig. 1. A 'multi-pathway' mechanism for insulin's action. Insulin receptors are shown schematically as consisting of 2α plus 2β subunits[2], where phosphorylation (P) occurs on the transmembrane β-subunit. However, there is evidence[3] that a further subunit (δ) forms part of the receptor.

effect on protein phosphatase activity[17]. Certainly such a system could provide both the sensitivity, rapidity and necessary amplification[1] to mediate many of the metabolic effects of insulin. Current evidence thus suggests that such a system might involve the insulin receptor-kinase and specific plasma membrane-bound cyclic AMP-dependent[11,12] and independent[18] protein kinases regulated by insulin through a specific guanine nucleotide regulatory protein. Although, clearly, the putative insulin-controlled guanine-nucleotide regulatory protein could exert other effects[16]. It is possible that the interaction between such species may explain why insulin elicits the incorporation of phosphate residues into predominantly serine residues when in the intact cell[6], rather than into tyrosine residues when a solubilized receptor preparation is used[7].

Mediation through a guanine-nucleotide regulatory protein is, however, unlikely to provide the whole answer to insulin's action. This can readily be gauged from observations on the activity of an intracellular 'dense vesicle' phosphodiesterase whose stimulation, in hepatocytes, by insulin was not blocked by prior exposure of the cells to glucagon[12]. Part of the explanation to this is undoubtedly the fact that glucagon itself activated the 'dense vesicle' enzyme. Nevertheless, exposure to glucagon and then insulin actually led to a synergistic activation of the enzyme. However, conditions which stopped the intracellular processing of insulin also blocked insulin's activation of the 'dense vesicle' enzyme, whilst leaving unaffected the activation of the plasma membrane enzyme[19]. This again suggests that internalization of the insulin–receptor complex may well trigger specific intracellular events.

A synthesis of this information suggests that there are at least three distinct, but undoubtedly very closely related, routes through which the insulin receptor can elicit effects on target cells. These are (1) the endocytosis of the insulin receptor, (2) the activation of the insulin receptor tyrosine-specific protein kinase and (3) the activation of a specific guanine nucleotide regulatory protein and associated protein kinase(s). This is summarized in Fig. 1, suggesting that an insulin receptor might trigger a variety of processes through either individual or coordinated routes. Such a proposal offers a means whereby insulin might exert effects on a wide variety of processes within the cell.

The activation of glucose transport, in adipocytes, by insulin may well offer an example of a process utilizing more than one of these routes. It has been demonstrated[20] that this occurs through a multistep mechanism; namely that insulin–receptor endocytosis triggers the transfer of inactive glucose carriers from an internal vesicle pool to the plasma membrane where they are subsequently activated by an, as yet, undefined insulin-dependent mechanism. It may well prove that the putative guanine-nucleotide regulatory protein associated with the insulin receptor and/or an insulin-controlled membrane protein kinase will provide the missing link for eliciting the activation of the carriers when they are inserted in the plasma membrane. Indeed, there is good evidence to suggest that GTP plays a key role in the regulation of insulin-stimulated glucose transport in the giant muscle fibres of the barnacle[21]. Certainly, this would seem to be an exciting period in research into the molecular mechanism of insulin's action.

Acknowledgements

Work in the authors' laboratory was supported by grants from the MRC, SERC, British Diabetic Association and California Metabolic Research Foundation. We wish to thank A. A. Eddy and R. M. Houslay for helpful comments on the manuscript.

References
1   Denton, R. M., Brownsey, R. W. and Belsham, G. J. (1981) *Diabetologia* 21, 347–362
2   Czech, M. P. (1981) *Am. J. Med.* 70, 142–150
3   Baron, M. D. and Sönksen, P. H. (1983) *Biochem. J.* 212. 79–84
4   Fehlmann, M., Carpentier, J-L., Van Obberghen, E., Freychet, P., Thamm, P., Saunders, D., Brandenburg, D. and Orci, L. (1982) *Proc. Natl Acad. Sci. USA* 79, 5921–5925
5   Houslay, M. D. (1981) *Bioscience Rep.* 1, 19–34
6   Kasuga, M., Zick. Y., Blith, D. L., Karlsson, F. A., Häring, H.-U. and Khan, C. R. (1982) *J. Biol. Chem.* 257, 9891–9894
7   Häring, H.-U., Kasuga, M. and Kah, C. R. (1982) *Biochem. Biophys. Res. Commun.* 108, 1538–1545
8   Roth, R. A. and Cassell, D. J. (1983) *Science* 219, 299–301
9   Avruch, J., Nemenoff, R. A., Blackshear, P. J., Pierce, M. W. and Osathanodth, R. (1982) *J. Biol. Chem.* 257, 15162–15166
10 Larner, J. (1982) *J. Cyclic Nucl. Res.* 8. 289–296
11 Houslay, M. D., Wallace, A. V., Wilson, S. R., Marchmont, R. J. and Heyworth, C. M. (1983) in *Hormones and Cell Regulation* (Dumont, J. E., Junez, J. and Denton, R. M., eds), vol. 7, pp. 105–120, Elsevier Biomedical Press
12 Heyworth, C. M., Wallace, A. V. and Houslay, M. D. (1983) *Biochem. J.* 214, 99–110
13 Houslay, M. D. (1983) *Nature (London)* 303, 133
14 Heyworth, C. M. and Houslay, M. D. (1983) *Biochem. J.* 214, 93–98
15 Heyworth, C. M., Rawal, S. and Houslay, M. D. (1983) *FEBS Lett.* 154, 87–91
16 Heyworth, C. M. and Houslay, M. D. (1983) *Biochem. J.* 214, 547–552
17 Cohen, P. (1982) *Nature (London)* 296, 613–620
18 Walaas, O., Horn, R. S., Lystad, E. and Adler, A. (1981) *FEBS Lett.* 128, 133–136
19 Wilson, S. R., Wallace, A. V. and Houslay, M. D. (1983) *Biochem. J.* 216, 245–248
20 Cushman, S. W., Wardzala, L. J., Simpson, I. A., Karneili, E., Hissin, P. J., Wheeler, T. J., Hinkle, P. C. and Salans, L. B. (1983) in *Hormones & Cell Regulation* (Dumont, J. E., Nunez, J. and Denton, R. M., eds), vol. 7. pp.73–84, Elsevier Biomedical Press
21 Baker, P. F. and Carruthers, A. (1983) *J. Physiol.* 336, 397–431

Miles Houslay is at the Molecular Pharmacology Group, Department of Biochemistry, University of Glasgow, Glasgow G12 8QQ, UK. Clare Heyworth is at the Paterson Laboratories, Christie Hospital, Manchester, UK.

Addendum – *M. D. Houslay*

Since writing the original article a number of important advances have been made in our understanding of the molecular mechanism of action of insulin. As expected it was only a matter of time before the gene for the receptor was cloned and sequenced. Thus two groups[22,23] have cloned the gene for the human placental insulin receptor. These have obtained similar, if not identical, results with the predicted structure of the insulin receptor proposed to contain some 1370 (Ref. 22) or 1382 (Ref. 23) amino acids. There is a single insulin receptor gene which codes for a pro-receptor having a signal sequence of some 27 residues followed by the information coding for the α- and the β-subunits. This data would agree with the biochemical studies performed on its biosynthesis (see Ref. 24). The α-sub-unit lacks any hydrophobic stretches long enough to provide a transmembrane domain and contains 15 out of the possible 21 sites for N-glycosylation on the receptor. The β-subunit has a well-defined transmembrane stretch of 23 amino acids, analogous to that seen with the EGF and LDL receptors. As expected there is considerable homology between the cytoplasmic domain of the insulin and EGF receptors as well as the v-*fms* oncogene. What we still need, however, is a mechanism. Searches for substrates of tyrosine kinase action have not proved overly successful so far[24] and it may be that it is the autophosphorylation of the receptor itself that provides a 'switch' to turn on another receptor-associated activity. Indeed, receptor autophosphorylation actually enhances the insulin receptor-associated tyrosyl kinase activity towards exogenous artificial sub-strates[25], an effect which can be mimicked when the insulin receptor is phos-phorylated by the src kinase[26]. Although serine phosphorylation has been difficult to demonstrate in intact cells[24] it would appear from studies on hepatoma cells that an extremely rapid phosphorylation of tyrosine residues on the receptor is followed by the phosphorylation of serine sites[27]. Since phorbol esters also elicit the serine phosphorylation of insulin receptors, whilst reducing their function-ing[28], it may be that serine phosphorylation actually decreases the functioning of the receptor itself. It will thus be of interest to identify the molecular basis for the reduced tyrosyl kinase activity seen in liver membranes from streptozotocin-diabetic rats[29].

Further evidence has come forth which suggests that the insulin receptor interacts in some way with the guanine-nucleotide regulatory protein system[13] in plasma membranes. This shows that certain of insulin's effects can be blocked by pertussis[30,31] as well as cholera[13] toxin and that only certain of insulin's actions are mediated through the G protein known as N_{ins}. This latter species appears to possess a 25 kDa subunit[31] which is a substrate for ribosylation for cholera toxin and can be affected by phorbol ester action and the induction of insulin resis-tance.

Thus a clear mechanism for insulin's action has yet to come to light, but at last we now seem to be making headway at a good pace.

References

22 Ullrich, A., Bell, J. R., Chen, E. Y., Herrera, R., Petruzelli, L. M., Dull, T. J., Gray, A., Coussens, L., Liao, Y. C., Tsubokawa, M., Mason, A., Seeburg, P. H., Grunfeld, C., Rosen, O. M. and Ramachandran, J. (1985) *Nature* 313, 756–761

23 Ebina, Y., Ellis, L., Jarnagin, K., Ou, J. H., Masiarz, F., Kan, Y. W., Goldfine, I. D., Roth, R. A. and Rutter, W. J. (1985) *Cell* 40, 747–758

24 Houslay, M. D. (1985) in *Molecular Mechanisms of Transmembrane Signalling*, vol. 4 of Molecular Aspects of Cellular Regulation (Cohen, P. and Houslay, M. D., eds), pp. 279–333, Elsevier Biomedical Press

25 Yu, K. T. and Czech, M. P. (1985) *J. Biol. Chem.* 259, 5277–5286

26 Yu, K. T., Werth, D. K., Pastan, I. H. and Czech, M. P. (1985) *J. Biol. Chem.* 260, 5838–5846

27 Pang, D. T., Sharma, B. R., Schafer, J. A., White, M. F. and Kahn, C. R. (1985) *J. Biol. Chem.* 260, 7131–7136

28 Takamaya, S., White, M. F., Lauris, V. and Kahn, C. R. (1984) *Proc. Natl Acad. Sci. USA* 81, 7797–7801

29 Kadowaki, T., Kasuga, M., Akanuma, Y., Ezaki, O. and Takaku, F. (1985) *J. Biol. Chem.* 259, 14208–14216

30 Heyworth, C. M., Grey, A. M., Wilson, S. R., Hanski, E. and Houslay, M. D.
    Biochem. J. (in press)
31 Heyworth, C. M., Whetton, A. D., Wong, S., Martin, B. R. and Houslay, M. D.
    (1985) *Biochem. J.* 228, 593–603

Glycosphingolipids as differentiation-dependent, tumor-associated markers and as regulators of cell proliferation

Sen-itiroh Hakomori

Glycosphingolipids alter their synthesis and membrane organization in association with cellular differentiation and oncogenic transformation. Many, if not all, tumor cells express aberrant glycosphingolipid markers which are defined by their monoclonal antibodies. Examples of human cancer markers are presented, which show typical oncofetal expression. In addition, a possible role of gangliosides in regulation of growth factor receptor function is discussed.

Since the first clear demonstration of glycolipid changes associated with oncogenic transformation in 1968[1], a great deal of effort has been made towards understanding the enzymatic basis of the phenomenon and its immunological and biological significance. There are three categories of change: incomplete synthesis, neosynthesis and organizational rearrangement of membrane glycolipids. These have been revealed, step-by-step, in a large variety of transformed cells induced by oncogenic DNA viruses, RNA viruses and chemical carcinogens, and in cells taken from spontaneous tumors, including a large variety of human cancers (see Refs 2–5 for reviews). Both a precursor which accumulates because of incomplete synthesis and a neoglycolipid resulting from neosynthesis can be recognized as 'tumor-associated' glycolipid antigens, not detectable on progenitor cell surfaces. Lacto*neo*tetraosylceramide in hamster NIL tumors[6,7] and gangliotriaosylceramide (Gg3; asialo GM2) in mice sarcoma[8] and lymphoma[9] are typical examples of experimental tumors. Since the monoclonal antibody approach was introduced by Köhler and Milstein, many tumor-associated antigens defined by this approach have been identified as the carbohydrate structures of glycosphingolipids and glycoproteins.* Thus, it has become increasingly clear that glycolipid changes contribute, at least in part, to the formation of tumor-associated antigens; this may represent retrograde expression of glycolipids present during fetal organogenesis. This review discusses briefly the biochemical mechanism and ontogenic properties of tumor-associated glycolipid antigens, and a possible role of glycolipids in cell growth regulation.

Structure and expression of tumor-associated glycolipid antigens

Gangliotriaosylceramide in L5178 lymphoma grown in DBA/2 mice or in KiMSV tumors grown in Balb/c mice behaves like a tumor-associated antigen

---

*The structures of glycolipids referred to in the text are as follows: Lacto*neo*tetraosylceramide, Galβ1→4GlcNAcβ1→3Galβ1→4Glcβ1→1Cer; gangliotriaosylceramide, GalNacβ1→4Galβ1→4Glcβ1→1Cer; globotriaosylceramide, Galα1→4Galβ1→4Glcβ1→1Cer. Other structures, see Ref. 5.

since: (1) the glycolipid is accumulated at the cell surface and can be surface-labeled, and (2) immunotherapy by the monoclonal IgG3 antibody directed to this glycolipid has been successful[9]. This model has been used extensively to study the mechanism of the expression of glycolipid antigens[10]. Rat sarcoma KMT-17 has a glycolipid antigen identified as globotriaosylceramide (Gb$_3$), and its hybridoma antibody was produced when syngeneic rat (WKA) was immunized with this tumor cell[11].

Glycolipid tumor antigens defined by monoclonal antibodies have been well established in a wide variety of human cancers. The GD$_3$ ganglioside in human melanoma[12,13], globotriaosylceramide in Burkitt lymphoma[14], and sialosyl Le^a[15,16], di- or trimeric Le^x[17,18], and sialosyl Le^x structure[19,20] in human gastrointestinal, pancreatic, lung, liver, and breast cancers are typical examples (see Table 1). Furthermore, the presence of blood-group antigens with incompatible specificity to the host has become increasingly clear over the last few years (see Refs 4 and 5 for review). Of particular interest is the presence of Forssman antigen in tumors arising from Forssman-negative tissue, A-like glycolipid antigen in tumors of blood group O individuals, and P-like and P$_1$-like antigens in the tumor of an individual with a rare blood group *pp* genotype as originally described by Levine[21,22].

Expression of glycolipid antigens during organogenesis, but not in the early embryo

Tumor-associated glycolipid changes, as described above and listed in Table 1, are generally assumed to originate in the fetus, although no clear evidence has been previously described. No glycolipid antigen is known which is expressed in both mouse tumors and early mouse embryo. Gangliotriaosylceramide, often expressed in mouse tumors, has not been found in the early mouse embryo or in mouse teratocarcinoma; and the Le^x determinant (SSEA-1), which is highly expressed in preimplantation mouse embryo[23], has not been found in many

Table 1. Typical glycolipid tumor-associated markers defined by monoclonal antibodies in human cancers

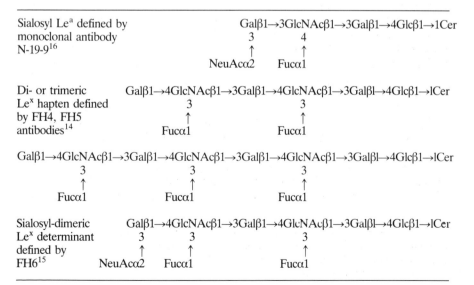

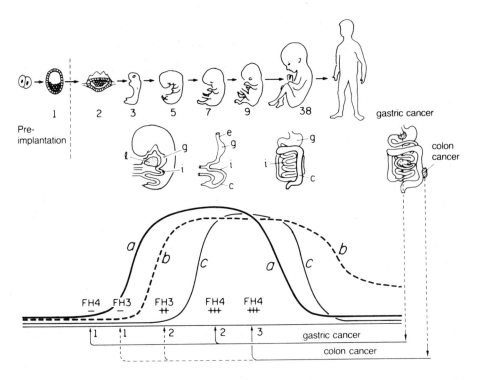

Fig. 1. Stage-dependent expression of the Le^x antigen (defined by FH3) and di- or trimeric Le^x antigen (defined by FH4; see Table 1) in gastrointestinal epithelia during human development, and retrogenetic expression of the antigens in gastrointestinal tumors. The Le^x and di- or trimeric Le^x antigens may not be expressed in preimplantation human embryo, as suggested by the absence of the Le^x antigen in undifferentiated human teratocarcinoma and the induction of antigen synthesis on differentiation. The antigens, however, are expressed in various tissues of postimplantation human embryos and fetuses. Curves a and c illustrate the change in FH4 antigen expression in gastric and colonic epithelia, respectively. Curve b represents the change in FH3 antigen expression in colonic epithelia. FH4 expression in colonic epithelia peaks between 7 and 9 weeks, then regresses almost completely, while the FH3 antigen does not regress and remains in the crypt cells. The FH4 antigen is strongly expressed in differentiated gastric cancer, suggesting that antigen retrogenesis occurs to the point when FH4 expression is at its maximum (arrow 2). However, FH4 antigen expression is negative in undifferentiated gastric cancer and may correspond to a very early stage of embryogenesis at which FH4 is not expressed (arrow 1). Both FH3 and FH4 antigen expression in colonic cancer could be strong if retrogenesis of the antigen expression occurs to the point at which the FH3 antigen is active. The numbers at each stage of development represent the number of weeks from fertilization. The scale showing the degree of antigen expression (ordinate) is arbitrary. g, gastric epithelia; l, liver; i, intestine; c, colon. Reproduced by permission from Ref. 25.

mouse tumors (Tsuchiya, S. and Hakomori, S., unpublished results), with the exception of B16 melanoma[24]. The gastrointestinal tumor antigen sialosyl Le^a has been found in human meconium, which represents fetal colonic epithelial cells, although the antigen is highly limited in adult gastrointestinal mucosa[15,16]. The localization and alteration of the Le^x determinant defined by the antibody FH3, and of di- or trimeric Le^x (see Table 1) defined by the antibody FH4 during human development and in human cancers, have been studied with the following results: (1) The Le^x determinant defined by FH3 showed a wider distribution than the multimeric Le^x defined by FH4. Both antigens were absent or present in relatively low concentration during early embryonic development (up to 35 days). They showed maximum expression at a specific stage of organogenesis in gastrointestinal, pulmobronchial, and urogenital epithelia, and regressed upon further differentiation and development (see Fig. 1). (2) The Le^x determinant was expressed about two weeks earlier than the di- or trimeric Le^x determinant defined by FH4, and the latter forms regressed more rapidly and more completely than the Le^x determinant on further development of epithelial tissue. Expression of the di- or trimeric Le^x antigen defined by FH4 was limited to specific types of cells in newborn and adult epithelial tissue, such as parietal cells of gastric epithelia and Paneth's cells of intestinal epithelia, and the antigen was absent from colonic epithelia, including the crypt cells. The antigen was strongly expressed in most tubular and papillary adenocarcinoma of stomach, adeno-carcinoma of colon, ductal carcinoma of breast, and their metastatic lesions. The antigen can be regarded as exhibiting retrograde expression to a certain stage of fetal organogenesis when there is maximum expression of the antigen, but retrograde expression does not extend to the earlier embryo[25] (see Fig. 1).

Factors affecting glycolipid expression at the cell surface
Many tumor-associated glycolipids, including those in Table 1, are character-ized as having unusual ceramide composition, i.e. phytosphingosine, long-chain fatty acids, and α-hydroxy fatty acids. Unusual ceramide composition may affect the degree of glycolipid exposure at the cell surface[10]. Steric hindrance due to neighboring proteins and longer-chain glycolipids, or sialosyl residues in adjacent molecules may alter the organization of glycolipids in membranes, affecting the degree of exposure[10,26]. Thus, the expression of glycolipid antigens is controlled not only by the level of glycosyltransferases, but also by critical factors affecting the state of glycolipid organization. Some glycolipid antigens, such as GD$_3$ in human melanoma and Gb$_3$ in Burkitt lymphoma, may be organized in such a way as to be highly exposed at the cell surface. A peculiar organization could be caused by aberrant ceramide composition (neoceramide) and other factors described above and illustrated in Fig. 2.

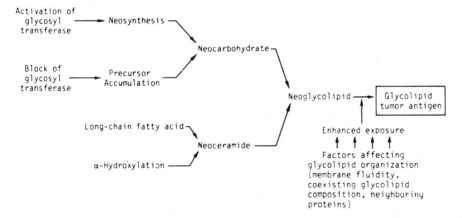

Fig. 2. A possible mechanism for the appearance of tumor-associated glycolipid antigens. Various factors affecting the change of glycolipid organization in membranes enhances exposure of the glycolipid.

Modulation of growth factor receptor by gangliosides and the loss of growth control in tumor cells through ganglioside changes

A possible role of gangliosides in cell growth regulation has been suggested by the following: (1) The synthesis of a specific type of glycolipid was greatly enhanced in association with 'contact inhibition' of cell growth. GM_3 synthesis was enhanced when cell growth was arrested and contact inhibition was induced in transformed cells by retinoids and butyrate. (2) Exogenous addition of glycolipid(s) incorporated into plasma membranes inhibited cell growth and induced contact inhibition. (3) Anti-GM_3 antibodies and Fab fragments inhibited cell growth, but anti-globoside did not inhibit growth (see Ref. 27 for review). The recent availability of purified growth factors and serum-free culture

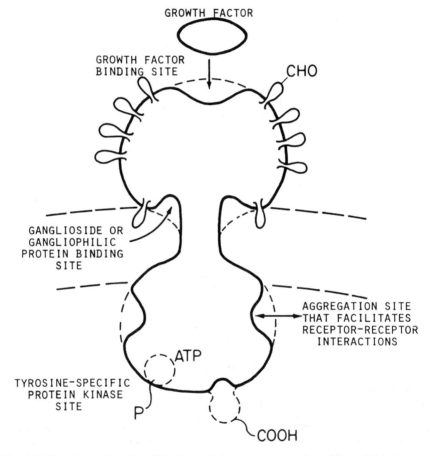

Fig. 3. 'Allosteric regulator' model of growth factor receptor, adapted from Schlessinger et al.[30]. The binding of the growth factor to the receptor may affect (1) tyrosine-specific protein kinase, which is independent of cyclic AMP-dependent kinase, (2) receptor–receptor aggregation, which facilitates clustering and internalization of the receptor–growth factor complex, and (3) direct binding to gangliosides or indirect binding through a gangliophilic protein. This model is based on the fact that growth factor-dependent tyrosine-phosphorylation of the receptor protein (M_r 170 000) as well as growth factor-dependent cell growth and mitogenesis were inhibited by exogenous enrichment of membrane gangliosides. This model also explains how ganglioside enrichment of membranes alters the affinity of cells to growth factors.

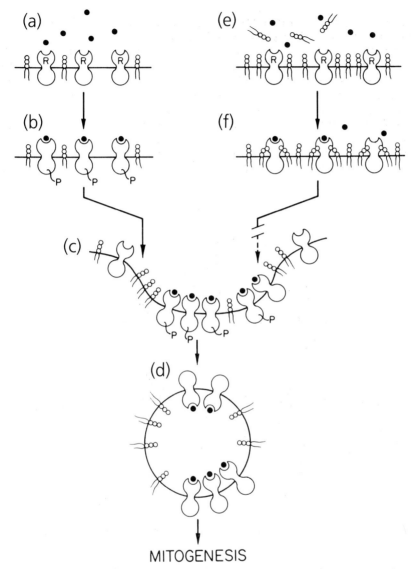

MITOGENESIS

Fig. 4. A possible mechanism of cell growth stimulation by growth factor, and inhibition of cell growth by gangliosides. Growth factor (●) added at the cell surface (a) is bound to the receptors (R). Subsequently, kinase activity of the cytoplasmic domain is activated, and receptors are phosphorylated (P). The phosphorylated receptors alter their conformation and aggregate together to form 'coated pits' (c), which are in turn internalized (d). The internalized receptor–growth factor complex will be utilized for mitogenesis. GM_3 and GM_1 gangliosides are capable of interacting directly or indirectly with epidermal growth factor receptor or platelet-derived growth factor receptor to inhibit their kinase activity and autophosphorylation. The concentration of GM_3 in cells growing normally, however, is not sufficient to strongly inhibit phosphorylation of the receptor (a–b). Therefore, internalization of the receptor–growth factor complex can proceed (c–d). When cells were grown in medium with exogenous addition of GM_3 ganglioside (e), GM_3 ganglioside incorporated in the lipid bilayer interacts strongly with the growth factor receptor, and subsequently, tyrosine phosphorylation of the receptor is inhibited (f). Therefore, internalization of the growth factor–receptor complex does not proceed (f–g).

A possible sequence of events in mouse cells
following a blocked synthesis of ganglioside

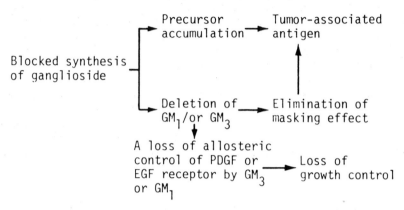

Fig. 5. A blocked synthesis of ganglioside results in accumulation of precursors which are recognized by antibodies and by the immune system as tumor-associated antigens. On the other hand, a blocked synthesis of ganglioside results in deletion of a specific ganglioside which causes a loss of allosteric control of the growth factor receptor and consequently results in loss of growth control. The deletion of higher gangliosides may eliminate the masking effect of precursor antigenicity, thus enhancing the antigenicity of glycolipid tumor antigens. The masking effect of tumor antigens by glycolipids having longer chains was recently described[10].

conditions has made it possible to study the phenomenon of growth inhibition of mouse 3T3 cells induced by GM_1 in greater detail, with the following results[28]: (1) Cell growth in serum-free medium was inhibited by the presence of GM_1 and to a lesser extent by GM_3, but not by sialosyllacto*neo*tetraosylceramide, although these gangliosides were incorporated equally well into the cell membranes. (2) The concentration-dependent binding of ^{125}I-labeled PDGF (platelet-derived growth factor) to cells indicated that cellular affinity for PDGF was altered by exogenous addition of GM_1 or GM_3. Thus, ganglioside-dependent cell growth inhibition is caused by altered affinity of the receptor to PDGF. (3) GM_1 and GM_3, but neither sialosyllacto*neo*tetraosylceramide nor globoside, inhibited the PDGF-stimulated tryosine phosphorylation of a M_r 170 000 protein which was identified as the PDGF receptor. These results suggest that the level of membrane GM_1 or GM_3 may modulate PDGF receptor function by affecting the degree of tryosine phosphorylation, and may alter the affinity of the receptor for PDGF. A similar inhibition of tyrosine phosphorylation of the EGF (epidermal growth factor) receptor (M_r 170 000 glycoprotein) by GM_3, and GM_3-induced cell growth inhibition in A431 cells have been observed[29].

Recently, Schlessinger *et al.*[30] proposed an 'allosteric regulator' model for the EGF receptor in which several binding sites on the receptor protein, in addition to the EGF binding site, were postulated. Since the chemical level and organization of gangliosides in plasma membranes may affect the allosteric configuration of the receptor, it is possible that one of the additional sites on the growth hormone receptor may bind GM_1 or GM_3 either directly or through an intermediate gangliophilic protein (see Fig. 3). Organization of gangliosides with such receptors may alter the receptor–receptor interaction which is necessary for internalization of the receptor–growth hormone complex (see Fig. 4). The model may be useful for further studies of cell growth regulation through membrane gangliosides. A loss or reduction of GM_3 or GM_1, caused by blocked synthesis of various oncogenic transformants, may result in loss of allosteric regulation through the growth factor receptor and may also induce precursor accumulation and cause enhanced antigenicity of the precursor glycolipid antigen. A possible sequence of events in mouse cells following a blocked synthesis of gangliosides by oncogenic transformation is illustrated in Fig. 5. The growth factor requirement of each normal and transformed cell is different. The mechanisms by which glycolipids regulate growth factor receptors may also be different. The model described above (and in Fig. 5) represents only one example. A large variety of growth factor requirements may be associated with a number of regulator glycolipids which are also 'sensors' of the external environment, such as cell–cell contact. This model may eventually fill the gap in our knowledge of how glycolipids regulate cell growth adapted to external environments.

Acknowledgement
The author's own studies cited in this article have been supported by grants from the National Institutes of Health (CA 19924, 20026) and the American Cancer Society (BC 9).

References

1 Hakomori, S. and Murakami, W. T. (1968) *Proc. Natl Acad. Sci. USA* 59, 254–261
2 Brady, R. O. and Fishman, P. (1974) *Biochim. Biophys. Acta* 335, 121–148
3 Critchley, D. R. and Vicker, M. G. (1977) in *Dynamic Aspects of Cell Surface Organization* (Poste, G. and Nicolson, G. L., eds), pp. 308–370, Elsevier/North-Holland Biomedical Press
4 Hakomori, S. and Young, W. W., Jr (1978) *Scand. J. Immunol. Supplement* 6, 97–117
5 Hakomori, S., and Kannagi, R. (1983) *J. Natl Cancer Inst.* 71, 231–251
6 Gahmberg, C. G. and Hakomori, S. (1975) *J. Biol. Chem.* 250, 2438–2446
7 Sundsmo, J. and Hakomori, S. (1976) *Biochem. Biophys. Res. Commun.* 68, 799–806
8 Rosenfelder, G., Young, W. W., Jr and Hakomori, S. (1977) *Cancer Res.* 37, 1333–1339
9 Young, W. W., Jr and Hakomori, S. (1981) *Science* 211, 487–489
10 Kannagi, R., Stroup, R., Cochran, N. A., Urdal, D. L., Young, W. W., Jr and Hakomori, S. (1983) *Cancer Res.* 43, 4997–5005
11 Ito, M., Suzuki, E., Naiki, M., Sendo, F. and Arai, S. (1984) *Int. J. Cancer* 34, 689–697
12 Pukel, C. S., Lloyd, K. O., Trabassos, L. R., Dippold, W. G., Oettgen, H. F. and Old, L. J. (1982) *J. Exp. Med.* 155, 1133–1147
13 Nudelman, E., Hakomori, S., Kannagi, R., Levery, S., Yeh, M.-Y., Hellström, K. E. and Hellström, I. (1982) *J. Biol. Chem.* 257, 12752–12756
14 Nudelman, E., Kannagi, R., Hakomori, S., Parsons, M., Lipinski, M., Wiels, J., Fellous, M. and Tursz, T. (1983) *Science* 220, 509–511
15 Magnani, J. L., Brockhaus, M., Smith, D. F., Ginsburg, V., Blaszczyk, M., Mitchell, K. F., Steplewski, Z. and Koprowski, H. (1981) *Science* 212, 55–56
16 Magnani, J. L., Nilsson, B., Brockhaus, M., Zopf, D., Steplewski, Z., Koprowski, H. and Ginsburg, T. (1982) *J. Biol. Chem.* 257, 14365–14369
17 Hakomori, S., Nudelman, E., Levery, S. B. and Kannagi, R. (1984) *J. Biol. Chem.* 259, 4672–4680
18 Fukushi, Y., Hakomori, S., Nudelman, E. and Cochran, N. (1984) *J. Biol. Chem.* 259, 4681–4685

19 Hakomori, S., Nudelman, E., Levery, S. and Patterson, C. M. (1983) *Biochem. Biophys. Res. Commun.* 113, 791–798
20 Fukushi, Y., Nudelman, E., Levery, S. B., Rauvala, H. and Hakomori, S. (1984) *J. Biol. Chem.* 259, 10511–10517
21 Levine, P. (1978) *Seminars in Oncology* 5, 28–34
22 Kannagi, R., Levine P., Watanabe, K., and Hakomori, S. (1982) *Cancer Res.* 42, 5249–5254
23 Gooi, H. C., Feizi, T., Kapaia, A., Knowles, B. B., Solter, D. and Evans, J. M. (1981) *Nature* 292, 156–158
24 Finne, J. (1983) *Biochem. Soc. Trans.* 11, 269–270
25 Fukushi, Y., Hakomori, S. and Shepard, T. (1984) *J. Exp. Med.* 159, 506–520
26 Urdal, D. L. and Hakomori, S. (1983) *J. Biol. Chem.* 258, 6869–6874
27 Hakomori, S. (1981) *Annu. Rev. Biochem.* 50, 733–764
28 Bremer, E. G., Hakomori, S., Bowen-Pope, D. F., Raines, E. and Ross, R. (1984) *J. Biol. Chem.* 259, 6818–6825
29 Bremer, E. G., Schlessinger, J. and Hakomori, S. (1986) *J. Biol. Chem.* 261, 2434–2440
30 Schlessinger, J., Schreiber, A. B., Levi, A., Lax, I., Liberman, T. and Yarden, Y. (1983) *CRC Rev. Biochem.* 14, 93–111

Sen-itiroh Hakomori is at the Fred Hutchinson Cancer Research Center, and Departments of Pathobiology, Microbiology and Immunology, University of Washington, 1124 Columbia Street, Seattle, WA 98104, USA.

Endosomes

Ari Helenius, Ira Mellman, Doris Wall and
Ann Hubbard

*Endosomes are a heterogeneous population of endocytic vacuoles through which
molecules internalized during pinocytosis pass* en route *to lysosomes. In addition
to this transport function, recent studies indicate that these organelles also act as
clearing houses for incoming ligands, fluid components and receptors.*

Historical view

The first observation that proteins internalized during endocytosis pass through
prelysosomal vacuoles before reaching secondary lysosomes, was made in the
early sixties. Werner Straus, working at the University of North Carolina,
investigated the endocytic uptake of intravenously administered horseradish
peroxidase by rat kidney epithelium[1]. He used a blue benzidine stain to localize
the internalized peroxidase and a red naphthol dye to stain lysosomes which
contain acid phosphatase. At early time points, Straus observed that the two
enzymes were in separate vacuoles, with the blue peroxidase-containing vacuoles
in the peripheral cytoplasm and with the red lysosomes in the perinuclear area.
Later, the peroxidase appeared in perinuclear vacuoles and ultimately in the acid
phosphatase-positive lysosomes, indicated by the formation of purple vacuoles.
Accordingly a function of these prelysosomal vacuoles, which Straus termed
'phagosomes', was to deliver newly internalized material to the secondary lysosomes for digestion. The 'phagosomes' were clearly part of the vacuolar apparatus of the cell – the system of membrane-bound bodies, vacuoles and vesicles
involved in the uptake and processing of endocytosed (and autophagocytosed)
material. Other components of the vacuolar apparatus include lysosomes, auto-
phagosomes, residual bodies, multivesicular bodies, endocytic coated vesicles,
certain Golgi elements, etc.[2]

Since the demonstration of plasma membrane recycling by Steinman *et al.*[3] and
receptor-mediated endocytosis of low density lipoproteins by Goldstein *et al.*[4] in
the mid-seventies, the field of pinocytosis and receptor-mediated uptake of
extracellular macromolecules has experienced a surge of activity. The role of
prelysosomal compartments has, in this context, become a focus of lively interest.
Prelysosomal vacuoles have now been described in a variety of cell types and
ligand–receptor systems. The old term phagosome (which is inappropriate since
the vacuoles do not arise by phagocytosis) has given way for terms such as
pinosomes, endosomes, intermediate vacuoles, and receptosomes. We will use
the term *endosome* because it does not assume specific compositional features
(such as the presence of receptors, which may be true only for a subpopulation of
prelysosomal vacuoles), and it does not emphasize a single function (such as
transport of substances into lysosomes).

The purpose of this review is to discuss the information available on endosomes, and to try to bring together a cohesive picture of this organelle and its
functions. The experimental systems used in our laboratories, the Fc-receptor of
macrophages, the galactose-specific receptor of hepatocytes, and the entry of
Semliki Forest virus into fibroblasts, will often be used for illustration.

Morphology

The cellular distribution and the morphology of endosomes has been studied in various cell types and tissues by electron and fluorescence microscopy. Since they do not have any obvious unique morphological characteristics, the identification of endosomes in such experiments depends on functional criteria. Commonly, their ability to be labeled following a brief exposure to some endocytosed marker is used. Such markers can be: (a) fluid phase components (such as the horseradish peroxidase used by Straus); (b) non-specifically adsorbed ligands (such as cationized ferritin); or (c) physiological ligands for receptor-mediated endocytosis coupled with ferritin, horseradish peroxidase, colloidal gold or fluorescent groups[5]. Endosomes can then be distinguished from lysosomes, which will also contain these markers, through the use of acid hydrolase cytochemistry. Staining for acid phosphatase or arylsulfatase activities is frequently used for this purpose. Alternatively the experiment can be performed at 16–20°C, at which temperature the passage of material from endosomes to lysosomes is blocked in several cell types[6,7].

Endosomes defined in this way display heterogeneous morphology and cellular distribution (Fig. 1). While the average size observed in thin sections is 0.3 μm, endosomes can often be as large as 1 μm. At least two populations of endosomes can be recognized. 'Early' or 'peripheral' endosomes are those which fill up first with the endocytosed marker and are usually located close to the plasma membrane. They often have an electron-lucent interior and plaque-like electron dense regions covering portions of the cytosolic surface[8]. In some cell types, these 'peripheral' endosomes consist partly of tubular elements which can form anastamosing networks (see Fig. 1). The second population of endosomes is often concentrated in the Golgi-lysosome region and tend to be spherical and somewhat larger. In some cases, however, they too seem tubular and it has been suggested that they are part of the so-called GERL, a Golgi-associated network of membranes[9]. These endosomes frequently have deep invaginations, and may contain internal vesicles derived from the limiting membrane ('multivesicular bodies'). The cellular location of the different endosomal populations are particularly clear in certain epithelial cells and other highly polarized cell types such as hepatocytes (Fig. 1). In most tissue culture cell lines, the distinctions are often difficult to ascertain.

In spite of continuous internalization of plasma membrane-derived vesicles during pinocytosis, the number of endosomes seems to remain roughly constant with time. It has been estimated that peritoneal macrophages contain about 240 endosomes per cell (in contrast to ~ 1000 secondary lysosomes) with a combined membrane area of at least 10–15% that of the plasma membrane[3]. However, the number (and size) of endosomes vary between individual cells and cell types, and with the physiological state.

Physical properties and composition

Endosomes have not yet been successfully isolated and hence, the available information about their properties and composition is sparse. Cells can, however, be homogenized so that the majority of endosomes remain intact and sediment in gradients as defined entities without loss of contents. A variety of density media including sucrose, Metrizamide and Percoll have been used to separate endosomes from secondary lysosomes. The buoyant density of the endosomal vacuoles varies between 1.02 and 1.12 g cm^{-3} depending on the gradient material. The endosome fractions also contain a variety of other smooth membrane

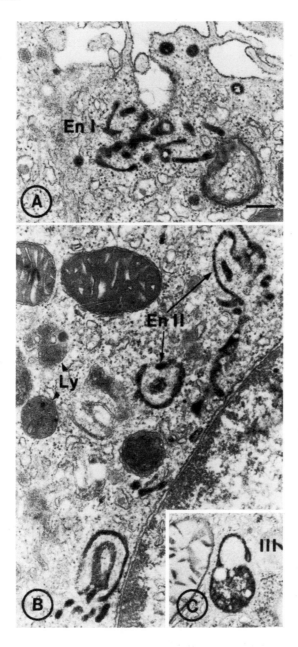

Fig. 1. Endosomes of rat hepatocytes. Three classes of endosomes can be distinguished in rat hepatocytes. Livers were perfused with the specific cytochemical conjugates, asialo-orosomucoid-horseradish peroxidase (A and B) or epidermal growth factor-peroxidase (C), at 16°C for 90 min prior to fixation and peroxidase cytochemistry[21]. Endosome–lysosome fusion is blocked at this temperature, leading to accumulation of ligands in endosomes in the peripheral cytoplasm (A, En I) as well as those in Golgi-liposome regions (B and C, En II and III). The tubular and vesicular nature of endosomes I and II is apparent. In liver, endosomes III are filled with lipid inclusions and small vesicles and are often in continuity with the tubular endosome II. Bar = 0.2 μm.

vesicles including plasma membrane, Golgi-derived membrane and endoplasmic reticulum. No more than a few percent of the membrane present in these fractions may be endosomes. Nevertheless, endosomes can be easily resolved from typical lysosomes, which are of greater density. Free flow electrophoresis studies have indicated that endosomes do not have as high a negative surface charge as lysosomes (M. Marsh and E. Harms, unpublished observations). In the electric field they migrate together with most of the other cellular membranes, well separated from the lysosome peak. No unique characteristic of endosomes is yet known which would help to isolate them on the basis of physical properties. Several laboratories are presently attempting to develop ligand-induced density modification procedures to isolate endosomes from the other smooth membranes.

The limited information available on the chemical composition of the endosome membrane seem to bear out at least a superficial similarity with the plasma membrane. Radioiodination studies performed using pinocytosed lactoperoxidase as a catalyst have shown that macrophage endosomes contain a set of proteins, accessible from the interior of the vacuole, which are similar to those on the plasma membrane[10]. The predominance of common labeled protein components in the endosomes and the plasma membrane was shown both by SDS-polyacrylamide gels and immune precipitation with a panel of monoclonal antibodies. Some clear-cut differences were, however, also observed. The only information concerning the lipid composition is based on two indirect experiments which argue for the presence of cholesterol: firstly, the buoyant density of endosomes shifts in the presence of digitonin[11]; secondly, Semliki Forest virus, which requires cholesterol in the target membrane in order to fuse with it, is able to fuse out of endosomes[7].

Endosomes are acidic

One of the most important of the endosome's known characteristics is its low internal pH. This trait was first suggested by experiments using intact cells. Tycko and Maxfield[12] took advantage of the pH-dependent fluorescence spectrum of fluorescein-conjugated α_2-macroglobulin to show that this ligand reached an acidic (pH 5–6) compartment rapidly (15–20 min) following its internalization. Subsequently, similar results were obtained using fluorescein-labeled transferrin (pH 5.3)[13] and using the low pH-dependent fusion activity of Semliki Forest virus as a biological pH probe (pH <6.0)[7]. The virus studies indicated that incoming virus reached acid vacuoles in BHK-21 cells no later than 5 min after leaving the cell surface. Although secondary lysosomes have long been known to have an acidic pH, the appearance of virus in the high density, hydrolytically active compartment was not detectable for >20 min.

Very recently, the suggestion that endosomes are acidic has received direct support from the work of Galloway *et al.*[14] who have demonstrated the acidification of endosomes *in vitro*. Endosomes and lysosomes (from fibroblasts and macrophages) were labeled with fluorescein-dextran and separated on Percoll gradients. Both fractions were then shown to decrease their internal pH in an ATP-dependent fashion. While final elucidation of the acidification mechanism will require further study, it appears that endosomes acidify, at least in part, due to the activity of a H^+-ATPase similar to that believed to operate in lysosomes and in secretory granules. Conceivably, the endosome ATPase is derived from the plasma membrane during endocytosis, since a similar enzyme also appears to be responsible for the acidification of isolated coated vesicles[15]. It thus seems well established that the vacuoles of the pinocytic pathway are acidified well before their coalescence with lysosomes. The teleological significance of low pH in endosomes, *vis à vis* receptor-mediated endocytosis, membrane recycling, and the entry of viruses and toxins will be discussed below.

Membrane recycling through endosomes

Werner Straus suggested that the endosomes he saw were not primary endocytic vesicles. Instead, he postulated a population of submicroscopic vesicles which provided for transport of solutes into the endosomal compartment. With great foresight he suggested that these could be related to the coated vesicles just discovered in 1962 by Roth and Porter (and Fawcett). There is today considerable evidence for the involvement of clathrin-coated regions ('coated pits') in pinocytosis of ligands bound to cell surface receptors. Most workers in the field favor a mechanism whereby these coated pits pinch off to form coated endocytic vesicles. These coated vesicles are, however, thought to exist only for a short time (15–60 s) before losing their coats and fusing with endosomes. An alternative view is advocated by Pastan and Willingham[9] (see p. 238), who suggest that endosomes arise directly from the plasma membrane by pinching off from the region adjacent to the coated pits. However, recent serial section analysis by van Deurs has unequivocally demonstrated the existence of endocytic coated vesicles as independent organelles[25].

It is often thought that fluid phase uptake, which can amount to 26% of a cell's total volume every hour[3], is mediated through the formation of small, uncoated vesicles – presumably without the participation of clathrin-containing coats. However, verification of such a separate pathway of pinocytosis has been difficult. The uncoated vesicles seen in many preparations may simply represent coated vesicles which have already defrocked. Our estimates based on virus uptake in BHK-21 cells suggest that a sufficient number of coated vesicles (about 2000 per min) are, indeed, formed to account for the measured fluid phase uptake[16]. Nevertheless, the possible contribution of uncoated pinocytic vesicles in traffic into endosomes must be considered. Whatever the nature of the primary endocytic vesicles, it is apparent that fluid phase markers can be channeled into many of the same endosomes as the ligands of receptor-mediated endocytosis[17]. In addition, ligands utilizing different receptors enter the same coated pits, and consequently the same endosomes[9,18].

From the time of their discovery, it has been clear that endosomes are involved in the transport of internalized substances into secondary lysosomes. This role has been amply confirmed with physiological as well as non-physiological marker substances. Delivery into lysosomes typically occurs after a lag the length of which varies depending on the system studied. In cultured fibroblasts it is 20–50 min, whereas in macrophages pinocytosed material begins to appear in lysosomes after only 5–10 min[5]. In oocytes, where the endosomes serve a storage function for yolk proteins, the delivery is almost indefinitely delayed.

However, endosomes are not merely transport or storage vacuoles. They display a variety of other elaborate functions which have received increasing attention in recent years. The most important of these is the sorting of the membrane of pinocytic vesicles from their contents. Whereas internalized solutes and receptor-bound ligands are typically routed with high efficiency into lysosomes, the membrane container is returned – 'recycled' – to the surface. The concept of membrane recycling was originally introduced to rationalize the enormous amount of plasma membrane continuously internalized during pinocytosis (up to 200% of the cell surface area/h)[3]. Several considerations suggest that recycling occurs mainly from endosomes: (a) the relatively long half-life of plasma membrane proteins and receptors implies that they are not exposed to lysosomal hydrolytic enzymes during recycling[3]; (b) the very rapid recycling times (<5 min) inferred for several receptors contrasts with the relatively slow delivery of substances into lysosomes[19,20]; (c) the receptor-mediated uptake of extracellular ligands and receptor recycling continues at intermediate temperatures (16–20°C) where traffic into lysosomes is inhibited[21,22]; (d) transferrin is internalized into endosomes and returned to the extracellular space without transit through high density secondary lysosomes[13] (see below). Hence, it seems likely that most membrane recycling occurs from endosomes. Some recycling can also occur at the lysosomal level, but the extent of this pathway may depend on cell-type or physiological state, as after the uptake of large, indigestible solutes[5].

How is the sorting of pinocytic vesicle membrane from contents accomplished during recycling? One possible answer may lie in simple geometric considerations. If the recycling vesicles are smaller than the incoming vesicles, the relative surface to volume ratios of these compartments will favor the retrieval of membrane over the internalized fluid[23]. Nevertheless, if the membrane returns in a vesicular form one would expect the reflux of some fluid. This has recently been documented by Besterman *et al.*[24] who used [^{14}C]sucrose as a marker of pinocytic vesicle content. In macrophages, the reflux amounts to about one fourth of the internalized volume. Interestingly, it is detectable only immediately after uptake, suggesting that recycling occurs primarily from an early endocytic compartment, i.e. endosomes. Again, kinetic and morphologic evidence suggest that this 'short-circuit pathway' is from peripheral endosomes. However, nothing is known about the mechanisms involved in the formation of recycling vesicles, or about the stringent controls which must exist to balance the amount of incoming and outgoing membrane during endocytosis.

Endosomes and receptor-mediated endocytosis

Animal cells bear a variety of receptors for distinct molecules or classes of molecules. Examples include receptors for hormones, growth factors, lipoproteins, lysosomal enzymes, viruses, and bacterial toxins. As a rule the ligands are efficiently internalized via coated pits/coated vesicles, localized transiently in endosomes, and finally delivered to, and degraded in, secondary lysosomes. In contrast, many receptors escape degradation and return to the cell surface to participate in subsequent rounds of ligand binding and uptake. As mentioned earlier, both the rapidity of receptor recycling and the observations that recycling continues at temperatures (16–20°C) which prevent fusion with lysosomes indicate that the return of free receptors occurs from endosomes. Thus, dissociation of the receptor–ligand complex must occur soon after internalization, in endosomes and/or endocytic coated vesicles. Electron microscopic evidence for dissociation in an endosome compartment has recently been presented[26].

One of the critical factors responsible for the dissociation of the receptor–ligand complexes in many cases appears to be low pH. Indeed, the affinity of many ligands to their receptors are known to be dramatically decreased when the pH is lowered to 5–6 (Table 1). Agents which increase the pH in endosomes and lysosomes inhibit receptor-mediated endocytosis by preventing the dissociation of receptor–ligand complexes and accordingly, receptor re-use.

There are several interesting variations to the theme. One is provided by the

Table 1. Receptor-bound ligands which are effected by low pH

Ligand	Cell type	Effect of low pH (5.5–6.0)
Phosphomannosylglycoproteins (e.g. lysosomal enzymes)	Fibroblasts	Dissociation from receptor
Mannosyl glycoproteins	Macrophages	Dissociation from receptor
Asialoglycoproteins	Hepatocytes	Dissociation from receptor (potentiated by low Ca^{2+})
Transferrin	Many	Loss of bound iron
Diphtheria toxin	Many	Membrane insertion
Enveloped viruses (e.g. Semliki Forest virus)	Many	Membrane fusion

receptor-mediated uptake of transferrin, a serum iron carrier. In this case, it is the binding of iron to the carrier protein that is acid-sensitive, and not the binding of the carrier to its membrane receptor. Internalized transferrin delivers its iron to cells, and then returns to the cell surface to be released into the medium. That the delivery of iron and recycling of apo-transferrin occurs in endosomes has recently been illustrated by the work of van Renswoude *et al.*[13] who used Percoll gradients to show that internalized transferrin is located only in the endosome fraction, and is never transferred to secondary lysosomes. Similar results have been obtained for the internalization and recycling of a monovalent anti-Fc receptor antibody in macrophages: i.e. internalized antibody rapidly returns to the cell surface without entering the secondary lysosome compartment[27]. In addition, lack of acid sensitivity of ligand binding may also be a crucial factor in the transepithelial transport of IgG in the brush border cells of newborn mammals, which depends on an intermediate endosome-like compartment[17].

There are several cases where receptors are not efficiently recycled and reutilized for ligand binding. One example is the macrophage Fc receptor. Upon binding a polyvalent ligand (IgG immune complex), *both* the ligand and the receptor are rapidly delivered to, and degraded in, lysosomes[27]. In this case, the receptor–ligand interaction does not appear to be acid-sensitive. It is not yet known, however, what provides the signal which prevents recycling of these receptor–ligand complexes, and directs them to the lysosomal compartment. At least in the case of Fc receptors, the state of receptor aggregation in endosome membranes may be a contributing factor, given that monovalent anti-receptor/ Fab receptor complexes appear to recycle. Analogous mechanisms may be responsible for mediating the 'down-regulation' of polypeptide hormone receptors.

Another important variation on the theme is provided by invasive agents such as enveloped viruses and bacterial toxins which introduce their genomes or their toxic subunits into the cellular cytosol. Diphtheria toxin and many of the enveloped animal viruses have been shown to enter via an endocytic pathway. In the virus systems (toga viruses, orthomyxoviruses and rhabdo viruses) the low pH of the endosomes induces a conformational change in the viral spike glycoproteins. This activates a membrane fusion activity which leads to the fusion of the viral membrane with the limiting membrane of the endosome[7]. In the case of diphtheria toxin, the low pH causes the insertion of the toxin into the lipid membrane, facilitating the passage of the toxic subunit into the cytosol[28,29].

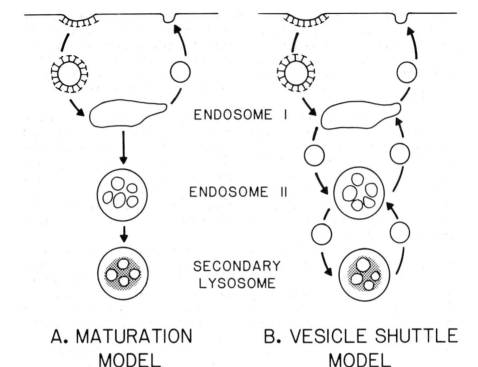

Fig. 2. The role of endosomes in pinocytosis. In this simplified view, pinocytosis is initiated at clathrin-coated regions of the plasma membrane which pinch off to form coated vesicles. These vesicles lose their coats and deliver their contents to endosomes. The transfer of endosome contents to lysosomes may occur by two possible mechanisms. According to the first view (left), an individual endosome matures and eventually fuses directly with lysosomes. The alternative view (right) maintains that contents are transferred from one endosome population to the next, and then to lysosomes, by specialized transport vesicles which shuttle between the compartments they interconnect.

Are endosomes stable or transient organelles?

While coated vesicles mediate the transport of extracellular markers into endosomes, it is not yet clear how the transport between the endosomes, and from endosomes to lysosomes occurs. Two possibilities are indicated in Fig. 2. To keep the picture simple and the discussion down to earth, we have ignored the possibility of parallel pathways.

According to the first view (the Maturation model, Fig. 2A) endosomes form *de novo* at the periphery of the cytoplasm by the fusion of incoming primary endocytic vesicles. After some time, during which they serve both as targets for further incoming vesicles and as sites of membrane recycling and sorting (Endosome I), they move into the perinuclear area with their contents of dissociated ligands and fluid phase components (Endosome II). Simultaneously they undergo changes in morphology through condensation, reciprocal fusions and by undergoing invaginations of their limiting membrane to form multivesicular bodies. Ultimately, fusion with primary or secondary lysosomes occurs, resulting in the degradation of endosome contents. Presumably, part of the endosome membrane is thereby degraded, accounting for the basal rate of plasma membrane protein turnover observed in many cells ($t_{1/2}$>20 h)[5]. The essential feature of this model is that the endosome and its contents move together as the organelle undergoes maturation, and eventually ends up in a lysosome. An individual endosome would thus be a transient structure. Such movement of endosome-like vacuoles from the cell periphery to the perinuclear region has been documented by time lapse photographs taken some years ago by J. Hirsch and Z. Cohn.

The second view (the Vesicle shuttle model, Fig. 2B) suggests that the endosomal vacuoles observed in cells are stable organelles with defined and constant functions, locations, and morphology. Internalized material passes through endosome compartments sequentially with little change occurring to the organelles themselves. Thus, transport of the content from one type of endosome to the next and finally into lysosomes, would occur by vesicle shuttle mechanisms resembling that operational between the plasma membrane and endosomes. This model implies a complex chain of vesicle formation processes, recognition reactions, and membrane fusions.

At present we know of no conclusive experiment which would allow a clear-cut choice between the two models. The problem is reminiscent of one which pertains to understanding the Golgi complex, where it is not yet clear whether the passage of secretory and membrane proteins occurs by vesicular traffic between different cisternal elements or whether cisternae themselves move from one side of the stack to the other. In the case of the endosomes, we suspect that the final answer will be somewhere between the two extremes shown in Fig. 2. For instance, it is unlikely that the tubular membrane networks which form the peripheral endosomes in some cell types can move intact within the cell. Here movement must occur in the form of detached vacuoles. On the other hand, there is not yet any evidence for discrete transport vesicles, which would operate between endosomes or between endosomes and lysosomes. Such carriers should be detectable particularly if they were involved in the transport of the contents of the multivesicular bodies from endosomes to lysosomes for degradation.

Conclusions

In this brief review, we have taken the liberty of leaving many issues untouched and many more unresolved. What we have attempted is to establish from a long and varied literature the existence of the endosome as a discreet, albeit still somewhat elusive, endocytic compartment which resides temporally between primary pinocytic vesicles and the ultimate delivery of their contents to acid hydrolase-rich secondary lysosomes.

Although a considerable amount of information must be obtained before a full understanding of the function, composition, and heterogeneity of these organelles is reached, some general concepts are emerging which may help explain the importance of endosomes in the endocytic pathway. One possible role of the endosome is to provide a compartment where vesicle traffic in and out can occur without continuous loss of lysosomal enzymes, which probably could not be avoided if recycling were to occur at the level of secondary lysosomes. More crucial, however, is the fact that endosomes, in effect, provide an 'acid bath' through which plasma membrane components continuously pass during recycling[30]. This has particular significance for a variety of receptors which are known to discharge their ligands at low pH. Not only will the dissociation of such receptor–ligand complexes occur almost immediately following internalization, but free receptors will be generated for return to the cell surface without requiring transit through the acidic, but perilous environment of the lysosome.

In addition to the 'crude' separation of contents material from the membrane container, endosomes appear to be involved in determining whether individual membrane components are to be recycled or delivered into the lysosomes for destruction. Endosomes may, in this way, provide an intracellular site where the cell can rapidly modulate expression of surface components. Furthermore, endosomes involuntarily serve as the portal of entry for bacterial toxins and viruses into the cytosolic compartment. Whether such an entry pathway exists for physiological ligands remains to be seen.

And what of the lysosome, whose prestige would appear to have been usurped and whose role in endocytosis diminished? Lest this discussion leaves such an impression, we would like to stress that secondary lysosomes still serve a variety of functions in the processing of internalized membrane and contents. This role has been most clearly documented by studies on serum low density lipoprotein uptake[4], where lysosomal function has been shown to play a crucial role in the regulation of cellular and organismal cholesterol metabolism.

References

1 Straus, W. (1964) *J. Cell Biol.* 21, 295–308
2 de Duve, C. and Wattiaux, R. (1966) *Annu. Rev. Physiol.* 28, 435–492
3 Steinman, R. M., Brodie, S. E. and Cohn, Z. A. (1976) *J. Cell Biol.* 68, 665–687
4 Goldstein, J. L., Anderson, R. G. W. and Brown, M. S. (1979) *Nature (London)* 279, 679–685
5 Steinman, R. M., Mellman, I. S., Muller, W. A. and Cohn, Z. A. (1983) *J. Cell Biol.* 96, 1–27
6 Dunn, W. A., Hubbard, A. L. and Aronson, N. N. (1980) *J. Biol. Chem.* 255, 5971–5978
7 Marsh, M., Bolzau, E. and Helenius, A. (1983) *Cell* 32, 931–940
8 Holtzman, E. (1976) *Lysosomes: a survey*, Cell Biology Monographs, Vol. 3, Springer-Verlag, New York
9 Pastan, I. H. and Willingham, M. C. (1981) *Science* 214, 504–509
10 Mellman, I. S., Steinman, R. M., Unkeless, J. C. and Cohn, Z. A. (1980) *J. Cell Biol.* 86, 712–722
11 Hubbard, A. L. (1982) in *Membrane Recycling, Ciba Symposium No. 92* (Evered, D., ed.), p. 109, Pitman Press, London
12 Tycko, B. and Maxfield, F. R. (1982) *Cell* 28, 643–651
13 Van Renswoude, J., Bridges, K. R., Harford, J. B. and Klausner, R. D. (1982) *Proc. Natl Acad. Sci. USA* 79, 6186–6190
14 Galloway, C. J., Dean, G. E., Marsh, M., Rudnick, G. and Mellman, I. (1983) *Proc. Natl Acad. Sci. USA* 80, 3334–3338
15 Forgac, M., Cantley, L., Wiedenmann, B., Altsteil, L. and Branton, D. (1983) *Proc. Natl Acad. Sci. USA* 80, 1300–1303
16 Marsh, M. and Helenius, A. (1980) *J. Mol. Biol.* 142, 439–454
17 Rodewald, R. and Abranamson, D. R. (1982) in *Membrane Recycling, Ciba Symposium No. 92* (Evered, D., ed.), p. 209, Pitman Press, London
18 Carpentier, J.-L., Gorden, P., Anderson, R. G. W., Goldstein, J. L., Brown, M. S., Cohen, S. and Orci, L. (1982) *J. Cell Biol.* 95, 73–77
19 Schwartz, A. L., Fridovich, S. E. and Lodish, H. F. (1982) *J. Biol. Chem.* 257, 4230–4237
20 Anderson, R. G. W., Brown, M. S., Beisiegel, V. and Goldstein, J. L. (1982) *J. Cell Biol.* 93, 523–532
21 Wall, D. A. and Hubbard, A. L. (1981) *J. Cell Biol.* 90, 687–695
22 Aulinskas, T. H., Coetzee, G. A., Gevers, W. and van der Westhuyzen, D. R. (1982) *Biochem. Biophys. Res. Comm.* 107, 1551–1558

23 Duncan, R. and Pratten, M. K. (1977) *J. Theor. Biol.* 66, 727–735
24 Besterman, J. M., Airhart, J. A., Woodsworth, R. C. and Low, R. B. (1981) *J. Cell Biol.* 91, 716–727
25 Petersen, O. W. and van Deurs, B. (1983) *J. Cell Biol.* 96, 277–281
26 Geuze, H. J., Slot, J. M., Straus, J. A. M., Lodish, H. F. and Schwartz, A. L. (1983) *Cell* 32, 277–287
27 Mellman, I. and Plutner, H. (1982) *J. Cell Biol.* 95, 446
28 Draper, R. K. and Simon, M. I. (1980) *J. Cell. Biol.* 87, 849–854
29 Sandvig, K. and Olsnes, S. (1980) *J. Cell Biol.* 87, 828–832
30 Palade, G. (1982) in *Membrane Recycling, Ciba Foundation Symposium No. 92* (Evered, D., ed.), pp. 293–297, Pitman Press, London

Ari Helenius and Ira Mellman are at the Section of Cell Biology, Yale University School of Medicine, 333 Cedar Street, PO Box 3333, New Haven, CT 06510, USA, and Doris Wall and Ann Hubbard are at the Department of Cell Biology and Anatomy, Johns Hopkins Medical School, 725 North Wolfe Street, Baltimore, MD 21205, USA.

Receptor-mediated endocytosis: coated pits, receptosomes and the Golgi

Ira Pastan and Mark C. Willingham

Many plasma proteins, hormones, viruses and toxins enter cells by a common pathway. After entry into receptosomes some ligands are delivered to the cytosol, some are carried on through Golgi elements to lysosomes and others are returned to the cell surface.

Large molecules such as plasma proteins, hormones and viruses enter cultured cells at vastly different rates. Some enter very efficiently by receptor-mediated endocytosis (RME). Others that do not bind to cell surface receptors enter much more slowly. Many molecules that enter cells by RME ultimately reach lysosomes; in this process it has been suggested that ligands were rapidly transferred from specialized surface structures termed coated pits to coated vesicles and then, after uncoating, directly to lysosomes (reviewed in Refs 1–3). However, the pathway of RME is considerably more complex. This review will focus on some of the new findings on the nature of the pathway.

The surface of a typical fibroblastic cell contains about one to two thousand indentations termed 'coated pits'. These specialized structures are characteristically 1400 Å diameter and occupy about 1 to 2% of the cell surface. On the cytoplasmic face of the pits is the protein clathrin that covers the pit with a basket-like structure. Early studies describing the role of coated pits in endocytosis are reviewed elsewhere[4,5]. In 1976, Pearse showed that clathrin was the major protein component of the coat[6]; since then the term 'clathrin-coated pit' has gained general acceptance.

In fibroblasts, low density lipoprotein (LDL) was observed to be concentrated in coated pits prior to its entry[1]; soon thereafter many ligands that bind to specific cell surface receptors were shown to enter cells through these organelles. Direct electron microscopic experiments have shown that LDL, α_2-macroglobulin (α_2M), epidermal growth factor (EGF), β-galactosidase, transferrin, interferon, *Pseudomonas* exotoxin, asialoglycoproteins, as well as viruses such as adenovirus. Rous sarcoma virus, vesicular stomatitis virus and Semliki Forest virus enter cells through the coated pit pathway (Ref. 7 and unpublished data).

How ligand–receptor complexes find their way to coated pits

Receptors are embedded in the plasma membrane of cells and diffuse randomly in the membrane with diffusion coefficients similar to those of many other membrane proteins. From these diffusion coefficients it has been calculated that at 23°C each receptor encounters a coated pit at least every 3–4 s (Ref. 7). Studies on the uptake of α_2M indicate that coated pits transfer ligands into intracellular uncoated vesicles about once every 20 s (Ref. 7). For cells to internalize ligands efficiently, coated pits must have an efficient mechanism for trapping and retaining ligand–receptor complexes.

Some receptors, such as those for EGF, are randomly distributed on the cell surface in the absence of ligand and only become concentrated (clustered) in coated pits in the presence of ligand[7,8]. This indicates that coated pits can distinguish certain ligand–receptor complexes from unoccupied receptors. To explain this discriminatory property it has been suggested that certain ligands induce an allosteric change in the receptor; it is this change in molecular shape that is recognized by the trapping mechanism in the pit (Fig. 1). Other receptors such as those for low density lipoprotein[1] and mannose 6-phosphate[7] have been found clustered in coated pits in the absence of added ligand. These occupied receptors may already be in a conformation recognized by the coated pits and, therefore, concentrated there.

When ligands such as EGF or α_2M are bound to the cell at 1°C and then the cells are rapidly warmed to 37°C, the ligand rapidly moves into the cell. Within 1 min or less, ligand is found to have moved through coated pits into intracellular vesicles that we have termed receptosomes[9]. Others have called these structures endocytic vacuoles or endosomes[3]. The term receptosomes was chosen when it was found that these organelles participate in receptor-mediated endocytosis. The term endocytosis was originally coined to cover all forms of internalization. Since cells also internalize molecules in macropinosomes generated from surface ruffles, which directly fuse with lysosomes (reviewed in Ref. 10), a more specific term was chosen.

How ligands are transferred from coated pits to receptosomes

It is widely believed that the mechanism of formation of receptosomes involves pinching off of coated pits to form 'coated vesicles'[1–3]. It is next suggested that the coated vesicles lose their clathrin coat and the clathrin moves back to the cell surface to form new coated pits[1–3,11,12]. The evidence for such a mechanism is primarily morphological. It is based on electron microscopy where ligand has been seen in coated pits communicating with the surface as well as in structures that have the appearance of coated vesicles because in the plane of section examined, no communication of the vesicular image with the cell surface was observed. However, in the last few years new data have raised the possibility that receptosomes may be formed by a different mechanism in which clathrin does not recycle to form new coated pits. On the basis of this data we have suggested that coated pits are stable structures always associated with the cell surface and that receptosomes form directly from coated pits as illustrated in Fig. 2. Evidence in favor of this mechanism is as follows:

(1) Determination of the location of clathrin in fibroblastic cells by electron microscopy using antibodies to clathrin failed to show a significant pool of soluble clathrin as predicted by the recycling model; instead, all the clathrin detected was associated with coated pits[13].

(2) Microinjection of antibodies to clathrin into cells failed to inhibit endocytosis or trap and precipitate clathrin in the cytosol as would have been expected if the clathrin of coated vesicles is removed from the coated vesicles and recycled to the surface every 20 s. In these experiments the injected antibody was detected attached to clathrin on the cytoplasmic face of coated pits[14].

(3) External labeling experiments in cells fixed at 1°C demonstrated that all coated structures which appeared morphologically in electron microscopic images to be coated vesicles located near the plasma membrane were functionally in communication with the cell exterior. The evidence for this was that large electron-dense markers, when added to the outside of a fixed cell, readily entered

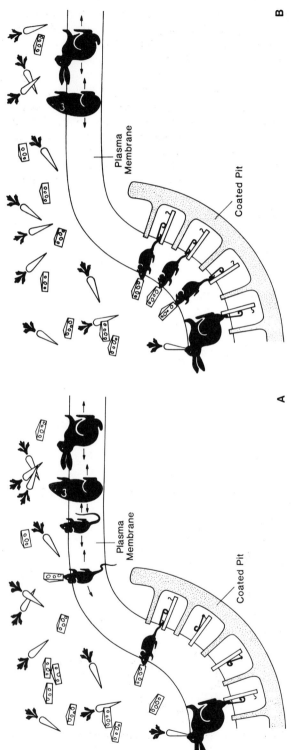

Fig. 1. Scheme of how ligand–receptor complexes may be trapped in coated pits. (A) The animals represent receptors diffusing in the plasma membrane. Cheese and carrots are ligands for mice and rabbits. Note the tail of the mouse and rabbits. Note the tail of the mouse has a different conformation when the mouse is occupied eating cheese. The mouse traps in the coated pit represent the biochemical basis of the clustering process. (B) The ligand–receptor complexes have clustered in preparation for endocytosis. Note that more than one type of receptor can be clustered in the same coated pit and some receptors lack the mechanism for efficient clustering (guinea pig).

and labeled these structures[15]. We believe the explanation for the entry of
electron-dense large molecules into these apparently isolated vesicular structures
from the cell exterior is that the necks connecting these coated pits to the cell
surface were out of the plane of section examined.

When cells kept at 1°C are raised to 37°C, about 30% of coated pits become
functionally inaccessible to an external label[15]. Electron microscopic studies
showed that many of these functionally inaccessible structures have narrow necks
which are attached to the plasma membrane; we believe that at 37°C the necks
are so narrow that materials cannot enter into the coated pits. In summary, we
suggest that coated pits remain permanently associated with the cell surface to
which they are connected by necks. At 1°C, these necks are open. At 37°C, they
periodically close and open. When a neck is closed, the coated pit with which the

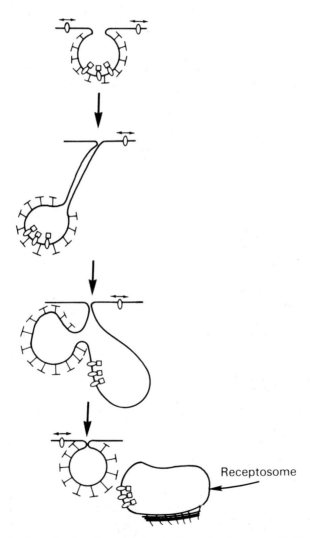

*Fig. 2. Postulated mechanism for receptosome formation from coated pits of the plasma
membrane.*

neck is associated is functionally sealed off but still physically connected to the cell surface (Fig. 2).

Recently, the existence of necks connecting coated structures to the surface has been investigated by serial sections[16,17]. In both studies, the authors found that they could not detect necks in 10–40% of the cases. However, it is still not clear that the contrast of tangentially sectioned membranes in such small necks would be sufficient to allow a clear image of these structures in every case. In unpublished studies, we have also attempted analysis of these connections using serial sections, but we have not been able to clearly interpret the shape of such small structures in every example. The interpretation of such experiments would be greatly improved by methods that might increase the contrast of the membrane structures compared to the surrounding cytoplasm and embedding material.

How receptosomes may form

The transfer of ligand from a coated pit to a receptosome is very rapid. Very few electron microscopic images have caught this process in transition. However, occasional images of vesicles forming from the base of coated pits have been observed (Fig. 3). Formation of such a vesicle must require a driving force. One possible driving force that could participate in vesicle generation is an osmotic gradient. It is possible that ion pumps present in the membrane of the coated pit perform this function[18]. Consistent with this notion is the finding that various monovalent ionophores and particularly proton ionophores slow EGF, α_2M, and VSV entry into cells[18,19].

In cultured cells, actin, myosin and other contractile proteins lie in a dense mat just under the plasma membrane. Coated pits often are seen protruding through this mat. The necks connecting these pits to the cell exterior pass through this mat and the opening and closing of these necks could be controlled by the contractile proteins in the mat.

Saltatory movement of receptosomes

After a ligand has entered a receptosome, it is carried from the cell periphery to the cell interior. Various ligands such as α_2M, EGF, insulin, and tri-iodothyronine have been labeled with rhodamine or fluorescein and their entry into living cells recorded using a sensitive technique termed video-intensification microscopy[7]. These studies showed that receptosomes move by saltatory motion and gradually accumulate in the Golgi region of the cell. Depending on the type of cell studied, the ligand was transferred into the Golgi system 10 to 20 min after its entry into the cell. Receptosomes probably reach the Golgi by following tracks of microtubules which direct them from the cell surface to the Golgi region. In fibroblasts, microtubule organizing centers are located in the Golgi region and from there the microtubules radiate to the cell periphery.

Properties of receptosomes

By phase-contrast microscopy receptosomes are invisible because they are small and their content of protein is low. They have only been seen in living cells by fluorescence techniques in which a receptosome containing labeled ligand appears as a point source of light. Receptosomes have a characteristic appearance by electron microscopy; they are 2000–4000 Å in diameter, have a continuous membrane with a frilled appearance at one edge and an apparently empty center often containing a single intraluminal vesicular structure[9]. Recepto-

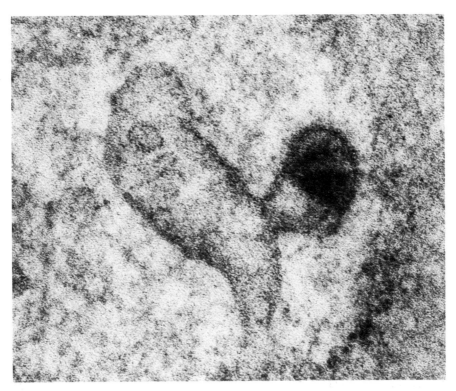

Fig. 3. An electron microscopic image which could represent the formation of a receptosome from a coated pit containing α₂M-peroxidase. Note the small intraluminal vesicle characteristic of a receptosome.

somes do not contain cytochemically detectable hydrolytic enzymes. Thus, they are different from lysosomes which are phase-dense and full of hydrolytic enzymes. However, receptosomes and lysosomes have two properties in common. Both move by saltatory motion and both have a low pH, about pH 5.0[20]. Using fluorescence microscopy in living cells, receptosomes often have been directly observed to undergo fusion with each other (manuscript in preparation), but do not fuse with mature lysosomes in the cytoplasm.

Transit through the Golgi

The Golgi system of fibroblastic cells consists of a series of stacks which are typically located near the nucleus, and a network of interconnecting tubules arranged in a reticular pattern that lie between the stacks and the plasma membrane[21]. This latter portion of the Golgi has been termed the reticular portion of the Golgi, the trans face of the Golgi, or the GERL complex (reviewed in Ref. 21). It is this portion of the organelle that may have been seen by Golgi himself[22]. In most cell types, the transit of molecules through various cellular compartments is not sufficiently synchronous to be able to trace their precise route through the Golgi system. However, in KB cells the entry of EGF is sufficiently synchronous so that the location of the EGF molecules can be followed. In these cells, EGF is first found in the reticular portion of the Golgi 10 to 12 min after entry. A few minutes later the ligand is found in small lysosomes. At no time is ligand detected in Golgi stacks[8].

The reticular portion of the Golgi contains coated pits, but the coated pits of the Golgi are only about half the diameter of those at the cell surface, averaging about 700 Å in diameter. When a ligand such as EGF or β-galactosidase enters the reticular portion of the Golgi, it is found both in the tubules and the coated pits of the Golgi[8]. When it is found in coated pits, the ligand is more concentrated in the pits than in the tubules to which the pits connect. This finding suggests that the function of the coated pits of the Golgi is similar to the coated pits of the cell surface, i.e. to concentrate ligands before transfer to the next compartment. For ligand present in the coated pits of the Golgi, the next compartment is the lysosomal compartment[8].

Some special features of the receptor-mediated endocytosis pathway

Many viruses also enter cells via coated pits and receptosomes. Among those found to use this pathway are adenovirus, Rous sarcoma virus, VSV and Semliki Forest virus[3,23]. Some of these viruses are not as rapidly internalized as protein ligands such as EGF, α_2M or LDL. Whether this is due to their large size, multivalency or other factors is not clear. Some lectins such as Con A also use the coated pit–receptosome pathway. Not all molecules that bind to the cell surface are transported selectively to coated pits. For example, when antibodies to various cell surface antigens bind to the plasma membrane, they can produce large patches outside of coated pits[10].

It has only been possible to determine the pathway of RME because some ligands can be bound to the cell surface at 1°C and followed stepwise through each compartment when the cells are raised to 37°C. This approach is not possible with molecules such as horseradish peroxidase (HRP) which enter by fluid phase endocytosis because they are not concentrated by specific binding to cell surface receptors. HRP only accumulates in sufficient quantities to be readily detected in cells on prolonged incubation at 37°C. When HRP is found in cells, it is located in receptosomes and lysosomes[24]. Its presence in receptosomes indicates it probably entered via coated pits, presumably not attached to a receptor. Surface ruffle activity may be a major form of endocytosis in specialized, actively motile cells such as macrophages and some cancer cells. However, the quantitative contribution of macro- and micro-pinosomes to overall endocytosis in flattened fibroblastic cultured cells is probably minor.

As discussed above, many ligands that have been studied enter cells via coated pits and receptosomes, but with quite different kinetics. Ligands such as EGF, α_2M, and LDL enter very rapidly by selectively clustering in coated pits within a few seconds at 37°C. Other ligands such as interferon (unpublished data) and adenovirus bind to specific receptors but enter cells much more slowly[25]. Nevertheless, they also enter via coated pits and receptosomes. Their failure to concentrate in coated pits could be due to their receptors not being recognized by the clustering mechanism in coated pits or due to relative immobility of the receptor in the plasma membrane. In some cases ligands such as human chorionic gonadotropin (HCG) have been observed to remain on the cell surface for many hours[26]. One possible explanation for the failure of HCG to be internalized is that its receptor is immobile.

Not all molecules that enter via coated pits reach lysosomes

Many viruses that enter cells via coated pits and receptosomes rapidly reach

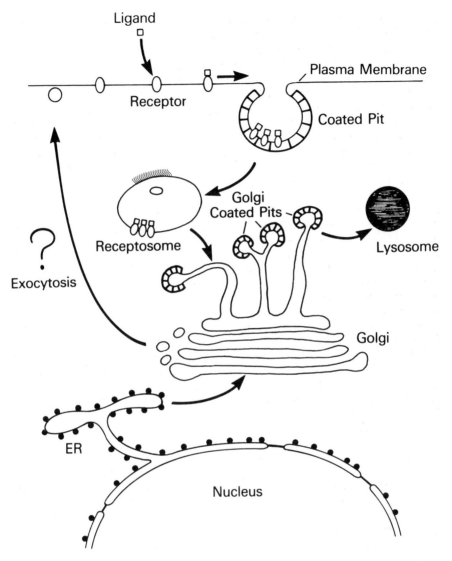

Fig. 4. Summary of the pathways of endocytosis, exocytosis and lysosomal delivery emphasizing the role of the Golgi in these processes.

the cytosol. Membrane-limited viruses such as Semliki Forest virus and VSV appear to do this by fusing their membrane with that of the receptosome, apparently promoted by the low pH of the receptosome[3,20]. Adenovirus which does not have a membrane disrupts the receptosome, releasing the virus and any other contents of the receptosome into the cytosol[23,25].

Most of the transferrin that enters cells does not end up in lysosomes; instead it rapidly returns to the cell surface depleted of its iron[27,28]. Within the cell even at low pH, transferrin remains associated with its receptor. It may be returned to the cell surface in the process of receptor recycling.

Receptor recycling

A comparison of the number of receptors present in a cell and the number of molecules taken up by a cell indicates that each receptor is used over and over many times. Although it had at one time been questioned as to whether or not receptors enter the cell with ligand, there is now convincing evidence that at least several receptors do enter the cell. In our laboratory highly purified receptosomes have been isolated from KB cells and shown to contain both transferrin and phosphomannosyl receptors (Dickson *et al.*, in preparation). Further, in intact cells the receptors for β-galactosidase and asialoglycoprotein have been directly demonstrated by electron microscopic methods to be in receptosomes[29,30]. Therefore, these receptors must separate from the ligand within the cell so that the ligand can go on to lysosomes and the receptor return to the cell surface. A logical place for this separation to begin is in the low pH environment of the receptosome[20]. In fibroblasts, newly synthesized membrane proteins pass through the Golgi stacks on their way through the exocytic pathway to the cell surface[31]. One way for receptors to reach the surface is to gain access to the exocytic pathway following fusion of receptosomes with elements of the Golgi. While the exact nature of this constitutive exocytic pathway is not understood, it clearly does not involve concentrative secretory granules, because these cultured cells do not contain such organelles. A scheme summarizing these steps is shown in Fig. 4.

This review has mainly focused on morphologic description of the organelles involved in RME. The biochemical basis of most of these steps remains to be determined.

References

1   Goldstein, J. L., Anderson, R. G. W. and Brown, M. S. (1979) *Nature* 279, 679
2   Pearse, B. M. F. and Bretscher, M. S. (1981) *Annu. Rev. Biochem.* 50, 85
3   Helenius, A., Marsh, M. and White, J. (1980) *Trends Biochem. Sci.* 5, 104
4   Bowers, B. (1964) *Protoplasma* 59, 351
5   Roth, T. F. and Porter, K. R. (1964) *J. Cell Biol.* 20, 313
6   Pearse, B. M. F. (1976) *Proc. Natl Acad. Sci. USA* 73, 1255
7   Pastan, I. and Willingham, M. C. (1981) *Science* 214, 504
8   Willingham, M. C. and Pastan, I. H. (1982) *J. Cell Biol.* 94, 207
9   Willingham, M. C. and Pastan, I. (1980) *Cell* 21, 67
10   Pastan, I. H. and Willingham, M. C. (1981) *Annu. Rev. Physiol.* 43, 239
11   Roth, T. F., Cutting, J. A. and Atlas, S. B. (1976) *J. Supramol. Struct.* 4, 527
12   Heuser, J. and Evans, L. (1980) *J. Cell Biol.* 84, 560
13   Willingham, M. C., Keen, J. H. and Pastan, I. (1981) *Exp. Cell Res.* 132, 329
14   Wehland, J., Willingham, M. C., Dickson, R. and Pastan, I. (1981) *Cell* 25, 105
15   Willingham, M. C., Rutherford, A. V., Gallo, M. G., Wehland, J., Dickson, R. B., Schlegel, R. and Pastan, I. H. (1981) *J. Histochem. Cytochem.* 29, 1003
16   Fan, J. Y., Carpentier, J.-L., Gorden, P., Obberghen, E. V., Blackett, N. M., Grunfeld, C. and Orci, L. (1982) *Proc. Natl Acad. Sci. USA* 79, 7788
17   Peterson, O. W. and van Deurs, B. (1983) *J. Cell Biol.* 96, 277
18   Dickson, R. B., Schlegel, R., Willingham, M. C. and Pastan, I. (1982) *Exp. Cell Res.* 142, 127
19   Schlegel, R., Willingham, M. C. and Pastan, I. (1981) *Biochem. Biophys. Res. Commun.* 102, 992
20   Tycko, B. and Maxfield, F. R. (1982) *Cell* 28, 643
21   Goldfischer, S. (1982) *J. Histochem. Cytochem.* 30, 717
22   Golgi, C. (1898) *Arch. Ital. Biol.* 30, 60
23   Dales, S. (1973) *Bacteriol. Rev.* 37, 103
24   Ryser, H. J.-P., Drummond, I. and Shen, W.-C. (1982) *J. Cell Physiol.* 113, 167

25 FitzGerald, D. J. P., Padmanabhan, R., Pastan, I. H. and Willingham, M. C. (1983) *Cell* 32, 607
26 Ahmed, C. E., Sawyer, H. R. and Niswender, G. D. (1981) *Endocrinology* 109, 1380
27 Karin, M. and Minz, B. (1981) *J. Biol. Chem.* 256, 3245
28 Octave, J.-N., Schneider, V.-J., Crichton, R. R. and Trouet, A. (1981) *Eur. J. Biochem.* 115, 611
29 Willingham, M. C., Pastan, I. H. and Sahagian, G. G. (1982) *J. Histochem. Cytochem.* 30, 104
30 Geuze, H. J., Slot, J. W., Strous, J. A. M., Lodish, H. F. and Schwartz, A. L. (1982) *J. Cell Biol.* 92, 865
31 Wehland, J., Willingham, M., Gallo, M. and Pastan, I. (1982) *Cell* 28, 831

Ira Pastan and Mark C. Willingham are at the Laboratory of Molecular Biology, National Cancer Institute, Bethesda, MD 20205, USA.

Protein kinases in signal transduction

Yasutomi Nishizuka

The biochemical basis of signal transduction across the cell membrane has long been a subject of great interest. The current excitement on protein kinases is focused on a wide variety of extracellular signals which induce phosphorylation of many cellular proteins.

The covalent attachment of phosphate to either seryl or threonyl residues of proteins was first identified by F. Lipmann and P. A. Levene in 1932. The importance of such modifications of proteins in cellular regulation was recognized as early as the 1950s by a series of studies developed by many investigators such as E. W. Sutherland, E. G. Krebs, E. Fischer and J. Larner who clarified the role of reversible phosphorylation in the control of several key enzymes in glycogen metabolism. In the late 1960s E. G. Krebs[1] discovered cAMP-dependent protein kinase (protein kinase A) and its definitive role in signal transduction. Around 1976, when the first issue of *TIBS* was published, several important investigations on protein kinases were started. In April 1978 R. L. Erickson[2] announced from Denver that the *src* gene product is a protein kinase; this was subsequently identified as a tyrosine-specific protein kinase by T. Hunter (1980)[3].

In parallel with these investigations, the studies on inositol phospholipids and receptor functions were initiated by M. R. Hokin and L. E. Hokin in the early 1950s. When inositol phospholipids are degraded, Ca^{2+} is mobilized simultaneously. In 1975, R. H. Michell postulated that this phospholipid breakdown might open the Ca^{2+} gate. At that time, it was becoming clearer from work carried out in Brussels and Nashville that Ca^{2+} is an even more important intracellular mediator in hormone actions such as hepatic glycogenolysis by α-agonists, angiotensin II and vasopressin (H. G. Hers, 1977; H. de Wulf, 1977; J. H. Exton, 1977). Incidentally, myosin light chain kinase (K. Yagi, 1977; D. J. Hartshorne, 1977), phosphorylase kinase (P. Cohen, 1978), and a protein kinase in the nervous tissue (P. Greengard, 1978) were found to be calmodulin-dependent enzymes. These enzymes were previously known to require Ca^{2+}, but the idea that several protein kinases are regulated by a common protein, calmodulin, had been missed for many years (for a review, see Ref. 4).

In 1977, when protein kinase C was first demonstrated in our laboratory as an undefined protein kinase present in many mammalian tissues, the enzyme was activated only by Ca^{2+}-dependent thiol protease and had no obvious role in signal transduction. Later, it was found that the enzyme could also be activated, without proteolysis, by a reversible association with phospholipid in the presence of Ca^{2+}. During the analysis of this protein kinase activation we noticed that the phospholipid prepared from erythrocyte ghosts required Ca^{2+}, while that prepared from brain membranes did not. This difference came from the diacylglycerol that contaminated the brain phospholipid. A small amount of diacylglycerol, one of the primary products of inositol phospholipid breakdown, increased the apparent affinity of protein kinase C for Ca^{2+} dramatically to the

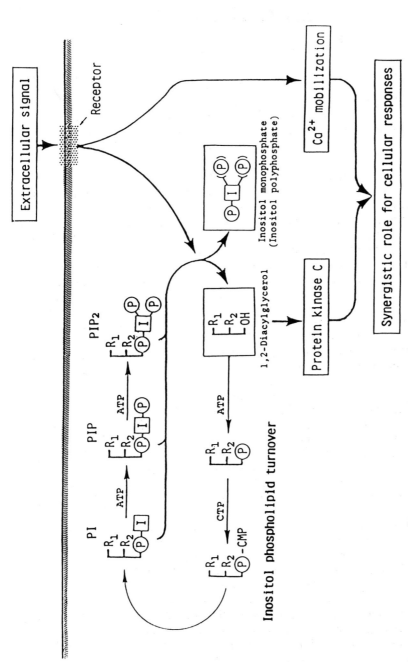

Fig. 1. Synergistic role of Ca^{2+} and protein kinase C for activation of cellular functions and proliferation. PI = phosphatidylinositol; PIP = phosphatidylinositol 4-phosphate; PIP_2 = phosphatidylinositol 4,5-bisphosphate; I = inositol; P = phosphoryl group; R_1 and R_2 = fatty acyl groups.

10^{-7} M range, and thereby activated this enzyme without further addition of this divalent cation (Fig. 1). A ubiquitous distribution of this protein kinase in mammalian and other animal tissues was soon confirmed by J. F. Kuo (1980) in Atlanta.

To identify further diacylglycerol as a 'go-between' of protein phosphorylation (American school) and inositol phospholipid turnover (European school), we developed a procedure to activate protein kinase C by applying synthetic diacylglycerols directly to intact cells. Diacylglycerols that have two long-chain fatty acids – such as diolein – could not be readily intercalated into the intact cell membrane. However, by replacing one of the fatty acids with acetyl group, the resulting diacylglycerols such as 1-oleoyl-2-acetyl-glycerol obtained some detergent-like properties, and could be dispersed easily into the phospholipid bilayer to activate protein kinase C directly. In the summer of 1981, we discussed a possible action of tumour-promoting phorbol esters for protein kinase C, since the tumour promoters have a structure in their molecule very similar to the diacylglycerol we employed. Before long we found that the phorbol esters could activate the enzyme directly as a substitute for diacylglycerol both *in vitro* and *in vivo*. The idea that a protein kinase C–phospholipid complex is the receptor of tumour promoters was presented first at Squaw Valley in March of 1982 (see Ref. 5). This proposal was immediately supported by a number of investigators such as J. E. Niedel (1983) and P. M. Blumberg (1983) who co-purified the phorbol receptor and protein kinase C. Our experiments suggested that, for each molecule of tumour promoters intercalated into the membrane to modify the phospholipid micro-environment, one molecule of protein kinase C moved to it and then produced a quaternary complex of phospholipid, Ca^{2+}, tumour promoter and protein kinase C, which was fully active for protein phosphorylation (a new concept of the 'mobile receptor')[6]. Indeed, in tissues such as brain, the amount of the phorbol receptor roughly matches the amount of protein kinase C. In physiological processes, it may be that one molecule of diacylglycerol produced from inositol phospholipids in membrane activates one molecule of protein kinase C. If so, four molecules of ATP should be consumed for one molecule of the enzyme activated (Fig. 1). Today, we obviously need new techniques to detect such a tiny change in the membrane, and to measure the precise hydrophobic interactions of lipid and protein.

Although both synthetic diacylglycerol and phorbol ester could fully activate protein kinase C, the release of serotonin from platelets was always incomplete. This raised the question of the relative importance of Ca^{2+} mobilization and protein kinase C activation, both of which are evoked by an extracellular signal such as thrombin. We already knew that, for physiological activation, protein kinase C was dependent on diacylglycerol but not on Ca^{2+}. Thus, we know that these two routes, by which information flows from the cell surface into the cell interior, can be opened selectively by a Ca^{2+} ionophore such as A-23187 and synthetic diacylglycerol or tumour promoter (Fig. 2).

On the way back from a Gordon Conference on Hormone Action in August 1982, I found myself seated next to H. Rasmussen on a non-stop PANAM flight from New York to Tokyo. Perhaps, it was the longest conversation on Ca^{2+} in my life! We were both extremely excited about 'calcium sensitivity modulation'; the sensitivity of platelet serotonin secretion to Ca^{2+} was greatly increased by the activation of protein kinase C. At the Royal Society meeting in London, organized by S. V. Perry and P. Cohen in December of 1982, we presented a synergistic role of Ca^{2+} and protein kinase C for the activation of cellular

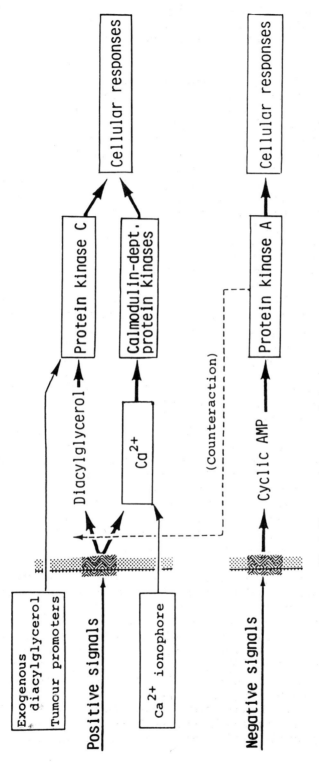

Fig. 2. Transmembrane control of protein kinases in signal transduction.

functions[7]. These two routes may exert differential control over different processes within a single activated cell. It is known for platelets, for instance, that the release reactions from different granules show different sensitivities to thrombin, even though all the release reactions show a similar sensitivity to Ca^{2+} concentrations (D. E. Knight and M. C. Scrutton, 1982). The synergistic role of the two routes was not confined to platelets, but also extended to mast cells and neutrophils for their exocytosis[7]. This proposal was soon supported by D. E. Knight and P. F. Baker (1983)[8] in London for catecholamine release from adrenal medullary cells, and by H. Rasmussen (1983)[9,10] in New Haven for aldosterone secretion from adrenal glomerulosa cells as well as for insulin release from pancreatic islets. By using an intracellular Ca^{2+}-indicator, quin-2, T. J. Rink (1983)[11] in Cambridge later confirmed that serotonin could be released partly from platelets without significant increase of Ca^{2+} when protein kinase C was activated. The synergistic role of the two routes is supported also by J. C. Garrison (1984)[12] in Charlottesville and subsequently by J. N. Fain (1984)[13] in Rhode Island by demonstrating that hepatic glycogenolysis can be provoked by simultaneous addition of Ca^{2+}-ionophore and phorbol ester. J. C. Garrison finds that the opening of these two routes in this way causes the phosphorylation of a full set of the polypeptides that can be phosphorylated by a single extracellular signal such as angiotensin II or vasopressin. The 'synergistic role of Ca^{2+} and protein kinase C' or 'Ca^{2+} sensitivity modulation' is important also for cell proliferation. Using macrophage-depleted lymphocytes treated with phyto-hemagglutinin, we can show that Ca^{2+} mobilization and protein kinase C activation act synergistically for their growth response[14].

The mechanism of increase in intracellular Ca^{2+} remains unclear. Originally, phosphatidylinositol was regarded as a prime target, but it now becomes clearer that phosphatidylinositol bisphosphate is degraded immediately after stimulation of the receptor (for a review, see Ref. 15). In the meetings at Zeist in September of 1983 and at Dallas in January of 1984, M. J. Berridge in Cambridge elicited a discussion on a possible role of inositol 1,4,5-trisphosphate, the other product of the phospholipid breakdown (A. A. Abdel-Latif and J. N. Hawthorne, 1977), for the mobilization of Ca^{2+} from its intracellular reservoir (see Ref. 16). This exciting possibility is currently examined further by many investigators, such as H. Streb in Frankfurt, J. Putney in Richmond, J. Williamson in Philadelphia and J. H. Exton in Nashville. On the other hand, the rise of diacylglycerol concentration in membranes is only transient, and this signal mediator disappears within a minute. It is attractive to imagine that the uncontrollable production of an active form of protein kinase C, of either cellular or viral origin, may promote oncogenesis just like tumour-promoting phorbol esters do. The tumour pro-moters cause the permanent activation of this protein kinase, since they are metabolized only slowly. We need to establish the time sequence and turnover rate of each biochemical event successively occurring after stimulation of receptor.

Although there are dramatic heterogeneities and variations in receptor functions, most tissues possess at least two major classes of receptors (Fig. 2). One class triggers cAMP formation, while the other provokes inositol phospho-lipid turnover, mobilizes Ca^{2+}, releases arachidonic acid and produces cGMP. Arachidonic acid is derived from inositol phospholipids, but in most tissues this fatty acid is released from other phospholipids as well. Some arachidonic acid metabolites such as prostaglandin endoperoxide may serve as activators for guanylate cyclase. Cyclic GMP-dependent protein kinase (protein kinase G), was first found by P. Greengard in 1970[17]. Because of their very similar properties it has been proposed that protein kinases A and G originated from a single ancestral protein (J. D. Corbin, 1977). We have postulated that, in intact platelets, cGMP may constitute an intracellular feedback control that prevents over-response (Refs. 5–7; also R. J. Haslam, 1980). Conversely, in the platelets permeabilized for low molecular substances, cGMP has been proposed to increase their sensitivity to Ca^{2+} (D. E. Knight and M. C. Scrutton, 1984)[18]. Still, it is possible that one of the functions of cyclic GMP is to decrease intracellular Ca^{2+} concentrations in a manner analogous to cAMP. Nevertheless, we still lack crucial information on the role of cGMP and protein kinase G.

The pleiotropic actions of protein kinase A are now firmly established (see Ref. 19). However, a major role of this protein kinase may be 'counteraction' of the signal-induced activation of cellular functions and proliferation. In some mammalian tissues such as liver, adipose tissue and some endocrine cells (*monodirectional control system*), the two classes of receptors mentioned above appear to function in similar directions. In contrast, in some other tissues such as platelets, lymphocytes and some neuronal cells (*bidirectional control system*), cAMP acts 'negatively' rather than 'positively'. The primary target of cAMP appears to be localized in the membrane. It is clear in these tissues that each of receptor-linked events such as inositol phospholipid breakdown, protein kinase C activation, Ca^{2+} mobilization, and arachidonic acid release is all blocked concurrently by an extracellular signal that increases cAMP[5–7]. The molecular basis of this 'counteraction' remains totally unknown. We suspect that this process is not due simply to the direct inhibition of phospholipases by protein kinase A.

An exciting problem is obviously the interaction or cascade of various protein kinases including tyrosine-specific enzymes. This class of enzymes are well known to be associated with the receptors of insulin and other growth-promoting factors such as EGF, PDGF and somatomedin C, and also with certain retroviral oncogene products. Unfortunately, however, no definite information is available as to any function of these protein kinases. At the Cold Spring Harbor meeting on 'The Cancer Cell' in September 1983, a possible cascade from protein kinase C to tyrosine-specific protein kinase was discussed. When cells were stimulated by phorbol ester or diacylglycerol, the amount of cellular phosphoryltyrosine was considerably increased within minutes (M. J. Weber, 1983; G. S. Martin, 1983) (see Ref. 20). However, it was recently suggested that protein kinase C phosphorylates the EGF receptor with a concomitant decrease in its both tyrosine-phosphorylating and EGF-binding activities (T. Hunter, 1984; M. R. Rosner, 1984)[21,22]. Phorbol ester was also shown, in intact cells, to stimulate the phosphorylation of insulin receptor (P. Cuatrecasas, 1983), that has a tyrosine-specific protein kinase activity (C. R. Kahn, 1982). It seems possible on one hand that protein kinase C is involved, directly or indirectly, in 'down-regulation' or 'desensitization' of various receptors, although in a manner as yet uncertain. On the other hand, it is worth noting that tumour promoter and growth factor generally act in concert and synergistically enhance cell proliferation in long term. In fact, the synergistic role of protein kinase C and tyrosine-specific protein kinase is a problem of immediate interest. For insulin, which does not provoke inositol phospholipid turnover, considerable progress has been made on the characterization of its soluble mediators (J. Larner, 1976; L. Jarett, 1979; M. P. Czeck, 1980) (see Ref. 23). However, more information is needed about the transmembrane control of various protein kinases whose intracellular mediators are not elucidated.

We are still far from full understanding of the physiological meaning of an extremely rapid turnover of the phosphate that is covalently linked to protein. However, we do realize that the protein kinases briefly outlined above are on the cross-over point of various pathways for exploring the roles of Ca^{2+}, cAMP, cGMP, diacylglycerol, arachidonic acid and prostaglandins, which all serve as indispensable mediators for signal transduction.

References

1 Walsh, D. A., Perkins, J. P. and Krebs, E. G. (1968) *J. Biol. Chem.* 243, 3763–3765
2 Collett, M. S. and Erickson, R. L. (1978) *Proc. Natl Acad. Sci. USA* 75, 2021–2024
3 Hunter, T. and Sefton, B. M. (1980) *Proc. Natl Acad. Sci USA* 77, 1311–1314
4 Cohen, P. (1982) *Nature* 296, 613–620
5 Nishizuka, Y. (1983) in *Evolution of Hormone-Receptor Systems* (Bradshaw, R. A. and Gill, G. N., eds), pp. 425–439, Alan R. Liss Inc., New York
6 Nishizuka, Y. (1984) *Nature* 308, 693–698
7 Nishizuka, Y. (1983) *Phil. Trans. R. Soc. Lond.* B 302, 101–112
8 Knight, D. E. and Baker, P. E. (1983) *FEBS Letters* 160, 98–100
9 Kojima, I., Lippes, H., Kojima, K. and Rasmussen, H. (1983) *Biochem. Biophys. Res. Commun.* 116, 555–562
10 Zwalich, W., Brown, C. and Rasmussen, H. (1983) *Biochem. Biophys. Res. Commun.* 117, 448–455
11 Rink, T. J., Sanchez, A. and Hallam, T. J. (1983) *Nature* 305, 317–319
12 Garrison, J. C., Johnsen, D. E. and Campanile, C. P. (1984) *J. Biol. Chem.* 259, 3283–3292
13 Fain, J. N., Li, S.-Y., Litosch, I. and Wallace, M. (1984) *Biochem. Biophys. Res. Commun.* 119, 88–94
14 Kaibuchi, K., Sawamura, M., Katakami, Y., Kikkawa, U., Takai, Y. and Nishizuka, Y. (1985) in *Inositol and Phosphoinositides* (Bleasdale, J. E., Eichberg, J. and Hauser, J., eds), pp. 385–398, Humana Press
15 Downes, P. and Michell, R. H. (1982) *Cell Calcium* 3, 467–502
16 Streb, H. D., Irvine, R. F., Berridge, M. J. and Schulz, I. (1983) *Nature* 306, 67–69
17 Kuo, J. F. and Greengard, P. (1970) *J. Biol. Chem.* 245, 2493–2498
18 Knight, D. E. and Scrutton, M. C. (1984) *Nature* 309, 66–68
19 Rosen, O. M. and Krebs, E. G., eds (1981) *Protein Phosphorylation, Cold Spring Harbor Conf. Cell Prolif. Vol. 8*, Cold Spring Harbor Laboratory
20 Levine, A. J., Topp, W. C., Vande Woude, G. F. and Watson, J. D. eds (1984) *The Cancer Cell, Cold Spring Harbor Conf. Cell Prolif. Vol. 11*, Cold Spring Harbor Laboratory
21 Cochet, C. C., Gill, G. N., Meisenhelder, J., Cooper, J. A. and Hunter, T. (1984) *J. Biol. Chem.* 259, 2553–2558
22 Friedman, B., Frackelton, A. R., Ross, A. H., Connors, J. M., Fujiki, H., Sugimura, T. and Rosner, M. R. (1984) *Proc. Natl Acad. Sci. USA* 81, 3034–3038
23 Larner, J., Cheng, K., Schwartz, C., Kikuchi, K., Tamura, S., Creacy, S., Dubler, R., Galasko, G., Pullin, C. and Katz, M. (1982) *Fed. Proc.* 41, 2724–2729

Yasutomi Nishizuka is at the Department of Biochemistry, Kobe University School of Medicine, Kobe 650, Japan.

Receptor phosphorylation and signal transduction across plasma membranes

Beverly Packard

The sites of phosphorylation on signal transducing receptors in plasma membranes appear to have two specificities – the hydroxyls of tyrosine and of serine and threonine. Several recent papers have presented evidence that, upon occupation, some receptors phosphorylate some of their cytoplasmic tyrosine residues as well as tyrosines on other cellular molecules[1-3]. The time between binding and increased phosphorylation suggests that the latter may be involved in signal transduction. Tyrosine kinase activity also seems to be associated with a class of oncogene products[4].

Increases in the numbers of serine and threonine residues of receptor molecules phosphorylated have been measured in cells exposed to transforming agents such as the tumor-promoting phorbol esters[5-7]. These increases appear to result from activation of the enzymic activity of the M_r 77 000 peptide protein kinase C (Ref. 8). This type of phosphorylation may be accounted for by alterations in the affinities of receptors for their respective ligands and changes in absolute numbers of receptors per cell[9,10].

The efficiency of signal transduction may be associated with the degree and type of phosphorylation of the cellular receptors. A property of the transformed state is its autonomy from normal control mechanisms. Signal transduction seems to be associated with the physical state of the receptor; for example, occupation by the ligand may just be a mechanism for inducing a conformational change of the receptor. Cells require receptors in their plasma membranes because the peptide molecules which control essential cellular activities such as growth and differentiation are, being hydrophilic/lipophobic, unable to enter cells which are covered with a coat containing a lipid core, i.e. the plasma membrane. Thus, it is likely that the natural ligands, by binding on the extracellular side of the receptor, can transmit information through the bilayer. This would involve inducing a conformational change on the cytoplasmic side of the receptor through the transmembrane segment of the receptor.

A transformed cell may have a similar but more efficient mechanism, as suggested by the observed autonomy. Perhaps phosphorylation can induce a similar conformational change but directly from the cytoplasmic side. Each phosphate group added to a serine or threonine introduces two negative charges to the molecule. This could give rise to electrostatic interactions and/or local pH changes, possibly leading to a reorganization of the architecture of the region containing plasma membrane–cytoplasmic junctions. One consequence of this could be an increase in the time that receptors stay in a transmitting mode. Using the A431 cells, a line of transformed cells, Rees et al.[11] have reported that the high-affinity class of EGF receptors, which is possibly the most important receptor population, is immobile. They suggest that lateral diffusion over a few hundred nanometers may not be required for the action of low concentrations of

EGF. Thus, a receptor may be locked into an immobile environment when it is transmitting information most efficiently; the cellular mechanism for locking may be phosphorylation of residues on the cytoplasmic side of the receptor. The two specificities observed on signal transducing receptors may represent degrees of effectiveness or efficiency, with phosphorylation of tyrosines being more transient than that of serines and threonines.

The biological response of the cell will depend on the effects which the 'activated' receptors have on molecular constituents around them, such as proteolytic enzymes and cytoskeletal components. For example, the type-beta transforming growth factor appears to be a bifunctional regulator of cellular growth – stimulation or inhibition of growth depends on the target cell and experimental conditions[12]. Furthermore, the phorbol esters can induce either differentiation or dedifferentiation, again the response depends upon the cell under examination and conditions used[13].

Thus, cells appear to have common general mechanisms with several effector routes; their operation in a multitude of environments may produce diverse biological responses. One such mechanism may be the transduction of information across membranes by phosphorylation of hydroxyls on the cytoplasmic sides of membrane receptors, with the observed biological response depending on the specific ligand, cellular receptor, and microenvironments of the cell.

References
1   Cobb, M. H. and Rosen, O. M. (1984) *Biochim. Biophys. Acta.* 738, 1–8
2   Downward, J., Parker, P. and Waterfield, M. D. (1984) *Nature* 311, 483–485
3   Hunter, T., Ling, N. and Cooper, J. A. (1984) *Nature* 311, 480–483
4   Hunter, T. (1984) *J. Natl Cancer Inst.* 73, 773–796
5   Davis, R. J. and Czech, M. P. (1984) *J. Biol. Chem.* 259, 8545–8549
6   Iwashita, S. and Fox, C. F. (1984) *J. Biol. Chem.* 259, 2559–2567
7   Jacobs, S., Sahyoun, N. E., Saltiel, A. R. and Cuatrecasas, P. (1983) *Proc. Natl Acad. Sci. USA.* 80, 6211–6213
8   Nishizuka, Y. (1984) *Nature* 308, 693–698
9   Lee, L.-S. and Weinstein, B. (1979) *Proc. Natl Acad. Sci. USA* 76, 5168–5172
10 Brown, K. D., Dicker, P. and Rozengurt, E. (1979) *Biochem. Biophys. Res. Comm.* 86, 1037–1043
11 Rees, A. R., Gregoriou, M., Johnson, P. and Garland, P. B. (1984) *EMBO J.* 3, 1843–1847
12 Tucker, R. F., Shipley, G. D., Moses, H. L. and Holley, R. W. (1984) *Science* 226, 705–7
13 Diamond, L., O'Brien, T. G. and Baird, W. M. (1980) *Adv. Cancer Res.* 32, 1–74

B. Packard is at the Biology Department, The Johns Hopkins University, Baltimore, MD 21218, USA.

Receptor-stimulated phosphoinositide metabolism: a role for GTP-binding proteins?

Suresh K. Joseph

The cellular response to a hormonal stimulus appears to involve at least three components – a receptor to recognize the hormone, an enzyme system to liberate messenger molecules into the cytoplasm and a third component which acts to couple the receptor to its messenger-generating system. The individual components of this signal transduction system have been extensively investigated in the case of receptors that produce changes in cellular cAMP concentration. These studies have shown that two distinct GTP-binding proteins allow the receptor to express either a stimulatory or inhibitory effect on adenylate cyclase activity. Current information on the structure and characteristics of these two proteins, referred to as N_s and N_i respectively, has been summarized recently in *TIBS*[1].

It has become apparent that a large group of hormones exert their biological effects on cells, not through cAMP, but by activating an enzyme (phospholipase-C) that specifically breaks down inositol phospholipids in the plasma membrane to produce inositol trisphosphate (an intracellular messengers that mobilizes Ca^{2+}) and 1,2-diacylglycerol (an intracellular messenger that activates a protein kinase referred to as protein kinase-C). [See Refs 2, 3 for recent reviews.] The nature of the proteins involved in the coupling of these receptors to phospholipase-C is completely unknown. However, growing experimental evidence strongly suggests that a GTP-binding protein is also involved. An early clue to this came from studies of the influence of GTP (or non-hydrolysable GTP-analogues) on hormone–receptor interactions. GTP decreased the affinity of receptors for their agonist. This was observed not only for receptors coupled to adenylate cyclase, but also for agonists whose physiological effects are now known to be mediated through inositol–lipid breakdown. Some examples are the receptors for chemotactic peptide in neutrophil membranes[4] and for vasopressin in liver membranes[5]. More recently, several groups have provided additional support for an involvement of GTP-binding proteins by making use of a bacterial toxin (derived from the whooping cough bacterium *Bortadella pertussis*). This toxin inhibits the activity of N_i by catalysing the ADP-ribosylation of the 41 kDa, α-subunit of this protein. Pretreatment of neutrophils[6,7], mast cells[8] and HL-60 promyelocytic leukemia cells[9] with this toxin supresses the response of these cells to agonists that initiate inositol–lipid breakdown. The inhibitory effects of the toxin do not appear to result from changes in cellular cAMP concentrations or inhibition of receptor binding. In mast and HL–60 cells it has been observed that pertussis-treatment decreases agonist-dependent production of inositol phosphates. On the basis of these results it has been proposed that the receptors in these cell types may be coupled to phospholipase-C by a GTP-binding protein that is a substrate for pertussis toxin[6–9]. What is not clear at present is whether the coupling protein involved is identical to N_i or is a unique, as yet unrecognized GTP-binding protein. An involvement of N_i would imply that this protein has a dual role as an inhibitor of adenylate cyclase activity and as an activator of phospholipase-C. However, a recent study by Masters _et al._[10] suggests that the protein is not N_i, at least in the chick heart and astrocytoma cells used by these workers. They find that concentrations of pertussis toxin that completely suppress the inhibitory effects of N_i on adenylate cyclase are without effect on inositol phosphate production mediated by muscarinic receptors.

Perhaps the most convincing evidence for an involvement of a GTP-binding protein would be the demonstation that the addition of GTP to an _in-vitro_ system can mimic the effect of adding an agonist. This goal has now been accomplished by several laboratories. Cockcroft and Gomperts[11] have shown that a non-hydrolysable GTP-analogue stimulates polyphosphoinositide breakdown in isolated neutrophil plasma membranes. Litosch _et al._[12] found that GTP-analogues greatly augment the accumulation of inositol phosphates promoted by the addition of an agonist to a cell-free system derived from insect salivary glands. Using platelets that have been made permeable to small molecules, Haslam and coworkers[13] reported that GTP-analogues promote 1,2-diacyl-glycerol formation and the secretion of 5-hydroxytryptamine. These data suggest that a novel GTP-binding protein may be involved in coupling receptors to phospholipase-C. This protein has been tentatively named N_p by Cockroft and Gomperts[11].

What are some of the alternatives regarding the identity of N_p? In late 1984, a new GTP-binding protein (designated N_o) was identified in brain[14,15]. This protein was present in high concentrations and was a substrate for pertussis toxin. However, so far it has not been identified in other tissues. N_o, N_s and N_i are all oligomeric proteins composed of three non-identical subunits. The α-subunits of these proteins have molecular weights of 39, 45 and 41 kDa respectively. The β and γ subunits of each of these proteins were thought to be the same but recent reports of size heterogeneity of these subunits suggest that this may not be the case[14]. Perhaps N_p represents a particular permutation of the known α, β, γ subunits. At meetings held this year at Cardiff and at Lucerne, two groups reported that the individual subunits may also be modified by phosphorylation. Northup and coworkers (University of Calgary) have found that a 35 kDa β-subunit is a substrate for phosphorylation stimulated by epidermal growth factor and Jakobs and colleagues (University of Heidelberg) have shown that that N_i α is a substrate for protein kinase C in platelets. Although the functional significance of these phosphorylations is not clear at present, it is an intriguing possibility that phosphorylation may serve to determine whether the same coupling protein interacts with adenylate cyclase or phospholipase C. Whatever the final outcome, these studies emphasize the importance of the family of GTP-binding proteins in transmembrane signalling and suggest that their involvement in all classes of receptor-linked responses may be the rule rather than the exception.

References

1 Houslay, M. D. (1984) _Trends Biochem. Sci._ 9, 39–40
2 Williamson, J. R., Cooper, R. H., Joseph, S. K. and Thomas, A. P. (1985) _Am. J. Physiol._ 248, C203–C216
3 Majerus, P. W., Wilson, D. B., Connolly, T. M., Bross, T. E. and Neufeld, E. J. (1985) _Trends Biochem. Sci._ 10, 168–171
4 Koo, C., Lefkowitz, R. J. and Snyderman, R. (1983) _J. Clin. Invest._ 72, 748–753
5 Cantau, B., Keppens, S., deWulf, H. D. and Jard, S. (1980) _J. Receptor Res._ 1, 137–168

6   Molski, T. P. P., Naccache, P. H., Marsh, M. L., Kermode, J., Becker, E. L. and
    Sha'afi, R. L. (1984) *Biochem. Biophys. Res. Comm.* 124, 644–650
7   Okajima, F. and Ui, M. (1984) *J. Biol. Chem.* 259, 13863–13871
8   Nakamura, T. and Ui, M. (1985) *J. Biol. Chem.* 260, 3584–3593
9   Brandt, S. J., Dougherty, R. W., Lapetina, E. G. and Niedel, J. E. (1985) *Proc.
    Natl Acad. Sci. USA* 82, 3277–3280
10 Masters, S. B., Martin, M. W., Harden, T. K. and Brown, J. H. (1985) *Biochem. J.*
    227, 933–937
11 Cockroft, S. and Gomperts, B. D. (1985) *Nature* 314, 534–536
12 Litosch, I., Wallis, C. and Fain, J. N. (1985) *J. Biol. Chem.* 260, 5464–5471
13 Haslam, R. J. and Davidson, M. M. L. (1984) *J. Receptor Res.* 4, 605–629
14 Sternweis, P. C. and Robishaw, J. D. (1984) *J. Biol. Chem.* 259, 13806–13813
15 Neer, E. J., Lok, J. M. and Wolf, L. G. (1984) *J. Biol. Chem.* 259, 14222–14229

*S. K. Joseph is at the Department of Biochemistry and Biophysics, Goddard Laboratory,
37 Hamilton Walk, Philadelphia, PA 19104, USA.*

Renewed interest in the polyphosphoinositides

Stephen K. Fisher, Lucio A. A. Van Rooijen and Bernard W. Agranoff

---

The significance of the enhanced cellular phosphatidate and phosphatidylinositol turnover which occurs in response to specific extracellular messengers has been the subject of much interest and speculation. Until recently, much less attention has been paid to the presence of two quantitatively minor phosphorylated derivatives of phosphatidylinositol, known collectively as the polyphosphoinositides. These lipids have an extremely rapid ^{32}P turnover rate and are presumed to be localized predominantly in the plasma membranes. Their turnover now appears to be linked with that of phosphatidate and phosphatidylinositol, and is discussed here in relation to the consequences of ligand–receptor interactions.

Polyphosphoinositides as cell membrane components

Phosphatidylinositol (PhI), as well as two phosphorylated derivatives, phosphatidylinositol 4-phosphate (PhIP) and phosphatidylinositol 4,5-bisphosphate (PhIP$_2$), are found in eukaryotic membranes (see Fig. 1). Because of the highly polar nature of these lipids, their quantitative extraction from tissues usually requires conditions of acidity or high ionic strength, and special thin layer chromatographic procedures are needed for their separation. These two factors may explain much of the past neglect of ligand-stimulated turnover of the polyphosphoinositides. An even more important factor is their rapid resynthesis, such that lipid breakdown can go unnoticed if it is not measured within seconds of ligand addition.

Subcellular distribution and metabolism

PhIP and PhIP$_2$ are synthesized from endogenous PhI via sequential phosphorylation by ATP at the D-4 and D-5 positions of the *myo*-inositol moiety, under the action of specific kinases. In turn, phosphomonoesterases can dephosphorylate PhIP$_2$ to PhIP and PhIP to PhI. The combined effects of the kinases and monoesterases result in the rapid equilibration of radioactivity in the gamma position of ATP with that of the inositide monoester functions. Alternatively, the entire headgroup of the polyphosphoinositides can be removed via phosphodiesteratic cleavage of the phospholipase C variety to yield the apolar product, diacylglycerol (DAG), together with inositol bis- or trisphosphate from PhIP or PhIP$_2$, respectively. Available information from subcellular fractionation studies suggests that most of the relevant enzymes of polyphosphoinositide metabolism are present in both the plasma membrane and in the cytosol[2]. The ability to form labeled PhIP$_2$ from endogenous PhIP and [γ-^{32}P]ATP is a convenient measure of PhIP kinase, and has been demonstrated in purified plasma membrane preparations, as well as in plasma membrane-enriched tissues, e.g. brain, kidney, polymorphonuclear leukocytes and erythyrocytes[2]. However, PhI kinase and/or PhIP kinase activity has also been documented in adrenal chromaffin granules, mitochondria, lysosomes, Golgi preparations and the nuclear envelope. PhI and PhIP kinases are Mg^{2+}-dependent, while the effects of Mg^{2+} and Ca^{2+} on the lipid phosphomonoesterase activities appear to vary with the tissue source of the enzyme. There is general agreement that Ca^{2+} ions at millimolar concentrations selectively activate the phosphodiesterase(s), although the optimal concentration appears to depend upon the assay conditions employed. The enzymatic potential for degradation of the polyphosphoinositides in brain exceeds that of synthesis by one or two orders of magnitude, the most active being an apparent 'phospholipase C' phosphodiesteratic activity. Other

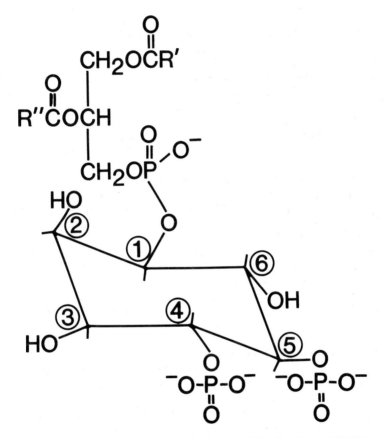

Fig. 1. The structure of phosphatidylinositol 4,5-bisphosphate (PhIP₂). Phosphatidylinositol (PhI) is phosphodiesterified at D-1 of myo-inositol, and has no phosphomonoester substituents, while phosphatidylinositol 4-phosphate (PhIP) is phosphorylated only at the D-4 position. PhI, PhIP and PhIP₂ are also commonly abbreviated as MPI, DPI and TPI (for mono-, di- and triphosphoinositide). The IUB–IUPAC recommended abbreviations are, respectively, PtdIns, PtdIns4P and PtdIns(4,5)P₂. These latter abbreviations, however, have been the subject of some confusion related to their correct structural assignments[1]. In each of the three inositides, the phosphodiesteratically-linked 1,2-diacyl-sn-glycero-3-phosphate is enriched in the 1-stearoyl, 2-arachidonoyl species. The possibility that the inositol lipids serve as a reservoir of arachidonate for prostanoid synthesis has been proposed, although it is not yet clear which inositide or inositide-related lipid is the donor. In this paper, myo-inositol D-1-phosphate, myo-inositol-D-1,4-bisphosphate and myo-inositol-D-1,4,5-trisphosphate are referred to as IP₁, IP₂ and IP₃.

possible pathways for polyphosphoinositide degradation, for example via phospholipase D or A_2 activity, are minor. It thus appears that the breakdown of polyphosphoinositides via a type C phosphodiesteratic cleavage is likely to be of most physiological significance.

Receptors coupled to polyphosphoinositide turnover

The Hokins first demonstrated that activation of certain receptors (e.g. muscarinic cholinergic or α_1-adrenergic) resulted in increased incorporation of added $^{32}P_i$ into phosphatidate (PhA) and PhI. It was subsequently reported that there was a net loss of PhI upon stimulation with the accumulation of an approximately equivalent amount of PhA[3]. This was thought to arise from an initial phosphodiesteratic breakdown of PhI, liberating DAG which was in turn rapidly rephosphorylated in the presence of [^{32}P]ATP to yield [^{32}P]PhA. The PhA was then proposed to be converted to PhI via (CDP–DAG)*, completing a 'phosphatidate–phosphatidylinositol cycle' (Fig. 2). The vast number of studies on stimulated incorporation of $^{32}P_i$ into PhA and PhI or of [^{3}H]inositol into PhI are thus several steps away from the presumed site of receptor–ligand action, i.e. phosphodiesteratic cleavage. In an early study, Durell *et al.*[4] noted a possible increased production of inositol bisphosphate, under conditions of stimulation of brain homogenate with acetylcholine. Despite this observation, and the known metabolic interrelationships between the inositol lipids, a direct effect of receptor activation on PhIP and PhIP$_2$ turnover was not proposed or examined further until 1977, when Abdel-Latif and colleagues demonstrated that exposure of the iris smooth muscle to acetylcholine resulted in increased breakdown of ^{32}P-prelabeled PhIP$_2$ (Ref. 5). These experiments, as well as a number of other indirect indications, led to intensified efforts to identify changes in polyphosphoinositides associated with receptor activation. There are by now numerous documented examples of receptor–ligand interaction linked to polyphosphoinositide turnover (Table 1). In most instances, this has been measured by loss of polyphosphoinositide radioactivity from [^{3}H]inositol or ^{32}P-prelabeled cells. Such studies indicate that radiolabeled PhIP$_2$, and in some instances PhIP as well, is rapidly diminished following addition of a specific ligand. For example, 20% or more of label in PhIP$_2$ is lost within 5–30 s of exposure of platelets to thrombin, of hepatocytes to vasopressin, or of parotid

*CDP–DAG = cytidine diphosphodiacyl glycerol.

Table 1. Receptors coupled to polyphosphoinositide turnover in target tissues

Tissue	Receptor	Refs
Iris smooth muscle	Muscarinic cholinergic, α_1-adrenergic	6
Hepatocytes	Vasopressin, angiotensin	7, 8
Parotid gland	Muscarinic cholinergic, α_1-adrenergic, substance P	9, 10
Platelets	Thrombin, ADP, platelet activating factor	11–14
Brain (nerve ending preparations or slices)	Muscarinic cholinergic, ACTH	10, 15, 16
Avian salt gland	Muscarinic cholinergic	17
Blowfly salivary gland	5-HT$_1$	10
Adrenal gland	ACTH	18
Pancreas	Muscarinic cholinergic, caerulein	19

gland slices to methacholine. There is evidence in the iris smooth muscle, in platelets, and in blowfly salivary gland for the simultaneous release of inositol trisphosphate, a result consistent with the phosphodiesteratic cleavage of PhIP$_2$ following receptor activation. The rapidity with which the lipid breaks down following ligand addition suggests that the cleavage of PhIP$_2$ rather than of PhI constitutes the initial event following receptor activation and that the disappearance of PhI is a secondary response which reflects the process of replenishment of the depleted polyphosphoinositide pool.

Of potential relevance are recent studies with isolated synaptic membranes. Gispen and colleagues have shown that the addition of adrenocorticotropin (ACTH) to these preparations results in an increase in polyphosphoinositide labeling[15]. The effects are interpreted to reflect increased phosphorylation of PhIP to PhIP$_2$. The presumed mechanism is inhibition by ACTH of the phosphorylation of a membrane protein of about M_r 48 000 ('B50') whose phosphorylated form inhibits PhIP kinase. The B50 kinase is thought to be similar or perhaps identical to protein kinase C, found commonly in the cytosol of a number of tissues, particularly brain. While the protein kinase C is isolated from the cytosol and the B50 kinase is membrane-bound, free and bound forms of protein kinase C have been found in cultured cells, and their ratio is reportedly altered by the presence of phorbol esters[20]. ACTH administration, both *in vivo* and *in vitro*, results in a rapid increase in the chemical amounts of both PhIP and PhIP$_2$ in the adrenal, with a time course similar to that reported for corticosterone production[18]. Direct additions of PhIP and PhIP$_2$ to adrenal mitochondria are reported to increase the rate of side chain cleavage of cholesterol to form pregnenolone, a result suggesting that the polyphosphoinositides play a significant role in steroidogenesis.

Calcium and the polyphosphoinositides

Since many receptor–ligand actions that affect polyphosphoinositide turnover exert their physiological effects by increasing intracellular Ca^{2+}, it is not surprising that a direct role for Ca^{2+} in the metabolism of these phospholipids has also been proposed. Central to this issue is the question of whether the increased lipid turnover either (1) is the consequence of an increase in cytosolic Ca^{2+}, (2) mediates the increase in Ca^{2+} permeability, or (3) parallels, but is independent of, Ca^{2+} mobilization. In support of the first possibility is the finding that the muscarinic cholinergic or α_1-adrenergic stimulated breakdown of PhIP$_2$ in iris smooth muscle requires added Ca^{2+}, is abolished in the presence of EGTA or inhibitors of Ca^{2+} translocation, and can be induced by the addition of Ca^{2+} ionophores[6]. In hepatocytes, vasopressin stimulation of PhIP$_2$ breakdown is abolished in the presence of EGTA[7]. Furthermore, the introduction of Ca^{2+} into a nerve ending preparation with the divalent cation ionophore A23187 stimulates the breakdown of PhIP and PhIP$_2$, under conditions in which inositol phosphates accumulate[21]. On the other hand, the stimulated breakdown of PhIP$_2$ in the parotid gland, platelet and pancreas appears insensitive to Ca^{2+} depletion, or is at least less so than the attendant physiological responses. This latter result supports the second possibility, namely that PhIP$_2$ breakdown reflects a molecular mechanism whereby cells gate Ca^{2+}, so that increased turnover of PhIP$_2$ is not regulated by the increase in intracellular Ca^{2+}. An alternative explanation is that these cells are not easily depleted of Ca^{2+} in the presence of extracellular EGTA. The various results, taken together, are compatible with the interpretation that polyphosphoinositide turnover is Ca^{2+}-dependent, but may not be Ca^{2+}-regulated.

Because of the known high affinity of polyphosphoinositides for binding Ca^{2+} ions, their plasma membrane localization and potential for rapid degradation upon receptor activation, these lipids have been considered as a possible reservoir of cell Ca^{2+}. It has been demonstrated that the Ca^{2+}-binding activity of erythrocytes increases directly with the state of inositide phosphorylation[22]. Similarly, phosphorylation of renal brush border membrane vesicles results in stimulation of Ca^{2+} intake, with increased phosphoinositide and PhA content[23]. It is less certain, however, that the chemical amounts of Ca^{2+} bound to polyphosphoinositides suffice to account for the increase in cytosolic Ca^{2+} resulting from receptor activation. Calculations of amounts of Ca^{2+} released from $PhIP_2$ in hormone-stimulated hepatocytes indicate that only a small fraction of the measured Ca^{2+} released from these cells could be derived from the polyphosphoinositide pool. In the case of platelets, the calculated amounts of Ca^{2+} released from $PhIP_2$ following ADP addition could, however, account for an increase in intracellular Ca^{2+} by 10 μM[13]. These observations must be tempered by considerations of conditions *in vivo*. For example, these various calculations assume that Ca^{2+} is the sole cation present. Although cytosolic Mg^{2+} is in fact present at greater concentration than Ca^{2+} and binds to the polyphosphoinositides with similar affinity, Mg^{2+} or Ca^{2+} salts of the polyphosphoinositides probably have different affinities for the enzymes for which they are substrates.

It is alternatively possible that products of phosphoinositide turnover trigger the rise in cell Ca^{2+}. For example, phosphatidate has been shown to have Ca^{2+} ionophore activity, as have arachidonate metabolites. Another candidate is IP_3, a product of $PhIP_2$ degradation. Preliminary reports indicate that IP_3 can increase Ca^{2+} efflux from cells under specified conditions[24]. In platelets, the physiological response resulting from a rise in intracellular Ca^{2+} can be mimicked by accumulation of DAG, this effect being mediated through activation of protein kinase C (Ref. 25). Thus, the production of both DAG and IP_3 may be necessary for expression of a full response. In fact, experimentally-induced increases in intracellular Ca^{2+} and DAG elicit synergistic rather than additive cell responses in the platelet[26].

Inositide turnover in the nervous system

While much of our present knowledge of the polyphosphoinositides has been obtained with non-neural preparations, it is likely that the role of these lipids in the central nervous system will come under increasing scrutiny. Brain contains high concentrations of polyphosphoinositides localized to two distinct pools: a metabolically stable pool associated with myelin and a more labile pool present in neuronal or glial plasma membranes[27]. Nerve ending preparations support a muscarinic cholinergic stimulation of PhA and PhI labeling, which has been localized post-synaptically[28]. Membranes from nerve ending preparations contain Ca^{2+}-activated phosphodiesterase, capable of the rapid degradation of endogenous $PhIP_2$ and $PhIP$[29]. Although there is evidence for a neurotransmitter-linked effect on PhIP and $PhIP_2$ turnover, direct stimulation of inositol lipid breakdown in the CNS and corresponding release of inositol phosphates is difficult to demonstrate. However, the observation by Allison *et al.*[30] that lithium administration to rats results in an intracerebral accumulation of IP_1, has been successfully exploited *in vitro*. A stimulated release of IP_1 can be detected following the addition of a number of neurohormones to brain slices incubated in the presence of Li^+ (Ref. 31). This effect of Li^+ is believed to be due to an

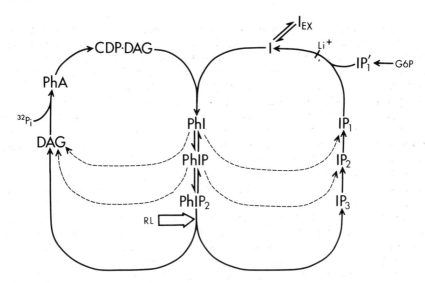

Fig. 2. Cyclic turnover of inositol lipids. The originally proposed cycle (upper left) of PhI–>DAG–>PhA–>CDP-DAG–>PhI is now extended to include the poly-phosphoinositides. While phosphodiesteratic cleavage of PhIP is indicated, there is better evidence for stimulated PhIP₂ breakdown following receptor–ligand (RL) activation. The cycle on the right demonstrates the sequential breakdown of IP₃ to inositol. The breakdown of IP₁ is blocked by Li⁺. Cellular inositol is supplied exogenously (I_{ex}) or produced by degradation of L-myo-inositol phosphate (IP'ᵢ) formed via cyclization of glucose 6-phosphate (G6P).

inhibition of the phosphatase that degrades IP_1 (Fig. 2). The increase in IP_1 could result from the phosphodiesteratic cleavage of PhI, but recent evidence favors an initial release of IP_3 (Ref. 10), followed by degradation to IP_1 by phosphatases. Whether this effect of Li⁺ can be related to its known psychotherapeutic effects remains an open question. However, its use as an experimental tool can be expected to provide much new information, both in the identification of new neurotransmitter systems which exert their effects through inositol lipid turnover and in the elucidation of the role of polyphosphoinositides in cell–cell communication in the brain.

References
1 Agranoff, B. W. (1978) Trends Biochem. Sci. 3, N283–285
2 Michell, R. H. (1975) Biochim. Biophys. Acta 415, 81–147
3 Hokin-Neaverson, M. R. (1974) Biochem. Biophys. Res. Commun. 58, 763–768
4 Durell, J., Sodd, M. A. and Friedel, R. O. (1968) Life Sci. 7, 363–368
5 Abdel-Latif, A. A., Akhtar, R. A. and Hawthorne, J. N. (1977) Biochem. J. 162, 61–73
6 Abdel-Latif, A. A. (1983) in Handbook of Neurochemistry, 2nd Ed., Vol. 3 (Lajtha, A., ed.), pp. 91–131, Plenum Press, New York
7 Rhodes, D., Prpic, V., Exton, J. H. and Blackmore, P. F. (1983) J. Biol. Chem. 258, 2770–2773
8 Creba, J. A., Downes, C. P., Hawkins, P. T., Brewster, G., Michell, R H. and Kirk, C. J. (1983) Biochem. J. 212, 733–747
9 Weiss, S. J., McKinney, J. S. and Putney, J. W., Jr (1982) Biochem. J. 206, 555–560
10 Berridge, M. J., Dawson, R. M. C., Downes, C. P., Heslop, J. P. and Irvine, R. F. (1983) Biochem. J. 212, 473–482

11   Agranoff, B. W., Murthy, P. and Seguin, E. B. (1983) *J. Biol. Chem.* 258, 2076–2078

12   Billah, M. M. and Lapetina, E. G. (1982) *Biochem. Biophys. Res. Commun.* 109, 217–222

13   Vickers, J. D., Kinlough-Rathbone, R. L. and Mustard, J. F. (1982) *Blood* 60, 1247–1249

14   Billah, M. M. and Lapetina, E. G. (1983) *Proc. Natl Acad. Sci.* 80, 965–968

15   Jolles, J., Zwiers, H., Dekker, A., Wirtz, K. W. A. and Gispen, W. H. (1981) *Biochem. J.* 194, 283–291

16   Fisher, S. K. and Agranoff, B. W. (1981) *J. Neurochem.* 37, 968–977

17   Fisher, S. K., Hootman, S. R., Heacock, A. M., Ernst, S. A. and Agranoff, B. W. (1983) *FEBS Lett.* 155, 43–46

18   Farese, R. V., Sabir, A. M., Vandor, S. L. and Larson, R. E. (1980) *J. Biol. Chem.* 255, 5728–5734

19   Putney, J. W., Burgess, G. M., Halenda, S. P., McKinney, J. S. and Rubin, R. P. (1983) *Biochem. J.* 212, 483–488

20   Kraft, A. S. and Anderson, W. B. (1983) *Nature* 301, 621–623

21   Griffin, H. D. and Hawthorne, J. N. (1978) *Biochem. J.* 176, 541–552

22   Buckley, J. T. and Hawthorne, J. N. (1972) *J. Biol. Chem.* 247, 7218–7223

23   Hruska, K. A., Mills, S. C., Khalifa, S. and Hammerman, M. R. (1983) *J. Biol. Chem.* 258, 2501–2507

24   Streb, H., Irvine, R. F., Berridge, M. J. and Schulz, I. *Nature* 306, 67–69

25   Nishizuka, Y. (1983) *Trends Biochem. Sci.* 8, 13–16

26   Michell, R. H. (1983) *Trends Biochem. Sci.* 8, 263–265

27   Eichberg, J. and Hauser, G. (1967) *Biochim. Biophys. Acta* 144, 415–422

28   Agranoff, B. W. (1983) *Life Sci.* 32, 2047–2054

29   Van Rooijen, L. A. A., Seguin, E. B. and Agranoff, B. W. (1983) *Biochem. Biophys. Res. Commun.* 112, 919–926

30   Allison, J. H., Blisner, M. E., Holland, W. H., Hipps, P. P. and Sherman, W. R. (1976) *Biochem, Biophys. Res. Commun.* 71, 664–670

31   Berridge, M. J., Downes, C. P. and Hanley, M. R. (1982) *Biochem. J.* 206, 587–595

The authors are at the Neuroscience Laboratory Building, University of Michigan, Ann Arbor, MI 48109, USA. The present address of L. A. A. Van Rooijen is Neurobiology Department Troponwerke, Berliner Strasse, 156 5000 Cologne 80, FRG.

Addendum – *S. K. Fisher, L. A. A. Van Rooijen and B. W. Agranoff*

That the phosphodiesteratic cleavage of phosphatidylinositol 4,5-bisphosphate (PhIP$_2$) represents an early biochemical consequence of receptor–ligand interaction continues to receive experimental support from studies in a diverse range of tissues (see Ref. 32 for review). In addition, progress has been made towards an understanding of the roles played in cell function by the two breakdown products, inositol 1,4,5-trisphosphate (IP$_3$) and diacylglycerol (DAG). Addition of IP$_3$ to detergent-permeabilized cells (pancreatic acinar[33], hepatocytes[34,35] and 3T3-fibroblasts[36]) results in mobilization of intracellular calcium, as determined either through an increased efflux of $^{45}Ca^{2+}$ from prelabeled cells or by an increased fluorescence of the intracellular Ca^{2+} indicator, quin-2. Preferential mobilization of calcium pools after IP$_3$ addition has been confirmed by demonstration of the release of calcium from microsomal but not from mitochondrial fractions of rat insulinoma cells[37]. While IP$_3$ is effective in calcium mobilization, inositol mono-

and bisphosphates are not. In some tissues, much of the inositol trisphosphate that forms is the 1,3,4-isomer rather than the expected 1,4,5-variety[38]. The origin of the 1,3,4-isomer is yet to be established with certainty, but one possibility is that it results from the dephosphorylation of inositol 1,3,4,5-tetrakisphosphate (IP$_4$), which is formed alongside IP$_3$ in stimulated tissues[39]. IP$_4$ itself may be formed from the 1,4,5-IP$_3$ via the action of an ATP-dependent kinase. While it could be formed by the cleavage of phosphatidylinositol 3,4,5-trisphosphate, there is no evidence for the existence of the lipid. DAG, the other product of PhIP$_2$ hydrolysis, is implicated in the activation of protein kinase C (PK-C)[40]. In platelets stimulated by thrombin[40], or hepatocytes by vasopressin[41], a rapid accumulation of DAG precedes the phosphorylation of certain cellular proteins. The effects of DAG on protein phosphorylation can be mimicked by the addition of phorbol esters, agents which possess a DAG-like structure, and like DAG, lower the affinity of PK-C for calcium. Activation of PK-C may also serve as a regulatory mechanism for inositol lipid turnover, since the addition of phorbol esters inhibits both receptor-mediated phosphoinositide turnover[42,43] and calcium mobilization[43].

The polyphosphoinositides have also been implicated in the proliferative response that some cultured cells undergo following the addition of growth factors and mitogens, e.g., platelet-derived growth factor (PDGF), vasopressin and bombesin[44]. Addition to 3T3 fibroblasts of PDGF, a product of c-*sis* proto-oncogene, results in both an elevation of intracellular calcium concentration and in the alkalinization of the cytoplasm. The latter event results from stimulation of a Na$^+$/H$^+$ antiporter system, which becomes fully functional after activation of PK-C. Both the increase in intracellular calcium and in pH appear to be pre-requisites for the initiation of DNA synthesis and cell proliferation. The possibility has been raised that the proteins encoded by v-*src* and v-*ros* oncogenes, both known to possess protein-tyrosine kinase activity, may themselves also act as inositol lipid kinases[45,46]. More recent evidence indicates that the two kinase activities reside on separate molecules[47]. However, the demonstration that the steady-state cellular levels of PhIP$_2$, DAG and inositol phosphates are raised in 3T3 and NRK fibroblasts transformed with three different *ras* genes[48], suggests that this oncogene product may indeed act to regulate phosphoinositide turnover, possibly through a GTP-binding protein mechanism[49].

References

32   Berridge, M. J. and Irvine, R. F. (1984) *Nature* 312, 315–321
33   Streb, H., Irvine, R. F., Berridge, M. J. and Schulz, I. (1983) *Nature* 306, 67–69
34   Burgess, G. M., Godfrey, P. P., McKinney, J. S., Berridge, M. J., Irvine, R. F. and Putney, J. R., Jr (1984) *Nature* 309, 63–66
35   Thomas, A. P., Alexander, J. and Williamson, J. R. (1984) *J. Biol. Chem.* 259, 5574–5584
36   Berridge, M. J., Heslop, J. P., Irvine, R. F. and Brown, K. D. (1984) *Biochem. J.* 222, 195–201
37   Prentki, M., Biden, T. J., Janjic, D., Irvine, R. F., Berridge, M. J. and Wollheim, C. B. (1984) *Nature* 309, 562–564
38   Burgess, G. M., McKinney, J. S., Irvine, R. F. and Putney, J. W., Jr (1985) *Biochem. J.* 232, 237–243
39   Batty, I. R., Nahorski, S. R. and Irvine, R. F. (1985) *Biochem. J.* 232, 211–215
40   Nishizuka, Y. (1984) *Science* 225, 1365–1370
41   Garrison, J. C., Johnsen, D. E. and Campanile, C. P. (1984) *J. Biol. Chem.* 259, 3283–3292

42 Labarca, R., Janowsky, A., Patel, J. and Paul, S. M. (1984) *Biochem. Biophys. Res. Commun.* 123, 703–709
43 Orellana, S. A., Solski, P. A. and Brown, J. H. (1985) *J. Biol. Chem.* 260, 5236–5239
44 Berridge, M. J. (1984) *Bio/technology* 2, 541–546
45 Sugimoto, Y., Whitman, M., Cantley, L. C. and Erikson, R. L. (1984) *Proc. Natl Acad. Sci. USA* 81, 2117–2121
46 Macara, I. G., Marinetti, G. V. and Balduzzi, P. C. (1984) *Proc. Natl Acad. Sci. USA* 81, 2728–2732
47 Thompson, D. M., Cochet, C., Chambaz, E. M. and Gill, G. N. (1985) *J. Biol. Chem.* 260, 8824–8830
48 Fleischman, L. F., Chahwala, S. B. and Cantley, L. (1986) *Science* 231, 407–410
49 Joseph, S. K. (1985) *Trends Biochem. Sci.* 10, 297–298 (and this book pp. 257–259)

Phosphoinositide turnover provides a link in stimulus–response coupling

Philip W. Majerus, David B. Wilson, Thomas M. Connolly, Teresa E. Bross and Ellis J. Neufeld

Much excitement has resulted from the discovery that phosphatidylinositol and its phosphorylated derivatives are storage forms of messenger molecules that can be released in response to specific extracellular signals. Signal molecules bind to cell surface receptors and the messenger molecules derived from the phosphoinositides couple the signal to a variety of responses within and between cells.

Phosphoinositides are minor phospholipids ($\sim 5\%$ of phospholipid) that turnover much more rapidly than other membrane lipids. Hokin and Hokin were the first to observe that acetylcholine accelerates this turnover rate[1]. Their results with pancreatic tissue have since been observed repeatedly in a myriad of tissues from yeast and insects to man[2]. Although many theories have been proposed, no clear function for the process was demonstrated until recently.

The production of icosanoid mediators (oxygenated derivatives of arachidonic acid and related polyunsaturated fatty acids such as prostaglandins, thromboxanes, leukotrienes) is limited by the release of arachidonate from phospholipids. In 1979, it was discovered that hydrolysis of phosphatidylinositol (PI) by phospholipase C resulted in transient accumulation of 1,2-diglyceride in platelets[3]. Diglyceride[4]- and monoglyceride-lipases[5] were found to be involved in sequential degradation of diglyceride in platelets to release arachidonate. This was the first evidence for phosphoinositide turnover as a signal-generating system. The mechanism for arachidonate release operates in many cells and tissues, although other mechanisms do exist. In platelets, it appears that the initial release of arachidonate after stimulation is from inositol phospholipids, while that released later is from phosphatidylcholine[6].

A second function for diglyceride was discovered by Nishizuka *et al.* who described a diglyceride-dependent protein kinase, designated protein kinase C, that phosphorylates serine and threonine residues of various cellular proteins[7]. This enzyme has a hydrophilic catalytic domain and a hydrophobic membrane-binding domain and is located in the cytosol of unstimulated cells where it is presumably inactive. According to a current hypothesis, when 1,2-diglyceride is produced, protein kinase C binds to the cell membrane (presumably to phosphatidylserine) and shifts the Ca^{2+}-dependence of the enzyme from mM to μM concentrations, thereby activating the enzyme. Protein kinase C activation has been studied most extensively in blood platelets where phosphorylation of a 40 kDa protein follows stimulation by physiological agonists. The functions of this and other protein substrates phosphorylated by protein kinase C are not yet known.

The third and most recently discovered signal molecule generated by phosphoinositide turnover is inositol 1,4,5-trisphosphate (IP_3), one of the products of phospholipase C hydrolysis of phosphatidylinositol 4,5-diphosphate (PI 4,5-P_2, see Fig. 1). Berridge *et al.*[8] proposed that IP_3 is the messenger that triggers intracellular calcium fluxes in cells on the basis (initially) of two observations: phosphatidylinositol turnover takes place in all tissues in which calcium fluxes occur upon cell activation[9]; and polyphosphoinositide turnover precedes phosphatidylinositol turnover and, therefore, could be the initial event of cell activation[10]. Numerous investigators have provided evidence to substantiate the hypothesis[8]; the most convincing is that IP_3 can be micro-injected into photoreceptor cells of *Limulus* to produce a transient rise in intracellular Ca^{2+} concentration[11] and a voltage response that mimics that produced by light[8]. The extracellular signal molecules that initiate phosphoinositide turnover have been reviewed recently, as have the roles of IP_3, diglyceride and arachidonate as messenger molecules[7,8,12]. Here, we ask several questions about phosphoinositide turnover.

Which phosphoinositides are broken down by phospholipase C?

Berridge[10] and Downes and Wusteman[13] noted that IP_3 appeared to be formed before inositol 1-phosphate (I 1-P) when blowfly salivary glands and rat parotid glands were stimulated by agonists; they proposed that phosphoinositide turnover proceeds by hydrolysis of PI 4,5-P_2 by phospholipase C. According to this now widely espoused idea, the apparent breakdown of PI involves conversion of PI to PI 4,5-P_2 before phospholipase C hydrolysis of the latter compound and then conversion of product IP_3 to I 1-P. In this scheme, I 1-P is derived from phosphatase action on IP_3 rather than from phospholipase cleavage of PI. This

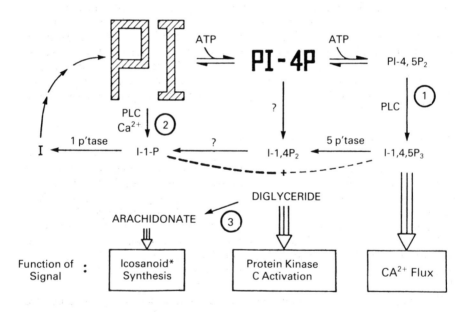

Fig. 1. *The proposed sequence of reactions in phosphoinositide signal transduction in thrombin-stimulated platelets. The sizes of the phosphoinositide letters reflect their molecular masses. Therefore, most diglyceride is derived from PI. The question marks indicate that neither the magnitude of phospholipase C (PLC) hydrolysis of PI 4-P nor the route of metabolism of I 1,4-P_2 is known. * Icosanoids include prostaglandins, thromboxanes, leukotrienes, and other oxygenated derivatives of arachidonate and related polyunsaturated fatty acids.*

seemed unlikely to us because all three phosphoinositides are substrates for the same phospholipase C enzymes[14]. We find that they are all readily hydrolysed by two different PI-specific phospholipase C enzymes isolated from ram seminal vesicles. Unstimulated platelets contain about 18, 3, and 1.3 nmol/10^9 cells of PI, PI 4-P and PI 4,5-P_2, respectively[15]. When platelets are stimulated with thrombin, there is a transient fall in PI 4,5-P_2 (with return to baseline by 90 s), no change in mass of PI 4-P, and ~50% breakdown of PI. If all PI hydrolysis proceeds via polyphosphoinositides, these moieties must turn over several times within 90 s after thrombin addition. It is possible to determine the magnitude of hydrolysis of each of the phosphoinositides in intact cells by measuring the flux or rate of conversion of PI to PI 4-P and PI 4,5-P_2 in response to cell stimulation. We measured these rates of conversion in thrombin-stimulated human platelets[15]. The conversion of PI to PI 4-P and PI 4,5 P_2 was estimated by $^{32}PO_4$-labeling of the monoester phosphates of polyphosphoinositides under conditions where the specific activity of the γ-phosphate of ATP is higher than the monoester phosphates of the inositol lipids. Under these conditions, an increase in the rate of formation of a polyphosphoinositide is reflected in the rate of increase in specific activity. When thrombin is added to the cells, there is a rapid increase in the rate of increase in specific activity of the 5-phosphate, indicating that increased turnover of PI 4,5-P_2 is associated with thrombin stimulation. (This type of experiment cannot distinguish dephosphorylation–rephosphorylation of PI 4,5-P_2 from phospholipase C cleavage coupled with increased net formation from PI 4-P, although in view of other results, the latter seems more likely.) In contrast, thrombin stimulation does not change the rate of labeling of the 4-phosphate of PI 4-P. During thrombin stimulation of platelets (90 s), there is very little net formation of polyphosphoinositides. In other words, PI breakdown in thrombin-stimulated platelets results from the direct action of phospholipase C on PI. This means that the production of IP_3 and diglyceride are separate events and much more diglyceride is produced than IP_3. This contrasts sharply with the scheme outlined previously where IP_3 and diglyceride are produced together in equimolar amounts.

Does breakdown of PI 4,5-P_2 stimulate flux?

We have isolated two distinct phospholipase C enzymes specific for phosphatidylinositol and find that all three phosphoinositides are good substrates for both of these enzymes, despite the apparently great differences between the head groups on these molecules. However, only PI hydrolysis is absolutely Ca^{2+}-dependent (K_m = 1–2 μM). Both PI 4-P and PI 4,5-P_2 are readily hydrolysed even in the presence of EGTA without added calcium ions[15]. Thus, PI hydrolysis is Ca^{2+}-dependent but polyphosphoinositide hydrolysis is not. This is consistent with the notion that IP_3 triggers intracellular calcium flux. Other work also suggests that hydrolysis of the polyphosphoinositide PI 4,5-P_2 is Ca^{2+}-independent[16,17].

We suggest the following sequence of generation of phosphoinositide-derived messengers (see Fig. 1). Upon activation of the cell, phospholipase C catalyses PI 4,5-P_2 hydrolysis and the IP_3 generated triggers an increase in intracellular Ca^{2+}. The Ca^{2+} signal allows phospholipase C to hydrolyse PI. Since the total amount of PI hydrolysed is ten times greater than that of PI 4,5-P_2, PI hydrolysis provides most of the diglyceride used to liberate icosanoid precursor fatty acids. The PI-generated diglyceride also activates protein kinase C which itself requires Ca^{2+} provided by the IP_3 mediated Ca^{2+} flux. This scenario differs from previous hypotheses[7,8] in that the production of the various messenger molecules is separated. IP_3 is the initial signal and is produced first, since diglyceride production requires Ca^{2+}. Our hypothesis also implies that the cellular level of PI 4,5-P_2 may be important, as outlined below.

What are the consequences of increased PI 4,5-P_2?

PI 4,5-P_2 represents less than 10% of phospholipid inositol, indicating limited production. Since little net formation of polyphosphoinositides occurs upon stimulation of platelets, the magnitude and/or duration of the Ca^{2+} flux produced could, in principle, be determined by the amount of PI 4,5-P_2 available for hydrolysis by phospholipase C at the time of cell stimulation. Recently, several protein tyrosine kinases have been found to catalyse the phosphorylation of PI to PI 4-P and in some cases PI 4-P to PI 4,5-P_2; they include the transforming protein of the Rous sarcoma virus, pp60[v−src] (Ref. 18), and that of the Avian sarcoma virus, UR 2 (Ref. 19). More recently tyrosine protein kinases of platelet-derived growth factor receptor (D. Porter, T. Deuel, and our unpublished results) and insulin receptor[20] have been shown to catalyse phosphorylation of PI. Tumor-promoting phorbol esters and a synthetic diglyceride, which activates protein kinase C, also lead to increased formation of polyphosphoinositides in platelets[21,22]. These studies have led to the speculation that lipid phosphorylation may influence the ability of these agents to stimulate cell growth. However, the PI kinase activity of these tyrosine protein kinases is meager, implying that a nonphysiological phosphate acceptor may be phosphorylated 'nonspecifically' at a low rate[12]. Furthermore, it has not been demonstrated that increased concentrations of PI 4,5-P_2 in cells are physiologically significant. However, high concentrations may be deleterious by analogy to the hypothesis obtained from studies of the tumor-promoting phorbol esters. The phorbol esters mimic diglyceride in activating protein kinase C but they differ from diglyceride in that they are not degraded rapidly and so provide a prolonged rather than a transient signal. These agents promote tumor formation, implying that overstimulation of protein kinase C is deleterious and results in deranged cell growth. A similar result might be produced from a prolonged or increased IP_3 signal derived from increased production of PI 4,5-P_2.

How is phosphoinositide turnover initiated?

When agonists occupy cell surface receptors, phospholipase C is activated. This activation may be controlled in a manner similar to that proposed for protein kinase C, i.e. the cytosolic phospholipase C enzyme is inactive until it is bound to a membrane-containing substrate PI. In fact, the enzyme will only cleave PI that is within a lipid bilayer. A dibutyryl phosphonate analog of PI that is hydrophilic and not incorporated into lipid bilayers does not inhibit PI-specific phospholipase C hydrolysis of PI, while a similar analog containing long-chain fatty acids, that is incorporated into membranes, is inhibitory[23]. Lipid membranes containing phosphatidyl choline are poor substrates for PI hydrolysis because the enzyme does not bind to them[14]. Thus, cell activation may result in protein or lipid rearrangement that allows PI-specific phospholipase C to bind to the membrane and initiate polyphosphoinositide breakdown. A membrane protein that may facilitate such a reaction is one of the GTP binding proteins known to be involved in adenylate cyclase regulation, designated G_i. It was shown recently that pertussis toxin treatment of neutrophils blocks agonist-induced arachidonate release[24,25]. This toxin catalyses the ADP ribosylation of the G_i protein, thereby inactivating it. Although not yet demonstrated directly, it may be that the inhibition of arachidonate release is a consequence of a lack of phospholipase C activation. In permeabilized platelets, nonhydrolysable analogs of GTP can stimulate phosphoinositide turnover directly, further indicating a role for GTP-binding proteins in the activation of the PI response[26]. More experiments are required to establish whether this hypothesis is valid.

How is the IP_3 signal controlled?

This discussion has focused mainly on factors controlling production of IP_3; however, factors affecting its destruction may also be important. The generation and destruction of IP_3 is analogous to the cyclic AMP system, with phospholipase C serving a function similar to that of adenylate cyclase. The presumed enzyme that converts IP_3 to IP_2 would therefore be analogous to cyclic AMP phosphodiesterase. Preliminary experiments using blowfly salivary glands[27], erythrocytes[28] and liver cells[29] suggested that IP_3 is converted to IP_2. In the case of erythrocytes, the enzyme is membrane-bound and converts I 1,4,5-P_3 to I 1,4-P_2 as well as glycerophosphorylinositol 4,5-P_2 to glycerophosphorylinositol 4-P. We have isolated a different enzyme from platelets that catalyses the conversion of I 1,4,5-P_3 to I 1,4-P_2 (Ref. 30). This enzyme is soluble and does not hydrolyse the glycerophosphorylinositol phosphates. It is a single polypeptide chain of ~38 kDa and its activity is inhibited by Ca^{2+}. Whether inhibition by Ca^{2+} plays a physiological role in Ca^{2+} signal generation remains to be seen. The exact pathway of degradation of IP_2 is also unknown (Fig. 1).

In summary we have addressed five questions concerning PI turnover; the first two have been answered, at least in part. Answering the last three questions and defining the role of this signal tranduction system in cell growth awaits further experiments.

Acknowledgements

The authors thank Joel Brown and also Denny Porter and Tom Deuel for their unpublished results showing Ca^{2+} fluxes in *Limulus* photoreceptors in response to IP_3 and PI kinase activity by the platelet-derived growth factor receptor, respectively. This research was supported by Grants HLBI 14147 (Specialized Center for Research in Thrombosis) and HL 16634 from the National Institutes of Health, and, in part, by National Institutes of Health Research Service Award, GM 07200, Medical Scientist, from the National Institute of General Medical Sciences.

References

1 Hokin, M. R. and Hokin, I. E. (1953) *J. Biol. Chem.* 203, 967–977
2 Mitchell, R. H. (1975) *Biochim. Biophys. Acta* 415, 81–147
3 Rittenhouse-Simmons, S. (1979) *J. Clin. Invest.* 63, 580–587
4 Bell, R. L., Kennerly, D. A., Stanford, N. and Majerus, P. W. (1979) *Proc. Natl Acad. Sci. USA* 76, 3238–3241
5 Prescott, S. M. and Majerus, P. W. (1983) *J. Biol. Chem.* 258, 764–769
6 Rittenhouse-Simmons, S. and Deykin, D. (1981) in *Platelets in Biology and Pathology II* (Gordon, J. L., ed.), pp. 349–372, Elsevier/North-Holland Biomedical Press
7 Nishizuka, Y. (1984) *Nature* 308, 693–697
8 Berridge, M. J. and Irvine, R. F. (1984) *Nature* 312, 315–321
9 Michell, R. H. and Kirk, C. J. (1981) *Trends Pharmacol. Sci.* 2, 86–90
10 Berridge, M. J. (1983) *Biochem. J.* 212, 849–858

11 Brown, J. E. and Rubin, L. J. (1984) *Biochem. Biophys. Res. Commun.* 125, 1137–1142

12 Majerus, P. W., Neufeld, E. J. and Wilson, D. B. (1984) *Cell* 37, 701–703

13 Downes, C. P. and Wusteman, M. M. (1983) *Biochem. J.* 216, 633–640

14 Wilson, D. B., Bross, T. E., Hofmann, S. L. and Majerus, P. W. (1984) *J. Biol. Chem.* 259, 11718–11724

15 Wilson, D. B., Neufeld, E. J. and Majerus, P. W. (1985) *J. Biol. Chem.* 260, 1046–1051

16 Michell, R. H., Kirk, C. J., Jones, L. M., Downes, C. P. and Creba, J. A. (1981) *Phil. Trans. R. Soc. London B* 269, 123–137

17 Billah, M. M. and Lapetina, E. G. (1982) *Biochem. Biophys. Res. Commun.* 109, 217–222

18 Sugimoto, Y., Whitman, M., Cantley, L. C. and Erikson, R. L. (1984) *Proc. Natl Acad. Sci. USA* 81, 2117–2121

19 Macara, I. G., Marinetti, G. V. and Balduzzi, P. C. (1984) *Proc. Natl Acad. Sci. USA* 81, 2728–2732

20 Machicao, E. and Wieland, O. H. (1984) *FEBS Lett.* 175, 113–116

21 Helenda, S. P. and Feinstein, M. B. (1984) *Biochem. Biophys. Res. Commun.* 124, 507–513

22 de Chaffoy de Courcelles, Roevens, P. and Van Belle, H. (1984) *Biochem. Biophys. Res. Commun.* 123, 589–595

23 Hofmann, S. L. (1983) PhD Dissertation, Washington University

24 Bokoch, G. M. and Gilman, A. G. (1984) *Cell* 39, 301–308

25 Okajima, F. and Ui, M. (1984) *J. Biol. Chem.* 259, 13863–13871

26 Haslam, R. J. and Davidson, M. M. L. (1984) *FEBS Lett.* 174, 90–95

27 Berridge, M. J., Dawson, R. M. C., Downes, C. P., Shelop, J. P. and Irvine, R. F. (1983) *Biochem. J.* 212, 473–482

28 Downes, C. P., Mussat, M. C. and Michell, R. H. (1982) *Biochem. J.* 203, 169–177

29 Storey, D. J., Shears, S. B., Kirk, C. J. and Michell, R. H. (1984) *Nature* 312, 374–376

30 Connolly, T. M., Bross, T. E. and Majerus, P. W. (1985) *J. Biol. Chem.* 260, 7868–7874

The authors are at the Division of Hematology–Oncology, Departments of Internal Medicine and Biological Chemistry, Washington University School of Medicine, St. Louis, MO 63110, USA.

Cell cycle control genes in yeast

Paul Nurse

Two major cell cycle controls have been identified in yeast; one acting in the G1 phase of the cell cycle results in commitment to the mitotic cycle and the second acting in G2 leads to the initiation of mitosis. Recent genetic and molecular analyses suggest that a protein kinase which may be regulated by phosphorylation is involved in both controls.

Yeasts are being used increasingly to study eukaryotic cell biology because of their convenience for both classical and molecular genetic analysis. For example, the control of the mitotic cell cycle has been investigated in both the budding yeast *Saccharomyces cerevisiae*[1,2] and the fission yeast *Schizosaccharomyces pombe*[3]. Here I review some recent developments concerning the two major cell cycle controls in yeast, one responsible for commitment to the mitotic cycle and the other for initiation of mitosis.

Mitotic cycles in fission and budding yeast

The mitotic cycles of the two yeasts are illustrated in Fig. 1. That of fission yeast is typically eukaryotic with discrete G1,S,G2 and M phases (pre-DNA synthesis, DNA synthesis, post-DNA synthesis and mitotic phases respectively). G1 is short in rapidly growing cells but is extended at slower growth rates. During mitosis a microtubular spindle forms[4], and the three chromosomes condense and become

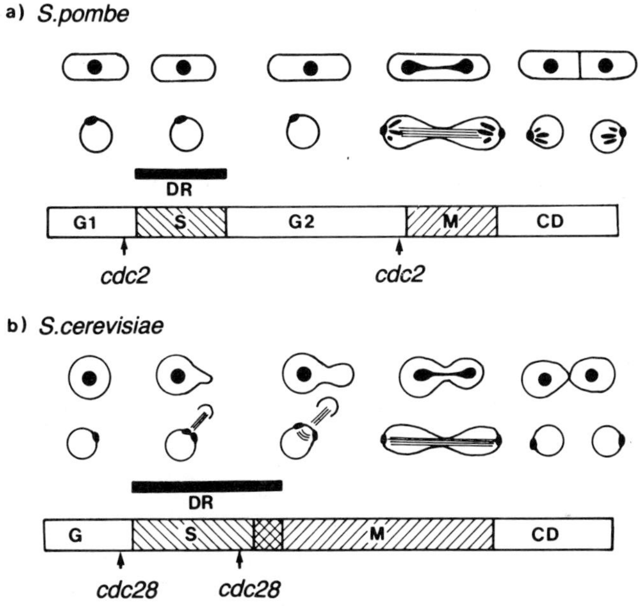

Fig. 1. Mitotic cell cycles of fission and budding yeast, showing the G1 S, G2, M and CD (cell division) phases. Upper row (a) and (b) shows behaviour of the cell and nucleus during the cell cycle; below is an enlargement of the nucleus showing the spindle pole body, chromosomes and spindle. Arrows show when the cdc2 and cdc28 genes complete their functions.

visible in the light microscope. This condensation is particularly obvious in certain mutants which arrest in the middle of mitosis[5], as shown in Fig. 2. During mitosis the nuclear membrane remains intact. After mitosis cell division proceeds by septation and medial fission.

The budding yeast cell cycle also has a G1 phase which is extended at slow growth rates. However, the organization of the second part of the cycle differs from fission yeast. A short microtubular mitotic spindle forms early, probably during S phase, and this persists for most of the rest of the cycle[1]. This type of cell cycle can be considered as having an extended mitotic phase. Just before cell division the short spindle elongates and nuclear division takes place; no chromosome condensation is observed and the nuclear membrane does not break down. The failure to observe chromosome condensation is unlikely to be a result of the smallness of the chromosomes since the largest budding yeast chromosomes are similar in size to the smallest fission yeast chromosome which does become visibly condensed. Cell division occurs by budding, a bud being formed early in the cycle during late G1 or S, increasing in size during the rest of the cycle and abscissing from the mother cell at cell division. In my opinion the extended mitotic phase and lack of visible chromosome condensation may result from the budding mode of division. Bud formation occurs at the site of cell division and can be considered as the first stage of that process. In most organisms cell division begins either during or just after mitosis. Consequently early initiation of cell division at bud emergence would require early initiation of mitosis. Since the cell is not ready to divide, the nucleus is 'frozen' in the mitotic state with a short spindle. Extreme chromosome condensation cannot take place during this time as it would inhibit transcription for much of the cycle. This view of the budding yeast cell cycle predicts that the controls over the initiation of mitosis are likely to be different in the two yeasts, and as we shall see below this appears to be the case.

Start control

A G1 commitment control called 'start' was identified in budding yeast by the pioneering work of Hartwell, Pringle and their co-workers[1]. Start was defined as

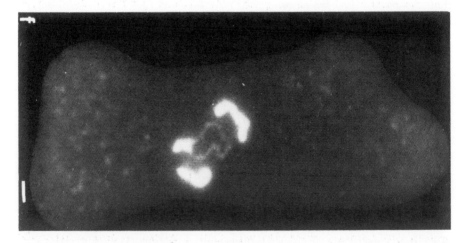

Fig. 2. Condensed chromosomes of the fission yeast mutant nda3-KM311 *of S. pombe. Three chromosomes are clearly seen with a loop probably made up of ribosomal DNA. Bar = 1μm.* Reproduced by permission from Ref. 5.

the earliest gene-controlled event in G1 and, more importantly, as the point when cells become committed to the mitotic cell cycle (Fig. 3). The other developmental pathway open to haploid cells is conjugation to a cell of opposite mating type. Cells which have not yet reached start in the cell cycle can undergo conjugation but once cells have passed start they are committed to the mitotic cycle and conjugation is not possible. Initial work established that temperature-sensitive mutants in four genes *cdc28, -36, -37* and *-39* were blocked at start when incubated at their restrictive temperatures[6]. The mating pheromone α-factor also blocks at the same point in the cell cycle[1]. Two of the start genes, *cdc36* and *-39,* may be directly involved in the block induced by α-factor. Mutations in these genes do not specifically arrest the cell cycle at start either in **a**/α diploids[6] or in mutants resistant to α-factor[7]. Cells in these situations cannot respond to α-factor. This suggests that the defects in the *cdc36* and *-39* gene products indirectly cause their block at start by activating the α-factor response pathway in the absence of the mating pheromone.

A similar start control has been identified in fission yeast[8]. In this case two genes have been identified, *cdc2* and *cdc10*. Mutations in these two genes block cells in G1 at a point when conjugation is still possible. By analogy with budding yeast this commitment point has also been called start.

In both yeasts, start occurs later in G1 at slow growth rates. This is because start is not usually passed until the cells attain a critical size. At slow growth rates, cell size at division is reduced (see next section) and consequently cells at the beginning of the cell cycle have to grow for a longer time before start can be completed[1,3]. Therefore, cells growing slowly remain uncommitted to the mitotic cycle for longer periods of time than cells growing rapidly. Once start has been passed the cell enters into the programme leading to S-phase, mitosis and cell division. The extension of G1 before start under poor growth conditions has led to confusion concerning the isolation of start mutants. Many mutants showing reduced growth rate will accumulate before start simply because they are growing slowly, and slow-growing cells expand their G1 before start. Thus, it is very important when identifying mutants that specifically block at start to ensure that they continue macromolecular synthesis and cellular growth under the block conditions. It is possible that mutations which reduce cell growth rate also have specific effects on the cell cycle, but it is difficult to establish this when cells are growing slowly.

It is very likely that the start controls in the two yeasts have a similar molecular basis since the genes *cdc28* in budding yeast and *cdc2* in fission yeast are similar. Both genes are required twice in the cell cycle, once in G1 at start and a second time later in the cycle for mitosis[8,9]. Also, the *cdc28* gene which has been cloned (see later) can substitute for a defective *cdc2* gene in *S. pombe*[10]. Finally, sequence comparisons have shown that the predicted amino acid sequences of the two genes have 62% identity. Because the two yeasts have diverged considerably in evolutionary terms, conservation of the *cdc2/28* function suggests that a similar function will be found in many other eukaryotic cells.

Another class of mutants is proving to be useful in examining start. These are *whi* mutants which advance cells into start at a reduced size[11]. They define two gene functions which are rate limiting in the processes determining when start takes place. Mutations in *whi1* are expressed throughout normal exponential growth, while the mutation in *whi2* is only expressed during the transition from exponential growth into stationary phase. The *whi2* mutant appears to be defective in the control which prevents start from being completed under starvation conditions, i.e. this mutation can be considered constitutive for cell proliferation even when growth conditions are inappropriate.

It is possible that the 'point'-like nature of start described above is an over-simplification[12]. *S. cerevisiae* diploid mutants of *cdc4* appear to be able to sporulate when blocked at their restrictive temperature. Since the *cdc4* gene functions after the α-factor block, cells blocked at this point should be past start, and yet they are still able to undergo the alternative developmental pathway of meiosis and sporulation[13]. Obviously this result blurs the 'point'-like nature of start. Presumably the operational definition of start depends on the alternative developmental pathway being considered. Cells may become committed to the mitotic cycle at an earlier stage when the alternative is conjugation than when it is meiosis and sporulation. Meiosis is a modified mitosis and the first stages of the two processes may be very similar. Thus, divergence of these two pathways might occur at a slightly later stage than the divergence between conjugation and the mitotic cycle.

Mitotic control
A second cell cycle control acting in G2 which determines the timing of mitosis has been extensively studied in the fission yeast[14] (Fig. 3). The *wee* mutants which divide at reduced cell size were found to map in two genes; *wee1* defines a negative element, and *cdc2* (already mentioned with respect to start) defines a positive element. There are two classes of *cdc2* mutant: temperature-sensitive lethals, which become blocked both at start and also just before mitosis; and *wee* mutants, which advance cells into mitosis at a reduced cell size and have a shortened G2. The *wee* mutants of *cdc2* are dominant and probably produce a modified protein of increased activity which is responsible for the advancement of mitosis. A third gene, *cdc25*, is also implicated in the control because its temperature-sensitive lethal phenotype is completely suppressed in a *wee1* mutant background[15]. A model which explains these observations is that *cdc2* initiates mitosis and is inhibited by the *wee1* gene product[14]. The *wee1* inhibition of *cdc2* is relieved by the *cdc25* product and as a consequence the *cdc25* function is not required for mitosis in the

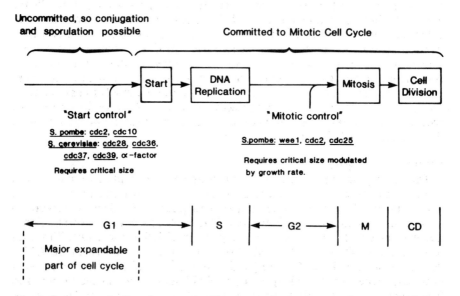

Fig. 3. *Summary of cell cycle controls. The start and mitotic controls are marked. Start divides the cell cycle into an uncommitted phase and a committed phase. The major genes involved are given under the respective controls.*

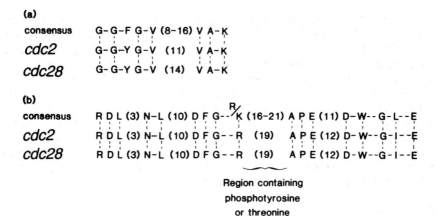

Fig. 4. Consensus sites surrounding ATP binding region (a) and phosphorylation receptor region (b) of kinase family (b). Site (a) taken from Ref. 19 is the consensus from CADPK and nine other kinases; site (b) taken from Ref. 20 is the consensus from CADPK and five other kinases. Phosphorylation receptor residue is either a tyrosine 7 residue after the R/K position in the consensus or an adjacent threonine. Both the cdc2 and cdc28 sequences contain a tyrosine at position 9 and a threonine at position 10 after the R/K residue.

absence of the *wee1* inhibitory element[15]. The mitotic control is modulated by the growth rate of the cells[3]. At slow growth rates the cell size required for mitosis is reduced and so cells are smaller when they undergo division. This explains why cells divide at a small size in poor growth conditions.

An equivalent control has not been found in budding yeast, which is not surprising if there is no real G2 phase. The second requirement for *cdc28* function occurs very early in the cell cycle soon after the first[9], a result consistent with the idea that mitosis is initiated early, probably during S phase. The control which determines when mitosis is completed in budding yeast can be described as a timer. A certain period of time must elapse after start before mitosis can be completed[1]. This means that at slow growth rates with extended generation times this period takes up less of the cell cycle, and at the end of the period cells will be small compared with faster growing cells. Consequently the cells are small after division and accumulate before start under poor growth conditions. Although the end result of reduced growth rates is the same in the two yeasts, the means by which they attain this result is quite different.

Cloning control genes

The *cdc28* gene and the other three *cdc* start genes of budding yeast have been cloned by Reed *et al.*[2], whilst *cdc2* and *cdc10* from fission yeast have been cloned in my laboratory[10,16]. The most interesting of these genes is *cdc2/28* which is required at both control points in the mitotic cycle. The *cdc28* gene codes for a transcript of about 1 kb and contains an open reading frame of 298 amino acids[2]. This open reading frame shows 21–25% identity with the sequences of cyclic AMP-dependent protein kinase (CADPK) and with several members of the *src* family of oncogenes, which are also likely to be protein kinases[17]. This has led Lorincz and Reed to propose that *cdc28* codes for a protein kinase. Support for this has come from Hindley and Phear who recently sequenced *cdc2*[18]. After allowing for the presence of four introns the *cdc2* gene was found to contain an open reading frame of 299 amino acids, indicating 62% identity with the sequence of *cdc28*. The regions conserved between *cdc2* and *cdc28* were compared to assess the significance of the 21–25% similarity of *cdc28* with the protein kinases. This comparison showed only 8% identity between the sequences of *cdc2, cdc28*, CADPK and v-*mos* (v-*mos* is one of the *src* family of oncogenes). However, this 8% similarity contains two functionally important regions, one surrounds an ATP-binding site of the type found in protein kinases[19] and the other surrounds a putative phosphorylation receptor site[20]. Both *cdc2* and *cdc28* contain almost the exact consensus sequences for these two sites (Fig. 4). This suggests that the *cdc2/28* gene codes for a protein kinase and that it is phosphorylated. The similarity between *cdc2/28* and v-*mos* can be mostly accounted for by these two sites. Therefore, it is unlikely that the *cdc2/28* gene protein resembles the oncogene, apart from having the ATP binding site and the phosphorylation receptor site.

The start gene *cdc36* from budding yeast has also been sequenced and contains an open reading frame which shows some similarity with *cdc4* and the *ets* oncogene[21]. An open reading frame found after sequencing the *cdc10* start gene in fission yeast also shows slight similarities to a variety of other genes[16]. However, the functional significances of these various comparisons is not yet clear.

The finding that the *cdc2/28* gene probably codes for a phosphorylated protein kinase has implications for the molecular basis of cell cycle control. It suggests that phosphorylation may play a key role at both the start and the mitotic controls. A similar situation has been described in vertebrate cells. A factor called maturation promoting factor (MPF) determines entry into mitosis in *Xenopus* eggs at the early cleaving stage[22]. This factor is stabilized by phosphatase inhibitors and so its activity may be altered by phosphorylation[23]. After partial purification, MPF is found in a fraction containing protein kinase activity[23]. These observations suggest that protein kinase activities are important in the cell cycle of vertebrate cells and it is possible that these phenomena have some relationship with the *cdc2/28* gene functions in yeast. The substrates of the *cdc2/28* protein kinase remain unknown but important clues may be provided by the dual role of the gene during the mitotic cycle. Presumably only a limited range of processes will be required at both the G1/S- and G2/M-phase boundaries.

cAMP-dependent protein kinase

In the work described above, mutants were isolated which have phenotypes suggestive of an involvement in cell control; the genes have been isolated and attempts made to work out their molecular function. A second approach is to work from known biochemical functions and to determine if alterations of these affect cell cycle control. This approach has recently been used to investigate the effects that CADPK and other related enzymes may have on the budding yeast cell cycle[24,25]. Mutants have been isolated which are conditionally defective in adenylate cyclase (*cyr1*) and the catalytic (*cyr3*) and regulatory (*bcy1*) subunits of CADPK. The kinase activity of the catalytic subunit is inhibited by the regulatory subunit, and can be restored by increases in cAMP level. Adenylate cyclase is the enzyme which produces cyclic AMP within the cell. Defects in *cyr1* or *cyr3* reduce CADPK activity and also result in cells accumulating in G1. Mutations in *bcy1* suppress the phenotypes of the *cyr1* and *cyr3* mutants. Interestingly when *cyr1* or *cyr3* mutant diploids are grown in rich growth medium they initiate meiosis and undergo some sporulation; normally such rich medium inhibits sporulation. A similar phenotype has been observed with *pat1* and *ran1* mutants of *S. pombe* which also undergo sporulation in rich medium[26,27]. The *pat1/ran1* gene is thought to code for an inhibitor of sporulation with relief of this inhibition being brought about by nutritional starvation and heterozygosity at the mating-type locus. However, the effects of these mutations in fission yeast on CADPK and other related enzymes are not known.

The *S. cerevisiae* data suggest that CADPK may have a key role at start. If the enzyme is inactivated cells are arrested at start and enter meiosis. This is an interesting hypothesis since one of the CADPK substrates could be the *cdc2/28* gene product and phosphorylation of this protein could activate the processes which lead to the completion of start. However, it is possible that CADPK acts indirectly on the cell cycle. The *cyr1* and *cyr3* mutants reduce overall cell growth rate and so the G1 arrest and derepressed sporulation observed could be consequences of the cells being starved of nutrients in the absence of the CADPK activity. Further work should settle this point and should also establish the relationship between these observations on CADPK and those concerning *cdc2/28* discussed earlier.

References
1 Pringle, J. and Hartwell, L. (1981) The *Saccharomyces cerevisiae* cell cycle, in *The Molecular Biology of the Yeast Saccharomyces* (Strathern, J., Jones, E. and Broach, J., eds), pp. 97–142, Cold Spring Harbor Laboratory, New York
2 Reed, S. (1984) Genetic and molecular analysis of division control in *Saccharomyces*, in *The Microbial Cell Cycle* (Nurse, P. and Streiblova, E., eds) pp. 89–107, CRC Press, Florida
3 Fantes, P. (1984) Cell cycle control in *Schizosaccharomyces pombe*, in *The Microbial Cell Cycle* (Nurse, P. and Streiblova, E., eds) pp. 109–125, CRC Press, Florida
4 McCully, E. and Robinow, C. (1971) Mitosis in the fission yeast *Schizosaccharomyces pombe*: a comparative study with light and electron microscopy. *J. Cell Sci.* 9, 475–507
5 Umesono, K., Hiraoka, Y., Toda, T. and Yanagida, M. (1983) Visualisation of chromosomes in mitotically arrested cells of the fission yeast *Schizosaccharomyces pombe*. *Curr. Genet.* 7, 123–128
6 Reed, S. (1980) The selection of *S. cerevisiae* mutants defective in the start event of cell division. *Genetics* 95, 561–577
7 Connolly, B., Bugeja, V., Piggot, J. and Carter, B. (1983) Mating factor dependence of G1 cell cycle mutants of *Saccharomyces cerevisiae*. *Curr. Genet.* 7, 309–312
8 Nurse, P. and Bissett, Y. (1981) Gene required in G1 for commitment to cell cycle and in G2 for control of mitosis in fission yeast. *Nature* 292, 448–460
9 Piggott, J., Rai, R. and Carter, B. (1982) A bifunctional gene product involved in two phases of the yeast cell cycle. *Nature* 298, 391–393
10 Beach, D., Durkacz, B. and Nurse, P. (1982) Functionally homologous cell cycle control genes in budding and fission yeast. *Nature* 300, 706–709
11 Sudbery, P., Goodey, A. and Carter, B. (1980) Genes which control cell proliferation in the yeast *Saccharomyces cerevisiae*. *Nature* 288, 401–404
12 Nurse, P. (1981) Genetic control of the yeast cell cycle: a reappraisal of 'start', in *The Fungal Nucleus* (Gull, K. and Oliver, S., eds) pp. 331–345, Cambridge University Press
13 Hirschenberg, J. and Simchen, G. (1977) Commitment to the mitotic cell cycle in yeast in relation to meiosis. *Expl. Cell Res.* 105, 245–252
14 Nurse, P. and Thuriaux, P. (1980) Regulatory genes controlling mitosis in the fission yeast *Schizosaccharomyces pombe*. *Genetics* 96, 627–637
15 Fantes, P. (1979) Epistatic gene interactions in the control of division in fission yeast. *Nature* 279, 428–430
16 Aves, S., Durkacz, B., Carr, A. and Nurse, P. Cloning, sequencing and transcriptional control of the *Schizosaccharomyces pombe cdc10* 'start' gene. (1985) *EMBO J.* 4, 457–463

17   Lorincz, A. and Reed, S. (1984) Primary structure homology between the product of
      yeast cell division control gene *cdc28* and vertebrate oncogenes. *Nature* 307, 183–185
18   Hindley, J. and Phear, G. (1984) Sequence of the cell division gene *cdc2* from *Schizo-
      saccharomyces pombe;* patterns of splicing and homology to protein kinases. *Gene*
      31, 129–134
19   Kamps, M., Taylor, S. and Sefton, B. (1984) Direct evidence that oncogenic tyrosine
      kinases and cyclic AMP-dependent protein kinase have homologous ATP-binding
      sites. *Nature* 310, 589–592
20   Groffen, J., Heisterkamp, N., Reynolds, F. and Stephenson, J. (1983) Homology
      between phosphotyrosine acceptor site of human *c-abl* and viral oncogene products.
      Nature 304, 167–169
21   Peterson, T., Yochem, J., Byers, B., Nunn, M., Duesberg, P., Doolittle, R. and
      Reed, S. (1984) A relationship between the yeast cell cycle genes *cdc4* and *cdc36* and
      the *ets* sequence of oncogenic virus E26. *Nature* 309, 556–558
22   Gerhart, J., Wu, M. and Kirschner, M. (1984) Cell cycle dynamics of an M-phase
      specific cytoplasmic factor in *Xenopus laevis* oocytes and eggs. *J. Cell Biol.* 98,
      1247–1255
23   Wu, M. and Gerhart, J. (1980) Partial purification and characterisation of matura-
      tion-promoting factor from eggs of *Xenopus laevis*. *Dev. Biol.* 79, 465–477
24   Matsumoto, K., Uno, I. and Ishikawa, T. (1983) Initiation of meiosis in yeast
      mutants defective in adenylate cyclase and cyclic AMP-dependent protein kinase.
      Cell 32, 417–432
25   Matsumoto, K., Uno, I. and Ishikawa, T. (1983) Control of cell division in *Saccharo-
      myces cerevisiae* mutants defective in adenylate cyclase and cAMP-dependent
      protein kinase. *Exp. Cell Res.* 146, 151–161
26   Iino, Y. and Yamamoto, M. Mutants of *Schizosaccharomyces pombe* which sporu-
      late in the haploid state. (1985) *Mol. Gen. Genet.* 198, 416–421
27   Nurse, P. Mutants of the fission yeast *Schizosaccharomyces pombe* which alter the
      shift between cell proliferation and sporulation. (1985) *Mol. Gen. Genet.* 198,
      497–502

*P. Nurse is at the Imperial Cancer Research Fund, PO Box 123, Lincoln's Inn Fields,
London WC2A 3PX, UK.*

Addendum – *P. Nurse*

Antibodies have been prepared against the *cdc2* and *cdc28* gene products and
used to establish that the genes do encode proteins that become phosphorylated
in vivo and have protein kinase activity[28,29]. The *cdc2* gene transcript level,
protein level and gross phosphorylation state do not change during the cell cycle
of rapidly growing fission yeast cells[29,30]. However, in cells arrested at start by
nitrogen deprivation the protein rapidly becomes dephosphorylated and loses its
protein kinase activity. This suggests that arrest at start by nutritional starvation
could be regulated by modulation of the *cdc2* protein kinase activity, possibly via
phosphorylation of the protein. The *cdc25* gene of fission yeast has now been
cloned and increasing its transcript level advances cells into mitosis, thus con-
firming its role as a positive-acting element in the control of mitosis[31]. Deletion of
the gene from the chromosome is only lethal in cells expressing the *wee1*
inhibitor, suggesting that *wee1* and *cdc25* work in an antagonistic fashion to
regulate the timing of mitosis within the cell cycle.

    The identification of *ras* oncogene homologues in budding yeast and the
characterization of *ras* mutants have provided a link with the enzyme CADPK.

The *ras* gene homologues appear to be important in regulating cAMP concentrations in the cell, probably by modulating adenylate cyclase activity[32]. Cells bearing a *ras* mutation equivalent to that which causes transformation in mammalian cells increases cAMP levels which could activate CADPK. However, this may not be the role of the *ras* gene function in fission yeast since in this organism equivalent mutations have no effect on cAMP levels[33].

References

28 Reed, S. I., Hadwiger, J. A. and Lorincz, A. T. (1985) *Proc. Natl Acad. Sci. USA* 82, 4055–4059
29 Simanis, V. and Nurse, P. (1986) *Cell* 45, 261–268
30 Durkacz, B., Carr, A. and Nurse, P. (1986) *EMBO J.* 5, 369–373
31 Russell, P. and Nurse, P. (1986) *Cell* 45, 145–153
32 Toda, T., Uno, I., Ishikawa, T., Powers, S., Kataoka, T., Broek, D., Cameron, S., Broach, J., Matsumoto, K. and Wigler, M. (1985) *Cell* 40, 27–36
33 Fukui, Y., Kozasa, T., Kaziro, Y., Takeda, T. and Yamamoto, M. (1986) *Cell* 44, 329–336

The Na$^+$,K$^+$ pump may mediate the control of nerve cells by nerve growth factor

Silvio Varon and Stephen D. Skaper

The survival of nerve cells, in vitro *and in* vivo, *is controlled by extrinsic agents called neuronotrophic factors. The best known among them, nerve growth factor, has been shown to control the performance of the Na⁺,K⁺ pump in the membrane of its target ganglionic neurons. In turn, the operation of the pump is essential for the survival of these neurons. Ionic control may be an important mechanism by which cell survival, growth and/or differentiation is regulated by certain extrinsic factors or hormones.*

Extrinsic influences have been invoked to explain the development of the nervous system: the orderly manner in which neuronal cells proliferate, migrate, extend axons to appropriate territories, and connect with the correct target cells (or die if they fail to do so). We believe that similar influences continue to apply in the mature organism, and play important roles in the capability or failure of neurons to perform their functions and to resist, or compensate for, pathological insults. Thus, the problem of identifying mechanisms which control the development and functions of nerve cells is important to both the neuroscientist and the clinical neurologist. To manipulate neuronal maintenance and repair to the best clinical advantage, it will be necessary to identify and understand the extrinsic factors which regulate survival and general growth (neuronotrophic factors), as well as the actions of nerve cells such as neuritic extension (neurite promoting factors). Such investigations are now under way in a number of laboratories (reviewed in Refs 1, 2).

The classical model for neuronotrophic and neurite promoting agents is nerve growth factor (NGF), a protein which specifically addresses sensory neurons in dorsal root ganglia (DRG) and sympathetic neurons in peripheral sympathetic ganglia. Three decades of investigation of NGF have contributed detailed information on the NGF protein itself, but nearly no knowledge on its mechanism of action[3-7]. In recent years, however, we discovered that NGF controls the movement of Na$^+$ and K$^+$ across the plasma membrane of all its target neurons, by controlling the performance of their Na$^+$,K$^+$ pump[8,9]. Ionic control is also of fundamental importance to many types of cell behavior, including proliferation[10], process elongation[11], and general growth and repair[12]. Thus, ionic control by NGF may be the key to its regulation of neuronal survival and, possibly, neurite extension[1,8,9].

The experimental system

We have taken the view that NGF, upon interaction with its known receptors on the neuronal membrane, alters a 'primary' cell function which in turn controls several 'secondary' functions, thereby setting in motion a number of cellular machineries, the composite results of which are the gross, longer-term consequences (survival, general growth, neurite extension) attributed to NGF. To investigate the early (primary and secondary) responses, we sought experimental systems in which: (i) measurable 'deficits' can be shown to develop during a short period of NGF deprivation; (ii) these deficits will be promptly and fully reversed by delayed administration of NGF; and (iii) more extended NGF deprivation will lead to irreversible damage and death of the target neurons.

Such requirements are met by ganglionic cell suspensions obtained by dissociation of the traditional NGF target tissues. The first deficit to be detected concerned the uptake of uridine in E8 (embryonic day 8) chick DRG cells[13]. The deficit develops over 6 h of NGF deprivation and is completely reversed within minutes of NGF administration. Other transport systems, e.g. glucose, display a similar dependence on NGF in these cells, and also share a dependence on Na^+ gradients across the plasma membrane[14]. These findings raised the question of whether NGF controls such nutrient transports in E8 DRG cells by controlling the transmembrane Na^+ gradient itself.

NGF regulates the Na^+,K^+ pump in E8 chick DRG cells

Incubation for 6 h with $^{22}Na^+$ demonstrates that NGF-deprived cells accumulate progressively more Na^+, and reach a plateau six- to eight-fold higher than cells incubated with NGF[15]. The plateau levels of Na^+ accumulation in the absence of NGF are strictly proportional to the external Na^+ concentrations, and are practically identical to those induced by blocking the Na^+,K^+ pump with either ouabain or dinitrophenol. This indicates that, at plateau time, intracellular Na^+ concentrations have become equal to the extracellular ones. Delayed presentation of NGF to cells deprived of NGF for 6 h promptly depleted them of their excess Na^+. The onset and rate of the restoration, in addition to its magnitude, are controlled by the concentration at which NGF is presented – reflecting the kinetics of the NGF binding to its cell surface receptors. Thus, a lack of NGF causes the development of a Na^+ control deficit, and the administration of NGF restores and sustains the Na^+ control competence of DRG neurons. Both responses are transcription- and translation-independent.

Converse types of behaviour are displayed by the K^+ ions of the DRG cells[16]. During 6 h incubation with NGF, the intracellular K^+ (traced with $^{86}Rb^+$) falls to the same low concentrations as the extracellular K^+, whereas it is maintained at its normally high level if NGF is present. NGF-deprived, K^+-depleted cells reaccumulate their K^+ within minutes of NGF administration, and both the amplitude and time of K^+ recovery depend on the NGF concentration. K^+ losses and Na^+ accumulation under NGF deprivation are passive events (i.e. they occur down the respective concentration gradients across the cell membrane), and they take place independently (e.g. the K^+ will be lost even in a Na^+-free medium). These features are consistent with a progressive inactivation in the absence of NGF of the Na^+,K^+ pump, which would no longer compensate for the inward Na^+ and outward K^+ 'leaks'. Speaking more directly for the involvement of a pump are the ionic events occurring under NGF administration, which are active ('uphill') ionic transport processes. Moreover, Na^+ extrusion and K^+ re-uptake under NGF are coupled processes: the restoration of normal Na^+ and K^+ concentrations inside the cell requires the presence of the complementary cation on the opposite side of the membrane. This Na^+ and K^+ dependence is typical of the Na^+,K^+ pump.

The traditional way to examine Na^+,K^+ pump activity in intact cells is to measure active K^+ influxes, i.e. that portion of unidirectional intake of K^+ (traced by an isotope such as $^{86}Rb^+$) which can be inhibited by ouabain. An analysis of active K$^+$ fluxes in NGF-deprived and NGF-reactivated E8 chick DRG cells[17] has confirmed both the dose-dependent control by NGF of their Na$^+$,K$^+$ pump, and the resumption of pump activity within seconds (at 50–500 units NGF-ml) or minutes (at 1–10 units NGF-ml) of NGF administration. Within these timeframes of reactivation by NGF, the reactivated pump perceives intracellular Na$^+$ levels which are much higher than normal, and responds to them by transient performances which exceed (by 20–30 times) those displayed at the NGF-supported steady state.

Regulation of neuronal Na$^+$,K$^+$ pump by NGF is a specific phenomenon
The ability to control pump performance in E8 chick DRG is specific for the NGF molecule[15,17]. Neither protection against pump inactivation in the absence of NGF, nor mimicry of the NGF action to restore pump performance, could be achieved by using: (i) molecules resembling, in charge or size, the mouse β-NGF (e.g. cytochrome *c*); (ii) other known growth factors (epidermal and fibroblast growth factors; a new ciliary neuronotrophic factor[1]); (iii) insulin, which has considerable analogies with NGF in its amino acid sequence [6]; (iv) the complete N1 supplement, which is required as an alternative to serum and in addition to NGF for the survival of neurons in monolayer cultures[18,25]; or (v) fetal calf serum itself.

The Na$^+$,K$^+$ pump response is also specific to neuronal preparations which traditionally respond to NGF in culture by either survival or neurite extension criteria[16,19]. Intact E8 chick DRG exhibit the same ionic responses as their dissociated cell suspensions to a lack of administration of NGF. E11 chick sympathetic ganglia, the other traditional NGF target tissue, also display the ionic responses both before and after dissociation. Neonatal mouse DRG dissociates require NGF for neuronal survival in culture, and also to sustain their pump performance; conversely, the undissociated mouse DRG display nearly the same fiber outgrowth with or without NGF in explant cultures, and develop no significant pump deficit when deprived of NGF. Chick ciliary ganglionic neurons are not sensitive to NGF in culture at all, and display the same pump perform-ances with or without NGF.

Chick DRG neurons *in vivo* have been traditionally assumed to lose their responsiveness to exogenous NGF as their age increases[3,6]. The Na$^+$,K$^+$ pump response to NGF correlates precisely with the dependence on developmental age of the NGF sensitivity in ganglionic neurons. The Na$^+$,K$^+$ pump performance of chick DRG neurons differs less and less in the presence and absence of NGF as the ganglionic age increases from E10 to E16[20]. This decline in an NGF-differen-tial, however, is not due to a decreasing effectiveness of NGF in controlling the ganglionic pump, but to an increasing ability of DRG neurons to control their pump performance independently from the availability of exogenous NGF. The same observations have been made with regard to chick embryo sympathetic ganglionic neurons, for which the independence from exogenous NGF begins to appear only after E13 (Ref. 26). Thus, in addition to revealing a parallel between ionic and traditional culture responses to NGF of DRG and sympathetic neu-rons, these observations stress ionic control as an important feature for neuronal performance even outside the obvious realm of NGF involvement.

NGF may use control of the Na$^+$,K$^+$ pump to control neuronal survival
The information accumulated in the above studies provides unequivocal evi-dence that NGF controls the performance of the Na$^+$,K$^+$ pump in its ganglionic

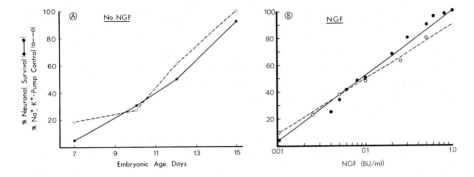

Fig. 1. Correlations between Na⁺,K⁺ pump control and neuronal survival. (Panel A) Survival and pump control of chick DRG neurons as a function of embryonic age. Enriched neurons were cultured as monolayers for 24 h in the presence or absence of NGF, and their survival expressed as a % of the number supported by NGF (● — ●). Neuronal suspensions were examined for their ability to exclude ²²Na⁺ in the absence of NGF with or without ouabain. Na⁺,K⁺ pump control (○---○) is expressed as a % of the maximal difference between the ouabain-sensitive sodium space and the NGF-independent (Na⁺,K⁺ pump controlled) space measured in the absence of ouabain. (Panel B) Survival and pump control as a function of NGF concentration. Embryonic day 8 chick DRG neurons were examined for 24-h survival in monolayer culture (○---○) and their ability to exclude ²²Na⁺ (● — ●) in suspension, over a range of NGF concentrations from 0.01 to 1.0 Biological Unit (BU)/ml. Note that the symbols are reversed from panel A.

target neurons. Could this be the way by which NGF effects its trophic functions, and in particular the control of neuronal survival? Arguments in favor of such a thesis rest on two kinds of considerations: (i) how strict and quantitative is the correlation between ionic control and cell-survival control?; and (ii) can one mimic the effect of NGF deprivation on neuronal survival by preventing the effect of NGF on the pump?

Chick ganglionic neurons can be collected at different embryonic ages, cultured in monolayers (with or without NGF), and examined in parallel for both ionic-pump performance and neuronal survival[27]. Quantitative correlations between pump control and neuronal survival are provided by two independent sets of data, shown in Fig. 1. One set (Fig. 1, A) concerns neuronal survival in the absence of NGF and, therefore, has more general implications than for the NGF phenomenon alone. For both DRG[20] and sympathetic[26], neurons, survival in the absence of NGF increases with developmental age in exact synchrony with NGF-independent control of the Na⁺,K⁺ pump in these neurons. The second set of data (Fig. 1, B) demonstrates the extent to which both the survival and the pump control regulated by NGF depend on the same NGF concentrations[21]. If a causal relationship lies behind such precise correlations, it can only be from pump control to survival control, since: (i) the failure to operate the pump without NGF precedes the survival failure by several hours; (ii) pump control is re-imposed within seconds of NGF presentation on cells which are still fully competent to survive; and (iii) pump restoration by NGF involves no transcription- or translation-dependent events. Nevertheless, it remains possible that the correlation between the two responses merely reveals their common dependence on a single, preceding event whose temporal and dose-dependent features are precisely reflected in the features of both responses, while pump and survival responses remain independent from each other.

If activity of the Na+,K+ pump is essential to neuronal survival, then blocking the pump activity by means other than NGF deprivation should lead to neuronal death even in the presence of NGF. Indeed, Fig. 2 shows that when 2×10^{-4} M ouabain is provided to E8 DRG neuronal cultures in the presence of NGF, neuronal-cell death develops over the next 30 h with exactly the same time course as if the cultures were deprived of NGF in the absence of the drug. The same holds true in NGF-supplemented but K+-free media[27]. Thus, neuronal survival requires the performance of the Na+,K+ pump. Since pump performance requires in turn the presence of NGF, one cannot but conclude that NGF control of the pump is an essential component of its action on neuronal survival and, possibly, the only component of it.

Additional investigations are required to assess the validity of this latter point, namely, whether the action of NGF on the Na+,K+ pump is the sole mechanism by which NGF controls neuronal survival. Such investigations will entail: (i) defining which of the immediate consequences of pump activity – transmembrane ionic gradients, intracellular ionic concentrations, and ATP hydrolysis – are essential for cell survival; and (ii) verifying whether achieving such consequence(s) (or, even better, activating the pump) in the absence of NGF could sustain neuronal survival, thereby bypassing altogether the need for the presence

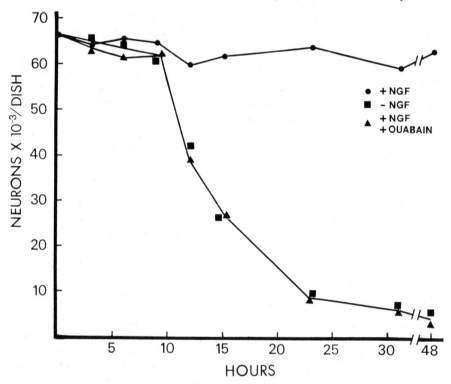

Fig. 2. Culture of E8 chick DRG neurons with NGF, without NGF, or with NGF plus ouabain. Enriched neurons (2×10^5) were seeded into polyornithine-coated 35 mm culture plastic dishes with 10 BU/ml NGF (●), no NGF (■), or 10 BU/ml NGF plus 0.2 mM ouabain (▲). The number of surviving neurons in each instance was determined at selected intervals over a 48 h period.

of NGF. There are, in fact, reports in the literature that survival in culture of DRG neurons is enhanced by external K^+ concentrations even in the absence of NGF (for example, see Ref. 22).

Where do we go from here?

The discovery of an action of NGF on the neuronal Na^+, K^+ pump, and of its link with the NGF action on neuronal survival, divides future NGF investigations into two distinct groups: (1) those concerned with the mechanisms by which NGF achieves its control of the pump; and (2) those probing into the regulation of neuronal survival beyond the control of the pump.

(1) The search for molecular events leading from the NGF-receptor binding step to the activation of the pump will largely reflect our views on what causes the progressive decline of pump activity in the absence of NGF, specifically whether pump decline involves: (i) loss of pump sites; (ii) reduction in traditional pump stimuli; or (iii) alterations in the pump molecule or its membrane domain. We already know that restoration by NGF of pump performance does not involve an increase in pump sites[23]. Ionic stimuli to the pump are not involved, since the external K^+ concentration is constant and the intracellular Na^+ concentrations vary in the wrong direction (i.e. they rise when the pump slows down without NGF, and drop when pump activity resumes under NGF). Moreover, unlike mitogens[10], NGF has been shown not to promote the influx of Na^+ (Ref. 15). It remains possible that NGF somehow controls the intracellular supply of ATP to the pump and thus restores activity to an ATP-starved, but otherwise entirely normal Na^+, K^+ pump. This speculation is compatible with the observation that cell-free membrane preparations from NGF-deprived, or NGF-supported, DRG display equal activity (and equal affinities for Na^+, K^+, or ATP) in their Na^+, K^+ stimulated, ouabain-sensitive ATPase[24]. An alternative view which remains equally plausible at present, however, is that the pump or its membrane domain are adversely affected in the absence of NGF via reversible processes which involve some intracellular constituent not residing in the plasma membrane itself. NGF can raise cyclic AMP contents in embryonic chick DRGs with time- and dose-dependencies similar to its pump effect, but cyclic AMP and Na^+, K^+ pump responses are independent of each other[24]. NGF also causes a rapid and transient increase in phospholipid methylation in embryonic chick DRG and sympathetic neurons, which precedes the other two responses but neither is needed by them nor fails to occur when the latter are blocked[28]. Thus, these three short-latency responses to NGF occur independently of one another although they appear to reflect at least one common step.

A clue to molecular events intermediate between NGF presentation and Na^+, K^+ pump protection has been recently provided by the observation that certain phorbol esters can replace NGF for the survival of DRG neurons[29]. Analysis of the Na^+, K^+ pump behavior has revealed that: (i) like NGF, phorbol ester prevents the decline in pump activity – yet another confirmation of the pump involvement in neuronal survival – but (ii) unlike NGF, phorbol ester fails to restore either pump performance or neuronal viability if the neurons have been allowed to lose pump competence over the NGF-reversible 6 h period[30]. Phorbol ester is known to operate via activation of a diacylglyceride- and phospholipid-dependent protein kinase C and it seems, therefore, that protein phosphorylation events sustained by this enzyme may be involved in the protection of the Na^+, K^+ pump by NGF as well.

(2) The search for molecular events leading from restored pump performance

to neuronal survival will, of course, be much more complex, since it involves an understanding of the intricate interconnections among a variety of cellular machineries through which survival of any cell is to be secured. Breaking those interconnections into more manageable fractions may be achieved by taking advantage of another set of recent investigations on neuronal survival. The survival of cultured ganglionic neurons requires a number of other exogenous agents, in addition to the appropriate neuronotrophic factor (NGF, here) and the nutrient and other constituents of the usual culture media. These additional survival requirements can be met by a chemically defined supplement, designated N1 and comprised of insulin, transferrin, putrescine, progesterone and selenite. We find that these requirements can be further reduced to insulin and transferrin for E7-16 chick DRG neurons[18], and to insulin, transferrin and selenite for E11-16 chick sympathetic neurons where the transferrin requirement is developmentally regulated[25]. These agents are not required for the action of NGF on the pump. Therefore, they must either: (i) control the execution of subsequent cellular events triggered by NGF via the pump, and hence, play a role subordinate to NGF; or (ii) control, in a manner totally independent of NGF, some other cellular machinery whose products are equally required for neuronal survival as those controlled by the pump. In either case, investigation of the molecular site of action of these other required agents will contribute considerably to our understanding of the consequences of NGF-controlled pump performance on neuronal survival. Such an understanding becomes even more urgent in view of recent findings that NGF can also protect against death certain cholinergic neurons in the adult CNS *in vivo*[31].

It seems appropriate to conclude by raising the speculation that monovalent cations may serve as 'second messengers' for several other agents regulating cell behaviour via binding to surface receptors. This is not an entirely novel speculation[10–12]. However, the present evidence for ionic involvement in the mode of action of NGF may prompt more serious consideration of its merits with regard to neural, as well as other cells.

References

1 Varon, S. and Adler, R. (1981) *Adv. Cell. Neurobiol.* 2, 115–163
2 Varon, S., Manthorpe, M., Davis, G. E., Williams, L. R. and Skaper, S. D. in *Physiological Basis for Functional Recovery in Neurological Disease* (Waxman, S. G., ed.), Raven Press (in press)
3 Levi-Montalcini, R. and Angeletti, P. U. (1968) *Physiol. Rev.* 48, 534–569
4 Varon, S. (1975) *Exp. Neurol.* 48 (No. 3, Part 2), 75–92
5 Bradshaw, R. A. and Young, M. (1976) *Biochem. Pharmacol.* 25, 1445–1449
6 Greene, L. A. and Shooter, E. M. (1980) *Ann. Rev. Neurosci.* 3, 353–402
7 Harper, G. P. and Thoenen, H. (1980) *J. Neurochem.* 34, 5–16
8 Varon, S. and Skaper, S. D. (1980) in *Tissue Culture in Neurobiology* (Giacobini, E., Vernadakis, A. and Shahar, A., eds), pp. 333–347, Raven Press
9 Varon, S. and Skaper, S. D. (1983) in *Somatic and Autonomic Nerve–Muscle Interactions* (Burnstock, G., Urbova, G. and O'Brien, R., eds), pp. 213–252, Elsevier/North-Holland, Amsterdam
10 Rozengurt, E. and Mendoza, S. (1980) *Ann. New York Acad. Sci.* 339, 175–190
11 Jaffe, L. and Nuccitelli, R. (1977) *Ann. Rev. Biophys. Bioengin.* 6, 445–476
12 Becker, R. U. (1981) *Mechanisms of Growth Control*, Thomas, New York
13 Horii, Z. I. and Varon, S. (1975) *J. Neurosci. Res.* 1, 361–375
14 Skaper, S. D. and Varon, S. (1979) *Brain Res.* 172, 303–313
15 Skaper, S. D. and Varon, S. (1980) *J. Neurochem.* 34, 1654–1660
16 Skaper, S. D. and Varon, S. (1981) *Exp. Cell Res.* 131, 356–361

17   Boonstra, J., Skaper, S. D. and Varon, S. (1982) *J. Cell. Physiol.* 113, 28–34
18   Skaper, S. D., Selak, I. and Varon, S. (1982) *J. Neurosci. Res.* 8, 251–261
19   Skaper, S. D. and Varon, S. (1980) *Brain Res.* 197, 379–389
20   Skaper, S. D. and Varon, S. (1983) *Dev. Biol.* 98, 257–264
21   Skaper, S. D. and Varon, S. (1982) *Exp. Neurol.* 76, 655–665
22   Chalazonitis, A. and Fischbach, G. D. (1980) *Dev. Biol.* 78, 173–183
23   Skaper, S. D. and Varon, S. (1981) *J. Neurosci. Res.* 6, 133–141
24   Skaper, S. D. and Varon, S. (1981) *J. Neurochem.* 37, 222–228
25   Selak, I., Skaper, S. D. and Varon, S. (1983) *Dev. Brain Res.* 7, 171–179
26   Selak, I., Skaper, S. D. and Varon, S. (1983) *J. Cell Physiol.* 114, 229–234
27   Skaper, S. D. and Varon, S. (1983) *Brain Res.* 271, 263–271
28   Skaper, S. D. and Varon, S. (1984) *J. Neurochem.* 42, 116–122
29   Montz, H. P. M., Davis, G. E., Skaper, S. D., Manthorpe, M. and Varon, S. (1985)
     Dev. Brain Res. 23, 150–154
30   Skaper, S. D., Montz, H. P. M. and Varon, S. *Brain Res.* (in press)
31   Williams, L. R., Varon, S., Peterson, G., Wictorin, K., Fischer, W., Björklund, A.
     and Gage, F. H. *Proc. Natl Acad. Sci. USA* (in press)

Silvio Varon and Stephen D. Skaper are at the Department of Biology, School of Medicine, The University of California at San Diego, La Jolla, CA 92093, USA.

The growth factor-activatable Na$^+$/H$^+$ exchange system: a genetic approach

Jacques Pouysségur

The membrane-bound Na$^+$/H$^+$ antiporter is a self-contained regulator of the pH within vertebrate cells (pH$_i$). Growth factors activate the antiporter in quiescent cells by modifying its 'pH$_i$-sensor', so that their cytoplasm becomes more alkaline. A genetic approach to this system opens the way to its molecular identification and its role in growth control.

Interest in intracellular pH (pH$_i$) as a possible ionic signal for cell activation arose from studies with sea urchin eggs. A rapid rise in pH$_i$ after fertilization was reported to result from an amiloride-sensitive exchange of extracellular Na$^+$ for intracellular H$^+$ (Ref. 1). These observations were the first to suggest a link between activation of Na$^+$/H$^+$ exchange and initiation of growth. Rapid stimulation of an amiloride-sensitive Na$^+$-influx now appears to be a 'universal' response of quiescent cells to growth-promoting agents (for reviews see Refs 2–4). The ubiquity of this mitogen/ionic coupled response has made the Na$^+$/H$^+$ antiport system an attractive model for analysing the mechanisms which transduce external signals into metabolic responses. Among the major questions arising are: (1) How does the growth factor–receptor interaction activate the antiporter? (2) Does the rise in pH$_i$ signal the initiation of growth? (3) What is the molecular structure of the antiporter?

Identification of the Na$^+$/H$^+$ antiporter

A simple way to find out whether a Na$^+$/H$^+$ exchange system is operating in a particular type of cell is to monitor external pH in response to manipulation of the Na$^+$-gradient across the plasma membrane. Addition of Na$^+$ to Na$^+$-depleted cells induces a rapid H$^+$ efflux and, conversely, removal of external Na$^+$ from a suspension of Na$^+$-loaded cells induces H$^+$ influx[1,5]. Na$^+$ and H$^+$ exchange with a coupling ratio of 1 and are specifically inhibited by amiloride or its analogs substituted in the 5-amino position[6]. Kinetic studies[7] using renal brush border membrane vesicles have shown that external H$^+$ interacts at a single site where Na$^+$, Li$^+$, NH$_4^+$ and amiloride all compete for binding. In contrast, internal H$^+$ interacts with the Na$^+$/H$^+$ antiporter at both a transport and an activator site[7]. A slightly different model with two mutually exclusive external binding sites for H$^+$ and Na$^+$ has been suggested from studies with cultured fibroblasts[5]. This transport system is reversible, electroneutral, driven by an ionic gradient, asymmetric at least with respect to its interactions with H$^+$, and operative in all vertebrate cells so far examined[4,8,9].

The Na$^+$/H$^+$ antiporter: a self-contained pH$_i$-regulator

When cells are acid-loaded, for example by using the NH$_4^+$-prepulse technique[8], pH$_i$-recovery (in HCO$_3^-$-free medium) is very fast; it is strictly dependent on the presence of external Na$^+$ or Li$^+$, and is prevented by amiloride. Studies are usually performed in HCO_3^--free medium to prevent the operation of an additional pH_i-regulating system, a Na^+-dependent Cl^-/HCO_3^- antiporter which is sensitive to stilbene derivatives[8,10]. Under physiological conditions, the Na^+/ K^+-ATPase of eukaryotic cell maintains an inward-directed Na^+-gradient, providing a constant powerful driving force for H^+-extrusion. However, the rate of H^+-efflux is self-controlled by the internal H^+-regulatory site. Indeed, when pH_i rises above a critical value ($>7.2–7.4$), the system virtually shuts off, and if the pH_i falls gradually, the rate of H^+-efflux increases in an allosteric manner[7,17] to reach a maximum around $pH_i = 6.0$ (Ref. 17). Thus, in response to an acute acid load, the Na^+/H^+ exchanger, which operates at a low rate under physiological conditions, is quickly turned on by the fall in pH_i and, as pH_i gradually rises and returns to the initial value, the Na^+/H^+ exchange activity slows down and stabilizes again at the basal level. With this 'pH_i-sensor' the Na^+/H^+ antiporter is devised for rapid and fine tuning of intracellular pH.

Growth factors activate the Na^+/H^+ antiporter

Considerable interest in this membrane-bound system arose when it was recognized that virtually all growth promoting agents (serum, epidermal growth factor, platelet-derived growth factor, α-thrombin, vasopressin, bradykinin, concanavalin A, etc.) stimulate an amiloride-sensitive Na^+-influx in many quiescent cells (human, mouse and hamster fibroblasts, lymphocytes, hepatocytes, neutrophils, platelets, etc.) (for reviews see Refs 3 and 4). Knowing the kinetic properties of the antiporter, two mechanisms could account for its activation: (1) growth factors could initiate a fall in pH_i or (2) growth factors could in some way induce a change in the kinetic constants of the antiporter. Evidence in favor of the second and most intuitively appealing mechanism came from studies on insulin action in frog muscle in which activation of Na^+/H^+ exchange is accompanied by alkalinization of the cytoplasm[11]. Subsequent studies using weak-acid distribution measurements or intracellularly-trapped fluorescent pH indicators with various G0-arrested cultured cells revealed that serum or purified growth factors induce a persistent rise in pH_i (0.15 to 0.3 pH units)[12–19]. This must be caused by the Na^+/H^+ exchanger because it is abolished in the presence of amiloride, in Na^+-free medium, and in mutants lacking Na^+/H^+ exchange activity[14].

More decisive evidence for the mechanism of activation emerged from three independent studies: serum in human fibroblasts[13], α-thrombin in hamster fibroblasts[17] and phorbol ester in T-lymphocytes[18] activate the Na^+/H^+ antiporter by increasing the affinity of the 'pH_i-sensor', the allosteric H^+-binding site. Thus, in the presence of growth factors the Na^+/H^+ antiporter operates at more alkaline pH_i values (0.2 to 0.3 pH units). Finally, recent studies[20] showed that a synthetic diacylglycerol and phorbol ester, two activators of protein kinase C (Ref. 21), activate Na^+/H^+ exchange. These results led to the conclusion that protein kinase C is a transducer of growth factor-mediated activation of the Na^+/H^+ antiporter (Fig. 1). Supporting this model is the evidence that a variety of extracellular signals stimulate inositol phospholipid breakdown, and therefore the formation of endogenous diacylglycerol[21,22]. However, this activating mechanism does not exclude other pathways of activation such as a phosphorylation step activated by Ca^{2+} calmodulin[19].

Strategy for a genetic approach

Advances in gene amplification and gene transfer techniques have made somatic cell genetics a powerful approach for studying the molecular biology of

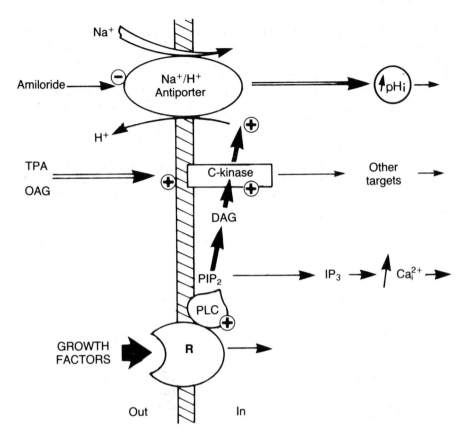

Fig. 1. Growth factor-induced rise in pH$_i$ – hypothetical sequence of events. TPA = 12-0-tetradecanoyl phorbol-13-acetate; OAG = 1-oleoyl-2-acetyl-glycerol; DAG = 1,2-diacylglycerol; PIP$_2$ = phosphatidylinositol 4,5-bisphosphate; IP$_3$ = inositol 1,4,5-tris-phosphate; PLC = phospholipase C; R = growth factor receptor. For more details see reviews in Refs 21 and 22.

proteins of low abundance. It was our premise that mutants lacking Na$^+$/H$^+$ exchange activity would be most useful in assessing the role of the rise in pH$_i$ in growth factor action. Taking advantage of the reversibility of the Na$^+$/H$^+$ exchange and the toxicity of high concentrations of H$^+$, our general strategy for mutant selection was to use the Na$^+$/H$^+$ antiporter as a specific and potent H$^+$-vector. By imposing a Na$^+$ or Li$^+$ gradient as a driving force and choosing the direction of the gradient, the antiporter can function either as a cell killer (H$^+$-uptake) or as a cell survival device (H$^+$-efflux). With this basic strategy we isolated: (1) mutants partially or totally defective; (2) mutants altered in Na$^+$, H$^+$ or amiloride binding sites; (3) mutants overexpressing the Na$^+$/H$^+$ exchange activity, revertants and transfectants.

Mutants lacking Na$^+$/H$^+$ antiport activity

Chinese hamster lung fibroblasts (CCL39) were loaded with Li$^+$ (Li^+_i ≃ 90 mM) and then exposed for 30 to 60 min to a Na$^+$, Li$^+$-free saline solution at pH$_o$ = 5.5. Under such conditions (Fig. 2a) cell viability dropped within a few minutes as a consequence of rapid H$^+$-uptake; pH$_i$ decreased below 5.0 within 5 min[23]. This H+-induced suicide occurs via the Na+/H+ antiporter since amiloride prevents cytoplasmic acidification and cell death. When mutagenized CCL39 cells were submitted twice to this H+-induced suicide test, 90% of the resistant clones were found to be defective in Na+/H+ exchange activity.

Mutant cells with no detectable activity display the following features: (1) when acid-loaded, pH_i-recovery is virtually abolished; (2) growth factors fail to stimulate the amiloride-sensitive Na+-influx and cytoplasmic alkalinization in quiescent mutant cells; (3) reinitiation of DNA synthesis and exponential growth is prevented at neutral and acidic pH_o (Refs 23 and 24). Adding HCO_3^- or greatly increasing the pH_o is required for the restoration of the pH_i defect and the parental growth phenotype in mutant cells[24]. These findings support the idea that pH_i is a key determinant in the commitment of G0-arrested cells to DNA replication.

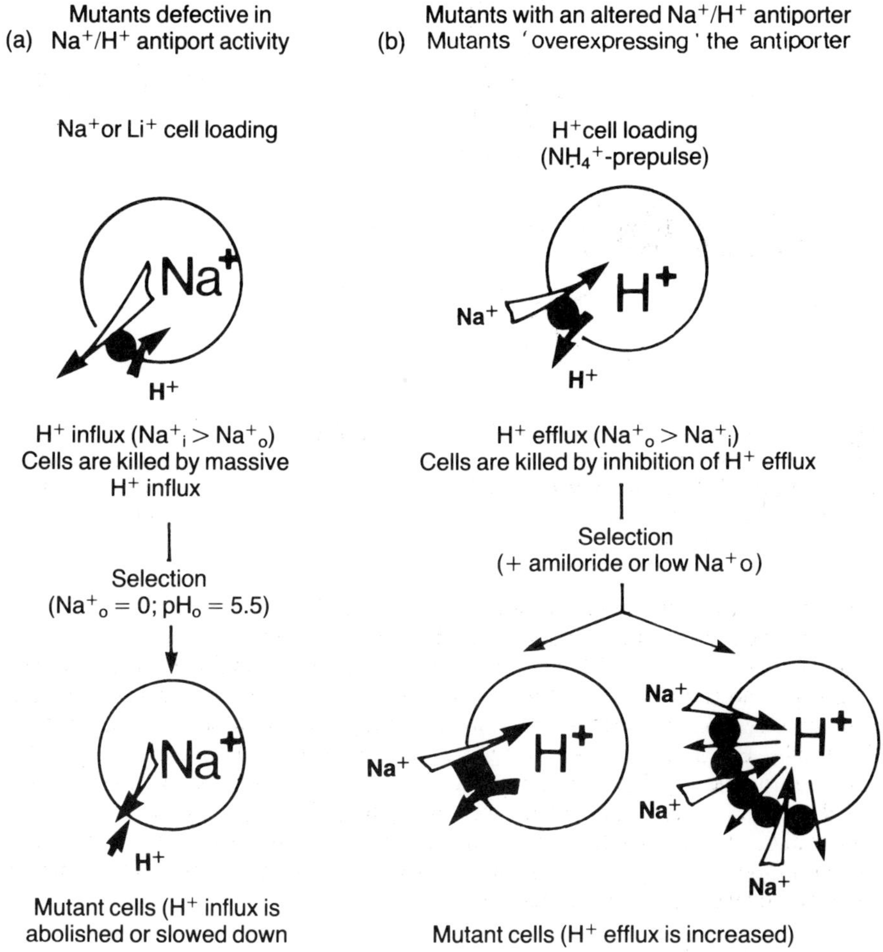

(a) Mutants defective in Na+/H+ antiport activity

Na+ or Li+ cell loading

H+ influx (Na+i > Na+o)
Cells are killed by massive H+ influx

Selection (Na+o = 0; pHo = 5.5)

Mutant cells (H+ influx is abolished or slowed down

(b) Mutants with an altered Na+/H+ antiporter
Mutants 'overexpressing' the antiporter

H+ cell loading (NH4+-prepulse)

H+ efflux (Na+o > Na+i)
Cells are killed by inhibition of H+ efflux

Selection (+ amiloride or low Na+o)

Mutant cells (H+ efflux is increased)

Fig. 2. Mutants of the Na+/H+ antiport system – schematic representation of the principles of selection. For selection of mutants lacking Na+/H+ antiport activity (a) the technical details are described in Ref. 23. For selection of mutants altered or 'overexpressing' the antiporter (b), cells are acid-loaded by using the NH4+-prepulse technique (incubation 60 min with 50 mM NH4 Cl)[8].

Mutants overexpressing an altered Na$^+$/H$^+$ antiporter

The principle of selecting mutants 'overexpressing' the antiport activity and those altered in ligand-binding sites is just the opposite to that for selecting cells deficient in the Na$^+$/H$^+$ antiporter. Cells are loaded with H$^+$ so that the full operation of the Na$^+$/H$^+$ antiporter is now essential for protecting the cells against the lethal acid-load (Fig. 2b). If H$^+$-efflux is slowed down during the first 60 min after acid-loading by low concentrations of 5-N-methyl,N-propyl amiloride (MPA[6]) the cells do not survive unless they 'overexpress' the antiporter or are endowed with a mutation which has a lower affinity for the amiloride analog. Resistant cells were progressively adapted to increasing concentration of MPA which was maintained only during the 60 min of the H$^+$-efflux test. A Chinese hamster variant, AR300 (which is 1000-fold less sensitive to MPA in the H$^+$-efflux test) 'overexpresses' a modified Na$^+$/H$^+$ antiporter (K_I for MPA is increased 20-fold, K_m for Na$^+$ or Li$^+$ is decreased 2.5-fold, and the V_{max} is increased 4- to 5-fold). The Na$^+$/H$^+$ exchange activity is so efficient in AR300 cells that when they are submitted to an acute acid-load, pH$_i$-recovery takes place within 5 s whereas it lasts more than 15 min in parental cells.

Alternatively, instead of adding an amiloride analog during the H$^+$-efflux selective test, external [Na$^+$] can be progressively reduced to decrease the rate of H$^+$-efflux (Fig. 2b). This selective procedure yielded another stable variant with a 6-fold increase in the rate of amiloride-sensitive Na$^+$-influx. This 'overexpression' of the Na$^+$/H$^+$ exchange activity results from a 3-fold increase in the affinity for Li$^+$ or Na$^+$ at external sites and a 2-fold increase in V_{max}. Interestingly, the affinities for H$^+$ or amiloride are unaltered, suggesting that the external Na$^+$, H$^+$ and amiloride binding sites do not completely overlap (Franchi and Pouysségur, unpublished).

Expression of a human Na$^+$/H$^+$ antiporter gene in mouse cells

The highly transfectable mouse cell line LTK$^-$ (thymidine kinase$^-$) was submitted to the H$^+$-suicide test (Fig. 2a) to select Na$^+$/H$^+$ antiporter deficient clones (AP$^-$). LAP cells (TK$^-$, AP$^-$) with no residual Na$^+$/H$^+$ antiport activity were isolated, and these served as recipients in a cotransfection experiment with a thymidine kinase$^+$ cloned gene and high-molecular-weight human DNA[25]. After an initial selection in HAT medium, the emerging TK$^+$ colonies (frequency $\simeq$ 10^{-3}) were submitted to an acid-load test to select only those expressing the Na$^+$/H$^+$ antiport activity (AP$^+$). AP$^+$ colonies, which arose among the TK$^+$ transfectants at a frequency of 10^{-3}–10^{-4}, express 20–30% of the parental Na$^+$/H$^+$ exchange activity. It is probable that these mouse transfectants (AP$^+$) express the human Na$^+$/H$^+$ antiporter gene because: (1) human Alu-repeated sequences are detected in all the primary and secondary AP$^+$ transfectants; (2) no AP$^+$ colony is obtained with the DNA of LAP cells (AP$^-$, TK$^-$) and (3) transfection of LAP cells with the DNA of AR300 mutant cells gives rise to AP$^+$ colonies expressing the altered Na$^+$/H$^+$ antiporter of the donor (Franchi, Perucca and Pouysségur, manuscript in preparation).

Prospects

After the rapid progress on the physiology and mechanistic aspects of the Na$^+$/H$^+$ antiporter, it is now desirable to obtain information about its molecular structure. The availability of radio-labeled high affinity amiloride analogs now allows the 'titration' of the Na$^+$/H$^+$ antiporter in solubilized membranes[26]. This approach, combined with the selection by gene amplification of 'overproducers', should soon give access to purification of the antiporter protein(s). Another approach towards the identification of the structure of this ionic transporter is the molecular cloning by DNA-mediated gene transfer. The preliminary results in that direction appear encouraging.

Acknowledgements

I am indebted to my colleagues Drs J. C. Chambard, A. Franchi, G. L'Allemain, S. Paris and D. Perruca for their collaboration and stimulating discussions. Thanks also to Dr M. Hosey for correcting the manuscript and to G. Clénet for secretarial assistance.

References

1 Johnson, J., Epel, D. and Paul, M. (1976) *Nature* 262, 661–664
2 Rozengurt, E. (1981) *Adv. Enzyme Regul.* 19, 61–85
3 Leffert, H. and Koch, K. in *Control of Animal Cell Proliferation* (Boynton, A. and Leffert, H. L., eds), Academic Press (in press)
4 Moolenaar, W. (1985) *Annu. Rev. Physiol.* 48, 363–376
5 Paris, S. and Pouysségur, J. (1983) *J. Biol. Chem.* 258, 3503–3508
6 L'Allemain, G., Franchi, A., Cragoe, E., Jr and Pouysségur, J. (1984) *J. Biol. Chem.* 259, 4313–4319
7 Aronson, P. S., Suhm, M. A. and Nee, J. (1983) *J. Biol. Chem.* 258, 6767–6771
8 Boron, W. (1983) *J. Membr. Biol.* 72, 1–16
9 Frelin, C., Vigne, P. and Lazdunski, M. (1985) in *Hormone and Cell Regulation* (Dumont, J., Hamprecht, B. and Nunez, J., eds), Vol. 9, pp. 259–268, INSERM
10 L'Allemain, G., Paris, S. and Pouysségur, J. (1985) *J. Biol. Chem.* 260, 4877–4883
11 Moore, R. (1981) *Biophys. J.* 33, 203–210
12 Schuldiner, S. and Rozengurt, E. (1982) *Proc. Natl Acad. Sci. USA.* 79, 7778–7782
13 Moolenaar, W., Tsien, R., van der Saag, P. and de Laat, S. (1983) *Nature* 304, 645–648
14 L'Allemain, G., Paris, S. and Pouysségur, J. (1984) *J. Biol. Chem.* 259, 5809–5815
15 Cassel, D., Rothenberg, P., Zhuang, Y., Deuel, T. and Glaser, L. (1983) *Proc. Natl Acad. Sci. USA.* 80, 6224–6228
16 Rothenberg, P., Glaser, L., Schlesinger, P. and Cassel, D. (1983) *J. Biol. Chem.* 258, 12644–12653
17 Paris, S. and Pouysségur, J. (1984) *J. Biol. Chem.* 259, 10989–10994
18 Grinstein, S., Cohen, S., Goetz, J., Rothstein, A. and Gelfand, E. (1985) *Proc. Natl Acad. Sci. USA* 82, 1429–1435
19 Villereal, M., Owen, N., Vincentini, L., Mix-Muldoon, L. and Jamieson, G. (1985) in *Cancer Cells* (Ferasmisco, J., Ozanne, B., Stiles, C., eds), 3, pp. 417–424, Cold Spring Harbor Laboratory
20 Moolenaar, W., Tertoolen, L. and de Laat, S. (1984) *J. Biol. Chem.* 259, 7563–7569
21 Nishizuka, Y. (1984) *Nature* 308, 693–698
22 Berridge, M. J. (1984) *Biochem. J.* 220, 345–360
23 Pouysségur, J., Sardet, C., Franchi, A., L'Allemain, G. and Paris, S. (1984) *Proc. Natl Acad. Sci. USA* 81, 4833–4837
24 Pouysségur, J., Chambard, J. C., Franchi, A., L'Allemain, G., Paris, S. and Van Obberghen-Schilling, E. (1985) in *Cancer Cells* (Ferasmisco, J., Ozanne, B., Stiles, C., eds), 3, pp. 409–415, Cold Spring Harbor Laboratory
25 Kühn, L., Barbosa, J., Kamarch, M. and Ruddle, F. (1983) *Mol. Biol. Med.* 1, 335–352
26 Vigne, P., Frelin, C., Audinot, M., Borsotto, M., Cragoe, E., Jr and Lazdunski, M. (1984) *EMBO J.* 3, 2647–2651

J. Pouysségur is at the Centre de Biochimie, CNRS, Université de Nice, 06034 Nice, France.

Programmable messengers: a new theory of hormone action

M. Rodbell

Many hormone receptors are linked to GTP-regulatory proteins in membranes. When these proteins are activated by hormones and GTP, the α-subunits are released from the membrane as soluble proteins. It is proposed that these α-subunits are modified by kinases, proteases and other protein-modifying enzymes to give new forms with differing functions. This provides a way of explaining the multiple actions of a hormone on its target cell, and the released α-subunits of GTP-regulatory proteins can be called 'programmable messengers'.

Two ideas have dominated the field of signal transduction over the past 25 years. One is that hormone/neurotransmitter receptors interact with various effector enzymes in the plasma membrane to generate signals in the form of small molecules. The classical example is the receptor-controlled adenylate cyclase system in eukaryotic cells. The other is that receptors exist either in membranes or in the cytosol as 'mobile' elements which, when combined with the activating hormone, induce the receptor to collide with or move to the site(s) of the effector systems. Examples of theories that have evolved from the mobile-receptor theory are the 'collision-coupling'[1] and 'two-step'[2] theories proposed for the coupling of β-adrenergic receptors to the adenylate cyclase system. Another example is the estrogen receptor; it has been thought that the receptor first reacts with the steroid in a cytosolic compartment, and that the activated receptor then enters the nucleus where it regulates gene expression.

There is ample evidence that cyclic AMP and other small molecules (cyclic GMP and inositol trisphosphates are recent examples) mediate some of the effects of hormones. The question is whether the pleiotypical responses induced by a hormone are due solely to any of these molecules. If not, what type of molecule might be more closely linked to receptors that could serve as primary messengers of hormone action? As for the concept of receptor mobility, there is evidence that membrane receptors can be induced by agonists to move about in the plane of the membrane. However, there is no compelling evidence that mobility is necessary or causal for signal transduction to take place. Indeed, there is a report that increasing the fluid environment to enhance receptor mobility in membranes is detrimental to hormone action[3]. For the estrogen receptor, recent studies indicate that most of the receptors are bound to the nuclear matrix prior to their occupation by hormone; receptor release into the cytosolic compartment is an artifact of the methods used for isolating the nucleus[4].

This article proposes an alternative view of the function of membrane receptors and develops a logical framework for a theory that the primary messengers of hormones acting on membrane receptors are proteins that bind and degrade GTP. These are the so-called GTP-regulatory proteins (G) that are linked to numerous receptor types in eukaryotic cells. The fundamental aspects were presented five years ago in a theory called 'Disaggregation Theory of Hormone Action'[5]. This theory is now extended and modified in the light of information acquired recently.

The disaggregation theory

Briefly, this theory suggests that various classes of receptors are complexed with a family of oligomeric GTP-regulatory proteins. When the receptors are occupied by agonists and the G units by GTP, the oligomers dissociate into monomers. In the process, the receptors are transformed from a high affinity state when they can bind physiological concentrations of hormones, into a low affinity state in which they are no longer active. At the same time, the G units are transformed to a 'monomeric' structure that reacts specifically with an effector unit (E) such as adenylate cyclase. The theory is thermodynamically sound[6]; it explains the apparent paradox of receptors undergoing transitions from high to low affinity states during concerted activation of G by hormone and GTP; it explains the findings of target analysis that the ground-state structure of receptors coupled to G exhibits a much higher molecular weight than the activated adenylate cyclase. This theory predicts that the putative monomeric form of G is the primary messenger of hormone action, whereas the product of the effector unit(s) is a secondary signal.

G units are oligomeric proteins

In recent years, G units have been purified and structurally analysed[7]. It is now clear that G units coupled to rhodopsin (termed transducin) and those coupled to receptors (R) that stimulate or inhibit adenylate cyclase (termed G_s and G_i, respectively), and a newly discovered G unit of unknown action (termed G_o) are composed of three distinct protein subunits, only one of which, the α-unit, binds GTP. The type of α-subunit coupled depends on the type of G unit (and associated R) to which it is attached. The other two subunits, designated β and γ, are highly conserved proteins – they are found in many cell types and species and have similar if not identical structures irrespective of the type of attached α-subunit.

Coupling to receptors

In reconstitution studies with purified components, G units interact with receptors when incorporated into lipid vesicles. The complexes formed exhibit the properties of R–G complexes in native membranes, i.e. hormones induce binding and degradation of GTP; R can take different affinity states, the higher affinity presumably linked to G; and GTP decreases the affinity of R for agonists[8,9]. Kinetically, the process of activation of G by agonists does not require hormone-induced associations between R and G, suggesting that the pre-formed complexes are the active species. Thus, there is no need to invoke the theories suggesting that hormones act by promoting such associations.

Reconstitution studies with rhodopsin and β-adrenergic receptors indicate that all three subunits of G are required for coupling between receptors and G. It follows that factors that disrupt the G unit must functionally uncouple R from this unit.

Disaggregation of G oligomers

In their purified, detergent-soluble form, G units dissociate when incubated with non-hydrolysable analogs of GTP (e.g. Gpp(NH)p or GTP-γ-S) or with aluminum fluoride in the presence of high concentrations of Mg^{2+} (Ref. 10). GTP is probably ineffective because GTP is hydrolysed to GDP as soon as the α-unit dissociates, and the subunits re-aggregate to form the holoprotein. This cyclical behaviour of the trimer may explain why GTP is relatively ineffective in the receptor-coupled systems within native membranes in the absence of hormones.

The observation most relevant to the 'disaggregation' theory is that G units are oligomers which, in the absence of activating ligands, cannot dissociate to release the 'active' GTP binding α-subunit. In this sense, the postulated monomer of G is equivalent to the activated α-subunit(s). Theoretically, activation of the R–G complex by concerted actions of hormone and GTP should lead to two interrelated phenomena: release of activated free α-subunits and conversion of receptors to a lower affinity, inactive form of R. Until α re-associates with the β/γ-subunits, R is desensitized, even if it is still linked to the β/γ-subunits.

Recently it has been reported that the α-subunits of G_i and G_o are water-soluble proteins whereas the combined β/γ-subunits are lipophilic and remain bound to liposomes after release of the α-subunits in response to guanine nucleotides[11]. This finding supports the conclusions drawn from studies with natural membranes that the α-subunit of G_s is released from membranes, a phenomenon that is crucial to the theory discussed below.

α-Subunits are released from membranes

Proof that α-subunits are released from R–G complexes in membranes by actions of hormones and GTP has been lacking. A possible means of testing release from native membranes arose from an apparently peculiar finding: co-incubation of membranes containing G_s units (rat liver, RL, and human

	HE* + cyc⁻	HE + cyc⁻	HE	cyc⁻
Adenylate cyclase (pmol/min)	92	0.9	0.1	0.8
Cholera toxin + ³²p NAD	+	–	+	+	+
Pertussis toxin + ³²p NAD	+	+	–	–	–

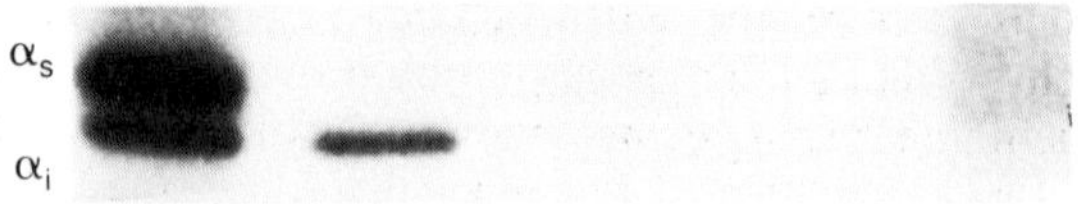

Fig. 1. Effects of pretreatment of human erythrocyte ghosts (HE) with pertussis toxin + NAD (HE*) on levels of adenylate cyclase activity and levels of $α_s$-subunit transferred to S49 lymphoma cyc− membranes. HE and cyc− membranes were co-incubated for 15 min at 30°C in presence of 0.1 mM Gpp(NH)p + 10 mM MgCl₂. The mixtures were layered over 30% sucrose and centrifuged for 20 min at 30 000 × g. The upper layer containing only cyc− membranes was assayed for adenylate cyclase activity (with 10 μM Gpp(NH)p, 5 mM MgCl₂, 50 μM ATP). Cyc− membranes were also treated with either cholera toxin or pertussis toxin, or both in presence of [³²P]NAD. Membranes were extracted and extracts electrophoresed (PAGE) for separation of $α_s$ (43 kDa) and $α_i$ (39 kDa) subunits, followed by autoradiography.

erythrocyte ghosts, HE), with membranes lacking this unit (isolated from a variant termed cyc− of S49 mouse lymphoma cells) rendered the cyc− membrane able to be activated by Gpp(NH)p or fluoride[12]. For this activation to occur, the cyc− membranes must be co-incubated with HE membranes which lack R units, or with RL membranes in the presence of glucagon plus GTP, or with donor membranes pretreated with cholera toxin and NAD (a procedure that ADP-ribosylates the α-subunit and which renders the G_s unit susceptible to activation by GTP).

Recently, we succeeded in separating donor and recipient cyc− membranes after co-incubation under various activating conditions[13]. Separation was achieved because the cyc− membranes have a lower density than either HE or RL membranes; layering the mixture of membranes over a sucrose gradient followed by centrifugation resulted in a layer of cyc− membranes free of donor membranes, as indicated by assays of various enzymes present in donor but not in cyc− membranes. When isolated after co-incubation with donor membranes under appropriate activating conditions, cyc− membranes acquired an active α_s-subunit (α of G_s) donated by HE or RL membranes. This was indicated by (1) the levels of Gpp(NH)p-stimulatable adenylate cyclase activity induced in cyc− membranes and (2) by the quantity of α_s transferred to cyc−. The latter was monitored by labelling α_s with [^{32}P]ADP-ribose catalysed by cholera toxin. A typical example of the relationship between transfer of α_s and the degree of activation of cyclase is illustrated in Fig. 1 using HE membranes co-incubated with cyc−.

This experiment also revealed, indirectly, that when G_i in HE membranes is activated by Gpp(NH)p and Mg^{2+} there is simultaneous activation of G_s. Activation of cyclase and transfer of α_s to cyc− membranes in HE membranes was slight unless the donor membranes were pre-treated with pertussin toxin plus NAD. This toxin ADP-ribosylates α_i and renders G_i inactive[14]. As shown in Fig. 1, toxin-treatment of HE causes cyc− membranes to acquire high levels of Gpp(NH)p-stimulatable cyclase activity with concomitant transfer of α_s (labelled with cholera toxin and [^{32}-P]NAD on re-isolated cyc−).

We interpret these findings as evidence that α_i released from G_i in the donor membranes influences the ability of α_s to interact with cyc− adenylate cyclase. We are investigating whether this is due to competition between released α_s and α_i for sites on adenylate cyclase or to some other process, such as the 'scavenging' of released α_s by exposed β/γ-subunits of G_i (Ref. 10). Irrespective of the mechanism, the thrust of these findings is that simultaneous activation of G_i and G_s, with consequent release of their respective α-subunits from the membrane, can dramatically affect the amount of α_s transferred to cyc−. Similar results are seen with liver membranes using combinations of hormones and GTP to induce activation.

Obviously, results obtained with a test system of two isolated membranes do not necessarily simulate what happens in an intact cell. Nonetheless, it is reasonable to speculate that release of α-subunits is the primary step leading to the pleiotropic effects of hormones on their target cells. If it is true that these proteins are primary messengers of hormone action, the present concepts of hormone action will have to be altered radically.

Programmable messengers

Perhaps the most significant difference between proteins and small molecules such as cyclic AMP is that a protein messenger is pluripotent in its capacity to react as a regulatory signal. Proteins can be phosphorylated, methylated, sulfated, oxidized, appended to other proteins via disulfide groups, and degraded to smaller forms by proteases, to name a few well known covalent modifications. Such modifications yield different structures with different functions. If α-subunits are modified after their release into the cytosolic compartments of the cell, and if some of the modifications lead to a different regulatory structure, then the α-subunit, the initial primary messenger, can be considered programmable. This concept of 'programmable messengers' is illustrated in Fig. 2.

In this scheme, each type of α-subunit released from the plasma membrane as a consequence of actions by hormone and GTP becomes exposed to different modifiers (M) that alter the structure and function of that unit. Each new form of α reacts selectively with an effector (E) which emits a signal (S) that can bring forth one or more responses. Possible examples of M include protein kinase C, insulin-receptor tyrosine kinase and calcium-activated protease. Examples of E are adenylate cyclase, guanylate cyclase, calcium transporters, phospholipases and glucose transporters. The central point of this thesis is that a single primary signal can give rise to an array of new signals which, in wave-like fashion, can propagate vast changes in the structure and metabolism of target cells. Specificity of response will depend on the types of receptor and G (or α-) units, and on the modifiers and effector of the cell phenotype. Given that there are various classes of receptors linked to G units and many potential signal-generating effector systems, a variety of cell responses can be envisaged.

The idea of programmable α-subunits as messengers provides an explanation for the frequently cited lack of correlation between hormone-stimulated AMP levels, for example, and other responses given by a hormone. Levels of activated cAMP-dependent protein kinase are also not correlated in all responses; a recent example is the discordance in the actions of β-adrenergic agonists on lipolysis and glucose transport in rat adipocytes[15]. There are examples of certain hormones inducing simultaneous rises in adenylate cyclase and cAMP-phosphodiesterases by apparently independent processes. Hormones that induce activation of G_i, while inhibiting the production of cAMP induced by a hormone operating through G_s, exert effects which are clearly unrelated to regulation of cAMP production.

Receptor desensitization

The programmable messenger theory can explain why receptor desensitization in intact cells can be reversed rapidly with low pulses of hormone and short times of exposure, but not with high concentrations and longer exposure to hormone. In the theory, only a fraction of the α-subunit would be released in a short pulse-type experiment with sub-maximal concentrations of hormone; during this brief interval, there may not be sufficient modification of α by modifiers to alter the equilibrium between bound and free α-subunit (Fig. 2) when the hormone is withdrawn. By the same reasoning, with higher concentrations of hormones and longer exposure times, more α-subunit is discharged from its union with β/γ-subunits and there is greater opportunity for modifiers to prevent α from re-associating with these β/γ. If this is so, reconstitution of functional receptors coupled to G units may require internalization of receptors (with or without attached β/γ), resynthesis of new α, and recycling of the units back to the plasma membrane.

Synergy

Perhaps the most interesting possible consequence of the programmable messenger theory is an explanation for the long-known synergism with which two hormones, operating through completely different mechanisms, exert effects on

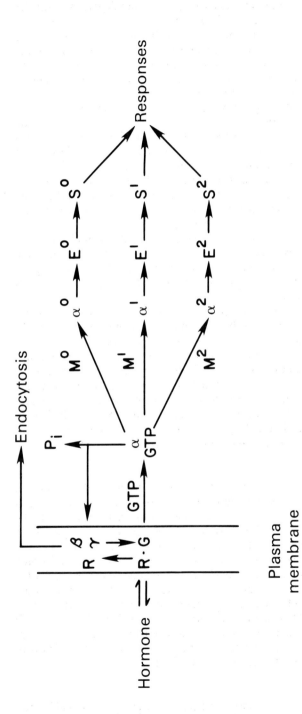

Fig. 2. Theory of 'Programmable Messengers'. Hormones interact with receptor/GTP-regulatory complexes (R·G) causing, in presence of GTP, release of the α-subunit of G from the interior face of the plasma membrane. R and β/γ-subunits of G remain in the membrane and can either re-bind α (-GTP) to re-form R·G or they are taken into cell by endocytosis. The released α-subunit is exposed to modifying enzymes (M) that transform α into new structures having affinities for different effector (E) units which, activated, yield signals (S) the combination of which give the pleiotypical responses of the target cell. Hydrolysis of GTP by a GTPase activity associated with the α-subunits is depicted by the liberation of inorganic phosphate (P_i). GDP, the other product is either liberated or remains bound to the α-subunits. In either case, the α-subunit preferentially binds to the β/γ-subunits in the membrane when the terminal phosphate of GTP is cleaved.

cells. A good example is the synergistic effect of insulin and adenosine on the metabolism of rat adipocytes[16]. Neither insulin nor adenosine alone have much effect at physiological concentrations. Combined at such concentrations, the hormones exert large effects on such metabolic processes as lipolysis and glucose transport. Since insulin activates a tyrosine kinase associated with the receptor[17], it is possible that the activated kinase phosphorylates a liberated α_i subunit (adenosine operates through a receptor linked to G_i in these cells) converting it from a weak or inactive regulatory signal into one that is very active. There are many examples of synergism between two hormones or neurotransmitters operating on the same cell through different primary mechanisms. The point to be stressed is that the search for the usual small molecule messengers, such as cAMP, as the primary agents of synergism has not yet been successful. Hopefully, the ideas put forth here will stimulate investigations along different, more productive lines of research.

Acknowledgement

The author thanks Professor Torben Clausen of Aarhus University for suggesting the expression 'programmable messengers'.

References

1   Tolkovsky, A. M. and Levitzki, A. (1978) *Biochemistry* 17, 3811–3817
2   Stadel, J., DeLean, A. D. and Lefkowitz, R. J. (1980) *J. Biol. Chem.* 255, 1436–1441
3   Salesse, R., Garnier, J., Leterrier, F., Daveloose, D. and Viret, J. (1982) *Biochemistry* 21, 1581–1586
4   King, W. J. and Greene, G. L. (1984) *Nature* 307, 745–747
5   Rodbell, M. (1980) *Nature* 284, 17–22
6   Minton, A. P. (1985) in *The Receptors* (Conn, P. M., ed.), Vol. 2, Academic Press
7   Gilman, A. G. (1984) *Cell* 36, 577–579
8   Cerione, R. A., Staniszewski, C., Benovic, J. L., Lefkowitz, R. J., Caron, M. J., Gierschik, P., Somers, R., Spiegel, A. M., Codina, J. and Birnbaumer, L. (1985) *J. Biol. Chem.* 260, 1493–1500
9   Brandt, D. R., Asano, T., Pedersen, S. E. and Ross, E. M. (1983) *Biochemistry* 22, 4357–4362
10 Northup, J. K., Smigel, M. D., Sternweiss, P. C. and Gilman, A. G. (1983) *J. Biol. Chem.* 259, 3560–3567
11 Sternwels, P. C. (1986) *J. Biol. Chem.* 261, 631–637
12 Nielson, T. B., Lad, P. M., Preston, M. S. and Rodbell, M. (1980) *Biochim. Biophys. Acta* 629, 143–148
13 Zaremba, T., Ngo, D. and Rodbell, M. (1985) *Fed. Proc.* 44, 700
14 Okajima, F., Katada, T. and Ui, M. (1985) *J. Biol. Chem.* 260, 6761–6768
15 Londos, C., Honnor, R. C. and Dhillon, G. S. (1985) *J. Biol. Chem.* 260, 15139–15145
16 Schwabe, U., Ebert, R. and Erbler, H. C. (1973) *Naunyn-Schmiedebergs Arch. Pharmakol.* 276, 133–138
17 Haring, H-V., Kasuga, M. and Kahn, C. R. (1982) *Biochim. Biophys. Res. Commun.* 108, 1538–1540

M. Rodbell is at the National Institute of Environmental Health Sciences, Research Triangle Park, NC 27709, USA.